Community Planning to Foster Resilience in Children

Community Planning to Foster Resilience in Children

Edited by

Caroline S. Clauss-Ehlers
Graduate School of Education
Rutgers, The State University of New Jersey
New Brunswick, New Jersey

and

Mark D. Weist
University of Maryland School of Medicine
Baltimore, Maryland

Kluwer Academic Publishers
New York, Boston, Dordrecht, London, Moscow

Library of Congress Cataloging-in-Publication Data

Community planning to foster resilience in children / edited by Caroline S. Clauss-Ehlers and
Mark D. Weist.
    p. cm.
Includes bibliographical references and index.
ISBN 0-306-48511-7 – ISBN 0-306-48544-3 (e-book)
1. Child psychiatry.   2. Community mental health services for children.   I. Clauss-Ehlers,
Caroline S.   II. Weist, Mark D.

RJ499.C597 2004
362.2′2–dc22   2004047310

$R J$
499
$C597$
2004

ISBN 0-306-48511-7

© 2004 by Kluwer Academic/Plenum Publishers, New York
233 Spring Street, New York, New York 10013

http://www.kluweronline.com

10 9 8 7 6 5 4 3 2 1

Permissions for books published in Europe: permissions@wkap.nl
Permissions for books published in the United States of America: permissions@wkap.com

Printed in the United States of America

To my dear husband, Julian, whose love, wisdom, and tenderness inspire resilience every day, and to our darling daughter, Isabel Seay, whose being was just a conversation as this project was planned and whose birth has touched our lives with awe and wonder ("CC").

To my father, Robert, the most resilient person I have ever known (MDW).

Contributors

Olga Acosta, DC Department of Mental Health, Washington, DC

Adeyinka M. Akinsulure-Smith, Bellevue/NYU Program for Survivors of Torture, New York, NY; Nah We Yone, Inc., New York, NY

Edith G. Arrington, University of Pennsylvania, Philadelphia, PA

Jennifer Axelrod, University of Illinois, Chicago, IL

Jason Barry, University of Rochester School of Medicine and Dentistry, Rochester, NY

Paul J. Brounstein, Substance Abuse and Mental Health Services Administration, Rockville, MD

Tanya N. Bryant, University of Maryland School of Medicine, Baltimore, MD

Robert Burke, Ball State University, Muncie, IN

Joanne Cashman, National Association of State Directors of Special Education, Alexandria, VA

Caroline S. Clauss-Ehlers, Rutgers, The State University of New Jersey, New Brunswick, NJ

Wendi Cross, University of Rochester School of Medicine and Dentistry, Rochester, NY

Charles G. Curie, Substance Abuse and Mental Health Services Administration, Rockville, MD

Nancy J. Davis, Substance Abuse and Mental Health Services Administration, Rockville, MD

Richard De Lisi, Rutgers, The State University of New Jersey, New Brunswick, NJ

Steven W. Evans, James Madison University, Harrisonburg, VA

Michael E. Faran, Tripler Army Medical Center, Honolulu, HI

Diane A. Faran, Hanahau'oli School, Honolulu, HI

James Garbarino, Cornell University, Ithaca, NY

Alina Camacho-Gingerich, St. John's University, Jamaica, NY

Isabelle M. Gremy, Observatoire regional de sante d'Ile-de-France, Paris, France

Alvin Hathaway, Pennsylvania AME Zion Church

Sylvia S. Huntley, University of Maryland School of Medicine, Baltimore, MD

Rafael Art. Javier, St. John's University, Jamaica, NY

Kimberly T. Kendziora, American Institutes for Research, Washington, DC

James Koller, University of Missouri, Columbia, MO

Teresa LaFromboise, Stanford University, Stanford, CA

R. Dwayne LaGrange, University of Maryland School of Medicine, Baltimore, MD

Jeannette M. Maluf, New York University Medical Center, New York, NY

Stephen Mathur, Columbia University, New York, NY

Lisa Medoff, Stanford University, Stanford, CA

Mickey C. Melendez, Rutgers, The State University of New Jersey, New Brunswick, NJ

Elizabeth Moore, University of Maryland School of Medicine, Baltimore, MD

Stephen M. Morris, Child Tripler Army Medical Center, Honolulu, HI

Edwin Morris, Missouri Department of Mental Health, Jefferson City, MO

Elizabeth Mullett, NYU Child Study Center, New York, NY

Carolyn Moore Newberger, Harvard University, Cambridge, MA

David M. Osher, American Institutes for Research, Washington, DC

Celeste C. Owens, University of Maryland School of Medicine, Baltimore, MD

Carl Paternite, Miami University of Ohio, Oxford, OH

Kay Rietz, Ohio Department of Mental Health, Columbus, OH

Tom Sloane, University of Maryland School of Medicine, Baltimore, MD

Hawthorne E. Smith, Bellevue/NYU Program for Survivors of Torture, New York, NY; Nah We Yone, Inc., New York, NY

Sharon Hoover Stephan, University of Maryland School of Medicine, Baltimore, MD

Saundra Tomlinson-Clarke, Rutgers, The State University of New Jersey, New Brunswick, NJ

R. Fox Vernon, Rutgers, The State University of New Jersey, New Brunswick, NJ

Mark D. Weist, University of Maryland School of Medicine, Baltimore, MD

Melvin N. Wilson, University of Virginia, Charlottesville, VA

Grace Wong, South Beach Psychiatric Center, Staten Island, NY

Peter A. Wyman, University of Rochester School of Medicine and Dentistry, Rochester, NY

Foreword
The Essential Quality of Resilience

The emergence of resilience as a central concept in discussions of child and adolescent development is encouraging to anyone who approaches the developmental issues of children and youth from an ecological perspective. Such a perspective requires that we acknowledge the central importance of context in all its cultural, social, historical, psychological, and biological dimensions. From an ecological perspective, the question, Does X cause Y? must be answered, It depends. For example, it depends on the context of those specific X and Y factors.

Does the presence of a particular risk factor predict the likelihood of developmental harm? From an ecological perspective, it depends on several important factors. The first is the overall accumulation of risk in the individual's life. Sammeroff's classic research demonstrated this with respect to the factors of poverty, parental absence, parental mental illness, large family size, parental substance abuse, parental low-educational attainment, rigid or punitive child-rearing style, and exposure to racism. This work demonstrates the critical importance of asking, Is this the first or the fourth risk factor? If it is the first, significant developmental damage for the average biological organism (i.e., child or adolescent) is unlikely; however, if a particular risk is fourth, damage to the average organism (even to most organisms) is likely.

Several studies[1] point to other elements of the context (e.g., neighborhood) as potential sites for risk accumulation. Why? Because human beings are not fragile—we can deal with adversity. If we were so delicate, the human species would have died out a long time ago. Research such as Sammeroff's supports this fact; however, this focus on human resistance to social risks is not enough.

Beyond the accumulation of risk at the social and psychological level are the risk factors within the organism—that is, the factors that create average and superior and risky individuals. Calculations of organismic risk amplify the impact

---

[1] e.g. Hampton, et al., community—Bronfenbrenner, 1975, society—Elder, 1974, culture—e.g. Rohner, 1975

of social and psychological risks. For example, research conducted by Caspi and his colleagues revealed that being an abused child does not automatically translate into subsequent problems with aggression and criminal behavior. Rather, the risk factors require that the organismic risk of deficient social information processing be linked to genetically-based neurotransmitter problems to produce the negative effects.

Although it is important to catalog risk factors, mapping developmental assets is also necessary, both for intellectual and moral reasons. If the prediction of outcomes is to proceed effectively and the intellectual imperative is to improve the variance accounted for, the developmental equation must include assessments of positive influences in conjunction with the negative. Adding social and psychological risks to organismic risks requires the addition of assets to accomplish this scientific goal. The moral imperative is to alert parents, educators, social workers, mental health professionals, and policy makers to the reality that it is possible to counterbalance risk accumulation with asset accumulation—that human beings individually and collectively are not passive victims of risk accumulation, but can resist harm themselves and receive assistance from others.

And this, I think, is why the theme of resilience is important both intellectually and morally. Intellectually, it offers a way of summarizing the reality that humans are not fragile beings. We are, to a greater or lesser degree, resilient. The more internal and external assets we possess, the more able we are to handle and even transcend risk factors in the environment—and even in ourselves.

A simplistic approach to resilience, however, is dangerous. Relying on resilience as a concept out of social context can become a recipe for rationalizing social deprivation and inequities. For example, relying solely on resilience, policy makers and the general public might conclude that worrying about poverty and abuse is unnecessary because kids are resilient. In a judgmental society like ours, however, it can lead to a form of blaming the victim (e.g., What's wrong with this child that he or she is not resilient?). And it can obscure real costs to people's sense of well-being and meaningfulness—Who cares how they feel about themselves and their joy in living? They are competent and prosocial.

If we are cognizant of these dangers and vigilant in opposing them in professional and public discussions, however, we can make effective use of resilience as a foundation for action on behalf of children. The chapters of this book succeed in doing so, with their special focus on the schools and community as a context for development and intervention. Whether it is children from diverse communities who deal with the nexus of poverty, racism, and violence, or those in military families struggling with the sources of instability in their lives, or children facing mental health problems, the authors offer well-grounded analyses and programmatic efforts to nurture resilience and defeat risks.

The authors keep faith with a complete concept of resilience in context. They refuse to accept simplistic answers to the questions of what happens and what works. By illuminating the complex and often subtle interplay of biological, psychological, social, and cultural forces in the lives of children and youth, they advance the field toward a more mature understanding of human strength and vulnerability.

JAMES GARBARINO
Elizabeth Lee Vincent Professor of Human Development
—*Cornell University*

Contents

Part 3. Areas of Special Need

Part 1

Foundations

Chapter 1

Introduction
Advancing Community Involvement and Planning to Promote Resilience in Youth from Diverse Communities

CAROLINE S. CLAUSS-EHLERS, Ph.D.[1] AND
MARK D. WEIST, Ph.D.[2]

Based on increasing awareness about the importance of preventing problems before they become crises, practitioners and educators are moving toward early intervention focused on children's strengths rather than weaknesses. At the heart of mental health promotion is the belief that exposure to factors that promote resilience ultimately helps children to cope with problems and succeed in life. The emphasis on strengths and the ability to overcome adversity is in direct contrast to traditional mental health approaches that seek to determine the nature of disease and the ensuing diagnosis. A focus on individual pathology too often locates the problem in the child alone rather than examining contextual stressors in families, schools, and the community at large. In addition, this practice risks overlooking community buffers that help children and their families cope with disabling situations.

[1] My work on this book was supported by funds from the Graduate School of Education, Rutgers, The State University of New Jersey, and a Research Council Grant from the Office of Research and Sponsored Programs at Rutgers, The State University of New Jersey.

[2] My work on this book was supported by cooperative agreement U93MC00174 from the Office of Adolescent Health, Maternal and Child Health Bureau (Title V, Social Security Act), Health Resources and Services Administration, with co-funding by the Center for Mental Health Services, Substance Abuse and Mental Health Services Administration. (NE810).

Increasingly, resilience-based interventions are expanding how we view mental health intervention by considering the internal strengths youth bring to a variety of situations, community and family resources that help children, and implications of cultural values for relevant care, all of which introduce a strengths-based framework to help children cope with stressors and succeed in life (Clauss-Ehlers & Lopez Levi, 2002). The overarching idea in the resilience approach is that while youth encounter a combination of stress and protective factors in their lives, more protective factors available to youth (both internal and external), will bring more skills and resources into their lives, making adversity more likely to be overcome.

Traditional psychological paradigms have placed an excessive emphasis on pathology and disease. The search to classify, categorize, and otherwise "know" the individual's problem dates back to 1833 with the publication of Emil Kraepelin's adult psychopathology classification, the first of its kind. Kraepelin (1833) assumed an organic etiology for each disease classification. Thus, from its initial beginnings, mental health began to conceptualize illness as an organic problem *located in the individual*. This *medical model* of psychotherapy was the dominant framework for mental health intervention through the 20th century, underpinning the works of leading psychodynamic practitioners and writers (e.g., Freud, Adler, Jung) and behavioral scientists (e.g., Pavlov, Jacobson, Wolpe; see Wampold, 2001). Indeed this medical model persists today, as shown in the relatively passive efforts of responding to problems of people with disorders seen in traditional outpatient mental health settings (see Weare, 2000; Weist, 2002).

While we are not arguing with the reality that mental illnesses do exist, or with the importance of understanding their etiology, the medical model will ultimately support the development of only a small number of the range of approaches and interventions that will reduce problems and help children and adolescents succeed in life. In this respect, a focus on resilience opens up horizons for assisting youth that go far beyond the focus on problems that "reside" within them. If we understand factors that promote resilience for children and adolescents, we can begin to look at how to construct, create, and otherwise cultivate environments that incorporate factors that help them thrive (Clauss-Ehlers, 2003).

This volume explores the question of health in the context of child and adolescent resilience. The chapters that follow attempt to broaden our approach by moving beyond risk, organicity, and pathology to examine both community and individual self-righting capacities (Werner & Smith, 1982). These self-righting capacities include processes that promote health and healing, processes that have a "profound impact on the life course of children who grow up under adverse conditions" (Werner & Smith, 1982, p. 202). It is an examination of these health-promoting behaviors, and the systems that support them, towards which this book is committed.

INCREMENTAL CONTRIBUTION OF THIS BOOK

Given that resilience has become an increasing focus of research and writing, we need to address the question, Why this book? To answer this question, we provide a brief review of books on resilience that have been written, then review incremental contributions the current volume makes to the resilience literature. This brief review is only on books that had resilience as the main concept being discussed and does not include those books that mention resilience in select chapters only (e.g., Csikszentmihalyi & Schmidt, 1998; James, Liem, & O'Toole, 1998; Eales, 1994; Grotberg, 2002; Masten & Reed, 2002). In addition, our review focuses on books published in the last 10 years (we apologize for any unintended omissions). The review reveals four general areas in which resilience is being written about. These areas include: 1) resilience in families, which explores how buffers and sources of resilience might have an impact on the lives of families (Brooks & Goldstein, 2001; Hetherington & Blechman, 1996; Walsh, 1998; Reynolds & Walberg, 1999); 2) resilience as an individual trait (Reivich & Shatte, 2002; Grotberg, 1999); 3) educational resilience (Brown, D'Emidio-Caston, & Bernard, 2001; Wang & Gordon, 1994); and 4) developmental/contextual aspects of resilience (Frydenberg, 1999; Glantz & Johnson, 1999; Cicchetti & Cohen, 1995; Taylor & Wang, 2000; Haggerty, Sherrod, Garmezy, & Rutter, 1996; Comunian & Gielen, 2000).

Each of the books referenced in these categories makes an excellent contribution to the resilience literature. The literature that focuses on families reviews implications of risk and resilience for family research (Cowan, Cowan, & Schulz, 1996), presents frameworks for therapeutic and preventive work for families in distress (Walsh, 1998), and explores how buffers and sources of resilience might have an impact on the lives of families (Brooks & Goldstein, 2001; Cowan, Cowan, & Schulz, 1996).

In the individual realm, one book outlines skills people can develop to overcome adversity, deal with self-criticism, cope with crisis and grief, and be resilient (Reivich & Shatte, 2002). Other work focuses on person-centered characteristics that can promote coping in difficult conditions (Frydenberg, 1999) and how to develop inner strength to combat obstacles (Grotberg, 1999). Still other books are specifically devoted to educational aspects of resilience. Foci here include: resilience education as a process that supports young people's ability to become knowledgeable and get involved in lifelong learning (Brown, D'Emidio, & Benard, 2001), and forging educational resilience in urban school settings (Freiberg, 1994).

Finally, a number of books on resilience emphasize a developmental/contextual approach, examining areas of resilience across contexts such as in families and schools (Taylor & Wang, 2000), and exploring social, cultural, and psychological adaptation (Haggerty, Sherrod, Garmezy & Rutter, 1996; Rumbaut,

2000). Other contributions locate the concepts of risk and resilience within a broader social context of war, racism, and poverty (e.g., Benard, 1999). Important contributions from the above literatures are included in this volume, and we add to these literatures in a number of ways. The book is divided into four sections: Foundations, Promoting Resilience in Diverse Communities, Areas of Special Need, and Promising Resilience-Promoting Developments. In the following, we highlight the central theme in each section, and briefly describe each chapter.

The first section of the book, "Foundations," reviews fundamental concepts from resilience research and suggests key future directions. In addition to this introductory chapter, R. Fox Vernon's chapter, *A Brief History of Resilience: From Early Beginnings to Current Constructions*, traces the roots of resilience research from child psychiatry and developmental psychology, reviewing definitional confusion, methodological issues, and public policy concerns. In the third chapter, *Re-Inventing Resilience: A Model of Culturally-Focused Resilient Adaptation*, the lead editor (CSCE) reviews culturally-focused resilience research and advocates for an inclusive understanding of resilience that incorporates diversity.

The second section of the book, "Promoting Resilience in Diverse Communities," responds to the reality that children and adolescents of color are the fastest growing group in the United States (U.S.), comprising 30 percent of the population in the year 2000 (Porter, 2000; U.S. Census Bureau, 2000). Moreover, a decade ago Martin and Midgeley (1994) estimated that almost 3,000 immigrants arrive in the United States each day, with immigration adding an estimated one million individuals to the population annually. These demographic changes have had a profound impact on life in the United States. Ours is a culturally pluralistic nation made up of diverse communities of children. While our multicultural society dictates the need for programs and services sensitive to the needs of diverse communities and cultures, research indicates that we fall short in this area. In the landmark publication entitled *Race, Culture and Ethnicity*, the Surgeon General found that people of color receive poorer quality mental health care and are less likely than Whites to use mental health services (U.S. Department of Health & Human Services, 2001). Hence, a primary purpose of this section is to provide an overview of stressors and supports that are of concern to youth from a range of diverse racial/ethnic backgrounds, with a view toward mental health promotion in the broadest sense.

The chapters presented in this section present unique resilience issues for youth from diverse backgrounds that include American Indians, Latinos, Asian and Asian Americans, African Americans, adolescents of color, and a global perspective of stressors that some youth face worldwide. We regret that we were not able to include a chapter for all racial/ethnic groups of children. This omission reflects some of the practical limitations in writing a book and is not meant to suggest a lack of interest or importance. To balance out this omission, we have encouraged all our contributors to incorporate aspects of resilience work with children across racial/ethnic groups in their chapters.

In *Sacred Spaces: The Role of Context in American Indian Youth Development*, Teresa LaFromboise and Lisa Medoff discuss particular stressors and strengths that American Indian youth face. The chapter highlights key elements of resilience for American Indian youth that include spirituality, family, traditional involvement, and economic development. In the next chapter, *Risk and Resilience in Latino Youth*, Rafael Art. Javier and Alina Camacho-Gingerich review the commonality of experience among Latinos as well as the great diversity in their experience that depends on factors such as immigration and acculturation, and present important strategies for promoting resilience among Latino youth.

Chapter 6, *Building on Strengths in Inner City African-American Children: The Task and Promise of Schools*, focuses on some of the unique stressors and strengths that inner city African-American children face. R. Dwayne LaGrange discusses the "double jeopardy" that exposes African-American youth to even greater risks and fewer resilience-promoting conditions, and reviews how schools can "harness the resources of the family and community to create an educational environment that supports student success." Grace Wong's chapter, *Resilience in the Asian Context*, describes how codes of behavior taught by Confucius promote skills that contribute to resilience such as self-discipline and interpersonal harmony as well as looking at stressors such as immigration that Asian children and their families face when they encounter American culture.

In Chapter 8, *Risk and Resilience During the Teenage Years for Diverse Youth*, Edith G. Arrington and Melvin N. Wilson review developmental trajectories that lead to unhealthy outcomes for youth, and how these may not always arise because of behavior youth engage in. Rather, these authors encourage us to look at larger contextual issues such as the educational and health disparities that youth of color experience. In the next chapter, *A Global Perspective on Youth Outreach*, Hawthorne E. Smith and Adeyinka M. Akinsulure-Smith review the severe stressors children face in the global climate that includes children in conflict areas exposed to violence, HIV/AIDS, war, death, torture, separation from family, and personal losses. Social-interpersonal engagement by caretakers with youth experiencing these stressors can assist them in making sense of their worlds and the hostile environments they experience.

The third section of this volume, "Areas of Special Need," addresses special problems and situations that call for an emphasis on resilience that so far has been limited. In Chapter 10, *Responses to Terrorism: The Voices of Two Communities Speak Out*, Caroline S. Clauss-Ehlers and colleagues document the experience of children living in New York City and Washington DC on September 11th, 2001 and review school and community-based approaches to prepare for these events and assist affected youth, families and community members. In the next chapter in this section, *Environmental Factors that Foster Resilience for Medically Handicapped*

Children, Jeannette M. Maluf discusses the interplay between the child's medical condition with pharmacological, behavioral, cognitive, educational, and family interventions that promote resilience.

In Chapter 12, *Fostering Resilience Among Youth in the Juvenile Justice System*, Kimberly T. Kendziora and David M. Osher review the high prevalence of mental health disorders among juvenile offenders that more often than not, do not get treated. They present insights in developing resilience focused treatment directions for diverse youth in the juvenile justice system. In the next chapter, *Clinical and Institutional Interventions and Children's Resilience and Recovery from Sexual Abuse*, Carolyn Moore Newberger, and Isabelle M. Gremy present a study that examines what interventions children receive after reporting sexual abuse, which children receive them, and how they influence children's resilience and recovery.

Chapter 14, *School Strategies to Prevent and Address Youth Gang Involvement*, by Sharon Hoover Stephan and colleagues reviews existing literature on gangs in schools such as predictors of gang membership, gang culture, and the impact on schools, and reviews school-based strategies to prevent and address youth gang involvement. Next, Michael Faran and colleagues discuss the unique challenges to resilience that youth of military personnel face in their chapter, entitled *Promoting Resilience in Military Children and Adolescents*. Stressors including deployments, family separation and moves, and financial difficulties combined with the critical role of the military in today's society call for resilience-promoting approaches for these families.

Section Four, "Promoting Resilience-Promoting Developments" reviews programs, educational strategies, and innovative partnerships that provide real life illustrations of resilience building in action. In Chapter 16, *Applying Research on Resilience to Enhance School-Based Prevention: The Promoting Resilient Children Initiative*, Peter Wyman and colleagues discuss how they applied core research findings into creating and implementing the Promoting Resilient Children Initiative (PRCI) using a sustainable school-based intervention delivery system, the Primary Mental Health Project (PMHP) model, an internationally renowned approach to promoting positive behavior and school success for elementary children. Next, Richard De Lisi in *Educational Resilience In Life's Second Decade: The Centrality Of Student Engagement* reviews the literature on educational resilience beginning with the reality that those who fall behind in school tend to stay behind the rest of their academic lives. This reality calls for a resilience-promoting approach and De Lisi provides key ideas for moving in this direction.

In Chapter 18, *Enhancing Child and Adolescent Resilience through Faith-Community Connections*, Celeste Owens and colleagues review literature that underscores the many protective influences of religious faith and involvement. In spite of the historical separation between faith-based and child serving organizations,

Owens et al. present how these partnerships can in fact develop, and review a range of promising outcomes from them. The next chapter, *A Whole-School Approach to Mental Health Promotion: The Australian MindMatters Program* by Elizabeth Mullett and colleagues provides an example of the paradigm change toward school-based mental health promotion that is occurring around the world. Lessons learned from this Australian program can help to escalate the pace of this paradigmatic change in the U.S.

In Chapter 20, *Home, School, and Community: Catalysts to Resilience*, Mickey C. Melendez and Saundra Tomlinson-Clarke discuss a proactive intervention model for youth who face stress that examines at-risk behavior within a cultural context. The authors illustrate the development of true systemic approaches, challenges in moving toward them and ideas for overcoming challenges. Next, in *Enhancing Student Resilience Through Innovative Partnerships*, Jennifer Axelrod and colleagues present national, state and local examples of child serving agencies (especially education and mental health) coming together to promote a full continuum of effective school-based programs and services, in ways that are driven by families and youth.

We close the book with an important chapter, *Resilience-Building Prevention Programs that Work: A Federal Perspective*, by Charles G. Curie and other leaders from the federal Substance Abuse and Mental Health Services Administration (SAMHSA) who present a comprehensive public health approach to the issue of risk and protection that attempts to "span the divide" between mental health problems and substance use disorders.

In 2004, there are major developments in the United States and globally that are transforming the way we approach child and adolescent health and learning. These include major reforms in U.S. systems of education (see www.ed.gov/nclb), mental health (as in the President's New Freedom Initiative; see www.mentalhealthcommission.gov) and juvenile justice (see http://ojjdp. ncjrs.org); and the development of international alliances focusing on the promotion of student, family and school success (see www.intercamhs.org) and the broader promotion of mental health and prevention of behavioral disorders (see www.charity.demon.co.uk). And this is just a sampling of the many activities occurring that reflect the reform and enhancement of public systems, especially those focusing on children and adolescents. At the core of these major initiatives is a focus on the promotion of strengths and resilience in youth and families. For these major initiatives to truly influence systems and powerfully shape the positive outcomes they aspire to, the most important action will occur at the level of the community, in ways that are responsive to diverse community members and their diverse strengths and needs. Our hope is that this book provides some assistance to local efforts to transform systems, programs, teaching and research agendas toward the promotion of resilience in children and adolescents.

REFERENCES

Benard, B. (1999). Applications of resilience: Possibilities and promise. In M.D. Glantz & J.L. Johnson (Eds.), *Resilience and development: Positive life adaptations. Longitudinal research in the social and behavioral sciences* (pp. 269–277). New York: Plenum Press.

Brooks, R., & Goldstein, S. (2001). *Raising resilient children: Fostering strength, hope, and optimism in your child.* New York: Contemporary Books.

Brown, J.H., D'Emidio-Caston, M., & Benard, B. (2001). *Resilience education.* Thousand Oaks, CA: Corwin Press.

Cicchetti, D., & Cohen, D.J. (Eds.). (1995). *Developmental psychopathology, Vol. 2: Risk, disorder, and adaptation. Wiley series on personality processes.* Somerset, New Jersey: Wiley, John & Sons.

Clauss-Ehlers, C.S. (2003). Promoting ecological health resilience for minority youth: Enhancing health care access through the school health center. *Psychology in the Schools, 40(3),* 265–278.

Clauss-Ehlers, C.S., & Lopez Levi, L. (2002). Violence and community, terms in conflict: An ecological approach to resilience. *Journal of Social Distress and the Homeless, 11(4),* 265–278.

Csikszentmihalyi, M., & Schmidt, J.A. (1998). Stress and resilience in adolescence: An evolutionary perspective. In K. Borman & B. Schneider (Eds.), *The adolescent years: Social influences and educational challenges: Ninety-seventh yearbook of the National Society for the Study of Educaiton, Part I.* (pp. 1–17). Chicago: NSSE: Distributed by the University of Chicago Press.

Eales, M.J. (1994). Adversity and resilience. In D. Tantam & M. Birchwood (Eds.), *Seminars in psychology and the social sciences. College seminars series* (pp. 224–237). England: The Royal College of Psychiatrists.

Frydenberg, E. (Ed.). (1999). *Learning to cope: Developing as a person in complex societies.* New York: Oxford University Press.

Grotberg, E.H. (1999). *Tapping your inner strength: How to find the resilience to deal with anything.* Oakland, CA: New Harbinger.

Grotberg, E.H. (2000). The international resilience research project. In A.L. Comunian & U.P. Gielen (Eds.), *International perspectives on human development* (pp. 379–399). Lengerich, Germany: Pabst Science Publishers.

Grotberg, E.H. (2002). From terror to triumph: The path to resilience. In C.E. Stout (Ed.), *The psychology of terrorism: A public understanding, Vol. 1. Psychological dimensions to war and peace* (pp. 185–207). Westport, CT, US: Praeger Publishers/Greenwood Publishing Group, Inc.

Haggerty, R.J., Sherrod, L.R., Garmezy, N., & Rutter, M. (Eds.). (1996). *Stress, risk, and resilience in children and adolescents: Processes, mechanisms and interventions.* Cambridge: Cambridge University Press.

Hetherington, E.M., & Blechman, E.A. (Eds.). (1996). *Stress, coping, and resiliency in children and families. Family research consortium: Advances in family research.* England: Lawrence Erlbaum Associates, Inc.

James, J.B., Liem, J.H., & O'Toole, J.G. (1997). In search of resilience in adult survivors of childhood sexual abuse: Linking outlets for power motivation to psychological health. In A. Lieblich & R. Josselson (Eds.), *The narrative study of lives* (pp. 207–233). Thousand Oaks, CA: Sage Publications, Inc.

Kraepelin, E. (1883). *Compendium der psychiatire.* Liepzig: Abel.

Martin, P., & Midgeley, E. (1994). Immigrants to the United States: Journey to an uncertain destination. *Population Bulletin, 49(2),* 1–47.

Masten, A.S., & Reed, M.J. (2002). Resilience in development. In C.R. Snyder & S.J. Shane (Eds.), *Handbook of postitive psychology* (pp. 74–88). London: Oxford University Press.

Porter, R.Y. (2000). Understanding and treating ethnic minority youth. In J. Aponte & J. Wohl (Eds.), *Psychological intervention and cultural diversity* (pp. 167–182). Boston: Allyn and Bacon.

Reivich, K., & Shatte, A. (2002). *The resilience factor: 7 essential skills for overcoming life's inevitable obstacles.* New York: Broadway Books.

Rumbaut, R.G. (2000). Profiles in resilience: Educational achievement and ambition among children of immigrants in Southern California. In R.D. Taylor & M.C. Wang (Eds.), *Resilience across contexts: Family, work, culture, and community* (pp. 257–294). Mahwah, NJ, London: Lawrence Erlbaum.

U.S. Census Bureau. *Census 2000.* Summary File 1.

U.S. Department of Health and Human Services (2001). *Mental health: Culture, race, and ethnicity—A supplement to mental health: A report of the Surgeon General.* Rockville, MD: U.S. Department of Health and Human Services, Public Health Service, Office of the Surgeon General.

Walsh, F. (1998). Strengthening family resilience. *The Guilford family therapy series.* New York: Guilford Press.

Wampold, B.E. (2001). *The great psychotherapy debate: Models, methods, and findings.* Mahweh, N.J.: Lawrence Erlbaum Associates.

Wang, M.C., & Gordon, E.W. (Eds.). (1994). *Educational resilience in inner-city America: Challenges and prospects.* Mahweh, N.J.: Lawrence Erlbaum Associates.

Wang, M.C., Haertel, G.D., & Walberg, H.J. (1999). Psychological and educational resilience. In A.J. Reynolds, H.J. Walberg, et al. (Eds.), *Promoting positive outcomes. Issues in children's and families lives.* Illinois: The University of Illinois at Chicago Series on Children and Youth.

Weare, K. (2000). *Promoting mental, emotional and social health: A whole school approach.* New York: Routledge.

Weist, M.D. (2002). Challenges and opportunities in moving toward a public health approach in school mental health. *Journal of School Psychology, 353,* 1–7.

Wenar, C., & Kerig, P. (2001). *Developmental psychopathology: From infancy through adolescence. (4th Ed.),* Boston: McGraw Hill.

Werner, E.E., & Smith, R.S. (1982). *Vulnerable but invincible: A study of resilient children.* New York: McGraw Hill.

Chapter 2

A Brief History of Resilience
From Early Beginnings to Current Constructions

R. Fox Vernon

As it enters a new age in its development, resilience research faces many growing pangs (Masten, 1999). It has introduced a hardy and original construct denoting the ability to rebound from acute or chronic adversity. Yet, as Glantz and Slobada (1999) warn, "There is no consensus on the referent of the term, standards for its application, or agreement on its role in explanation, models, and theories" (p. 111). It has been then impetus for an explosion of empirical research and has played a pivotal role in the origin of a new discipline, developmental psychopathology. Yet, in the view of some, it has left matters in disarray. Windle (1999), for example, argues that the resilience literature offers "no organizing framework for integrating studies, for evaluating common and unique findings across different subject populations, variable domains, or spacing interval, or for studying the impact of alternative operational definitions and classification procedures on the identification of resilient individuals" (p. 174). Resilience science has amassed a confident array of scholars who do research as its proponent (see, for example, Cicchetti & Garmezy, 1993; Masten, 2001), yet it has also provoked skepticism, represented in the words of Kaplan (1999), who suggests that it is "a concept whose time has come and gone" (p. 72).

The optimism and concern surrounding resilience research represents the inevitable turbulence that attends any young and ambitious field of study. These struggles speak not only to the auspicious beginnings of resilience research (as evidenced by the proliferation of studies) but also to its uncertain future, as critics emerge to question its potential. Excepting for these pains, the young science—if it is not presumptuous to label it such—has yet to face noteworthy adversity. This makes it difficult to predict its future. Will resilience research itself be resilient (Tolan, 1996), or will it fade into the background as have so many initially promising areas of psychological research? It certainly has displayed a bright start, having had seemingly effortless success in catalyzing innovative scientific investigation, inspiring clinicians and researchers alike with an optimistic view of human nature, and uniting disparate subdisciplines under its banner.

THE ROOTS OF RESILIENCE

Resilience science was initially brought forth into psychology as the serendipitous progeny of two parents, child psychiatry and developmental psychology. In their own ways, each had become intrigued by the negative aspects of adversity. In child psychiatry, this intrigue was based on the longstanding assumption, drawn largely from Freud, that early negative experiences give rise to adult psychopathology. Sir Michael Rutter, a British pioneer in the field, explains that the work of his compatriot, John Bowlby, ushered in the first era of systematic investigations addressing childhood adversity. Bowlby's famous World Health Organization (WHO) monograph (1951) stands as perhaps the earliest prominent signpost of this era. Bowlby's work had materialized from the earlier roots of child psychiatry, which were planted in the mental hygiene and child guidance movements of the early 20th century. "Mental hygiene" was the former term for what we now label mental health. In the United States, this movement emerged with the public's reaction to Clifford Beer's autobiography, *A Mind That Found Itself* (1908), in which Beer—who served as a leader of the movement until his death—detailed his harrowing experiences in institutions for the insane. On the crest of the public's outcry, the first of many societies for mental hygiene was established in 1908. The child guidance movement peaked later, in the 1920's and 1930's, and was marked by the founding of numerous clinics. These clinics implemented coordinated efforts to prevent mental health disorders in adults by addressing problematic child behaviors (Romano & Hage, 2000).

Bowlby, though trained as a classical psychoanalyst (Melanie Klein served as one of his supervisors), presented ideas about the mother-child bond that countered contemporary psychoanalytic theory, rankling eminent figures in psychoanalysis. Winnicott, for example, upon hearing Bowlby read his first formal paper on attachment theory (Bowlby, 1958) at the 1957 meeting of the British Psychoanalytic Society confided the following to a colleague, "It was certainly a difficult paper to appreciate without giving away everything that has been fought for by Freud" (as quoted in Bretherton, 1991, p. 18). Winnicott shared an even stronger reaction with Anna Freud, "I can't quite make out why it is that Bowlby's papers are building up in me a kind of revulsion" (as quoted in Bretherton, 1991, p. 20).

Bowlby's work clearly excited a stir. Theoretically speaking, he retreated from psychoanalysis's fascination with the fantasy life and presumed oral drive of the child, turning instead to the actual behaviors exhibited by mother-child pairs. Bowlby's research, inspired partly by ethological research on birds and primates, suggested that the primary need of the infant was not merely for the mother's breast (or its milk), but for the proximity and appropriate attention of the mother herself. This research brought a new focus to child psychiatry, and likely drew the attention of developmental psychologists as well, whose work Bowlby had drawn upon (Gullestad, 2001). Though Bowlby's research and theorizing ignited interest in early relational patterns, especially "the affectional components of mothering" (Rutter, 1985, p. 598), his claims were rather bold and all-encompassing, overreaching the available evidence. Given our modern understanding of attachment, Bowlby exaggerated the pervasiveness and irreversibility of the damage done by disruptive infant-caregiver relations (Rutter, 1985). This inflated view of early childhood attachment, though disagreeing with Freud's theories in its specifics, nonetheless agreed with Freud's general convictions about the pervasive, negative influence of childhood conflict. Today, such ideas have been tempered, and the views of Bowlby and Freud, especially where held zealously, have been derided as "infant determinism" (Kagan, 1996). Nevertheless, Bowlby's work—especially as it was operationalized in Ainsworth's tripartite of attachment styles: secure, avoidant, and anxious-ambivalent (Ainsworth & Wittig, 1969)—provided a powerful foundation and empirical model for the resilience research to come.

THE BIRTH OF RESILIENCE

Research into resilience proper began in the early 1970's, when the concept was first introduced. Following largely in the footsteps of Bowlby and Ainsworth, child psychiatry had begun to center much of its resources on accumulating data about the effects of various childhood traumas on later development. Examples of this type of work included Rutter's (1971) study of mother-child separation, and Hetherington (1980) and Wallerstein's (Wallerstein & Kelly, 1980) inquiries into parental divorce. Together, these types of studies signified an emerging appreciation for risk factors, those variables that appeared to correlate with later dysfunctional behavior. Indeed, the study of risk factors became a thriving area of research itself, eventually establishing the identification of multitudes of early stressors (poverty perhaps being the most global and prominent) and their associated sequela. Horowitz (1989) has distinguished five distinct strains of research on risk factors, including 1) research on infants who were born either prematurely or with prenatal complications, 2) research on children and adolescents with conduct disorders, 3) research on infants exposed to harmful environmental agents (lead and alcohol being prime examples), 4) research on animals to understand critical developmental periods, and finally, 5) research on the emotional and social maladjustment of children and adolescents.

As researchers began to refine and expand their appreciation of assorted stressors and risk factors, they stumbled across a rather unanticipated finding. Garmezy, widely acknowledged as the founder of resilience research (Masten & Coatsworth, 1998; Rolf, 1999), explains that at the time he was conducting research on people with schizophrenia. He and his mentor Eliot Rodnick observed that certain patients with schizophrenia were surprisingly functional in their daily lives (Rolf, 1999). These patients, labeled as having "reactive" schizophrenia (but whom today we would label as having schizophreniform disorder), drew a striking comparison to patients with "process" schizophrenia. Unlike their counterparts, people with reactive schizophrenia generally had much shorter hospital stays, were able to hold regular jobs, and often engaged in long-standing romantic bonds. In tracing the histories of individuals with schizophrenia, Garmezy and his mentor found that the backgrounds of individuals with reactive schizophrenia displayed impressive patterns of competence (Rolf, 1999). Piqued by these observations, Garmezy initiated a study of children whose parents suffered from schizophrenia. In a seminal article written in the early 1970s, he described the remarkably positive adjustment of these children, 90% of whom did not develop schizophrenia as had their parents (Garmezy, 1971). He reported that these children "bear the visible indices that are hallmarks of competence—good peer relations, academic achievement, commitment to education and to purposive life goals, [and] early and successful work histories" (Garmezy, 1971, p. 114). Calling for the field to shift its focus away from the study of risk factors, he suggested that future research be directed toward understanding "the forces that move such children to survival and to adaptation" (Garmezy, 1971, p. 114).

Garmezy's findings were repeated by several other researchers, most of whom establish the pantheon of pioneers in the field, including Sir Michael Rutter (1979), James Anthony (1974), Lois Barclay Murphy (Murphy & Moriarty, 1976), and Ruth Smith and Emma Werner (Werner & Smith, 1982). As these and other investigators closely examined the effects of early trauma and adversity, they were repeatedly impressed by the large number of children who displayed competence. Researchers found that even when exposed to the most horrific conditions—including war, incarceration in concentration camps, sexual and physical abuse, and parental drug abuse—50% to 70% of affected children survived, going on to lead developmentally normal lives (Lazarus, DeLongis, Folkman, & Gruen, 1985; Rutter, Maughan, Mortimore, Ouston, & Smith, 1979; Werner & Smith, 1982). The work of these pioneers launched the first generation of resilience research. Scientists began to focus not just on risk factors and stressors, but on what came to be termed protective factors, the hypothesized building blocks of resilience.

THE RISE OF DEVELOPMENTAL PSYCHOPATHOLOGY

Vitalized by the newly spawned investigations of resilience, developmental psychopathology coalesced into being in the 1970s as a bona fide subdiscipline of psychology. In its early years, this field—which includes resilience and other focus areas beneath its umbrella—was dominated not only by figures we have mentioned above—including Anthony, Garmezy, and Rutter—but also by such notables as Alan Sroufe and Edward Zigler, whose work cross-pollinated with that of resilience researchers, focusing as it did on like issues, including vulnerabilities, stressors, risk factors, competencies, and dysfunctional and functional adaptation. This new and aspiring field drew from two powerful research forces. The first was that of developmental psychology, which by this time had become more or less rooted within the academy, and the second was that of the combined clinical sciences of psychiatry and psychology. These intellectual forces carried highly polarized methodological and theoretical frames of reference. The more academic developmental psychology, for instance, was relatively wedded to the "experience-far" methodologies of quantitative empiricism, especially as espoused and practiced by behaviorism, which had reigned supreme within academic psychology since earlier in the 20th century. Clinical psychiatry and psychology, on the other hand, was rooted primarily in Freudian theories, and favored naturalistic, "experience-near" methodologies that culled and tested its ideas from the cauldron of clinical interviews and observations. Additionally, developmental psychology emphasized the cognitive aspects of human functioning, whereas the clinical sciences emphasized internal, emotional dynamics.

Historically, these differences (and likely others) "operated to keep the academic and clinical study of psychology almost totally isolated from each other" (Cicchetti, 1984, p. 3). This created obvious weaknesses. Academic psychology tended to ignore psychopathology, and clinical psychiatry and psychology tended to ignore human development (Cicchetti, 1984). The marriage of these two fields under the domain of developmental psychopathology brought together two types of minds that had rarely been formally joined, and it offered a fresh dialogue and perspective on both pathological and normative behavior. This may in part explain the openness and theoretical sensitivity of resilience researchers, who recognized the silver lining in what had initially been somewhat dour research on risk factors and vulnerabilities. The emergent communication between two diverse methodological outlooks also inspired researchers to expand their tools of inquiry. Masten, a scholar currently at the vanguard of research in developmental psychopathology and resilience, alludes to this when she proposes the utility of comparing data from "variable-focused" and "person-focused" investigations (Masten, 2001). This methodological openness allowed for research that was inspired by clinical questions, and vice versa, to the benefit of both research and practice. As Cicchetti (1984) remarks, "The clinician very often has an application for the results of academic research, and the academic can very often use the focus and direction in research that an attention to practical problems can provide" (p. 4). Taken as a whole, the resilience literature, especially as it has been influenced by the emergence of developmental psychopathology, deserves accolades for its integration of the "cumulative wisdom of clinical experience and research findings" (Guttman, 1989, p. 252).

HEADY OPTIMISM

Given its contribution to developmental psychopathology and its hopeful discoveries about the apparent elasticity of human functioning in the face of adversity, the initial wave of resilience research was understandably optimistic and ambitious in its claims. Anthony (1974), for example, coined the term "invulnerable" to describe the resilient children he studied. Following suit, the APA monitor soon printed a piece entitled, "In Praise of 'Invulnerables,'" shortly to be followed by a *Psychology Today* article inscribed with the headline "Superkids," both penned by the same author (Pines, 1975, 1979). In 1982, Werner and Smith published *Vulnerable but Invincible*, the first in a series of trailblazing reports, all based on an extensive longitudinal study of 698 children from the Kauai, Hawaii (Werner & Smith, 1982).

The initial heady outlook of the first generation of resilience research—marked by such terms as "invulnerable" and "invincible"—soon subsided. Subsequent research revealed there was no such reality as the absolutely invincible child. Indeed, a more sober Rutter (1985; 1991) commented that the terms invulnerable and invincible were "wrongheaded" in at least two ways. First, such terms implied that the basis of resiliency resided in the individual. Ongoing research suggested, however, that resiliency was based as much on contextual and situational variables as on individual characteristics (Rutter, 1987; Wolff, 1995). Second, these terms implied that resilience was a stable factor, a trait perhaps. The evidence, however, revealed that resilience varied over time. Further, resilience seemed to be affected by developmental factors, and thus might wax or wane depending on the individual's developmental trajectory (Rutter, 1987; Wolff, 1995). The data, as Rutter's qualifications revealed, were beginning to tell a less simplified tale than researchers had initially anticipated. Perplexed by the significant variations in individual's response to adversity, researchers began searching for the exact variables that might explain why some individuals succumbed to tragedy whereas others persevered.

This has brought the field to its current position, which might be compared to the bloom of early adolescence. In its present generation, resilience research can reflect upon its handsome track record of research drawing from such diverse disciplines as developmental psychology, social psychology, counseling and clinical psychology, child psychiatry, psychopathology, and epidemiology, amongst others.

Resilience science has also contributed to the reinvigorated interest in positive and adaptive aspects of human functioning, represented by such developments as the third revision of *The Diagnostic and Statistical Manual of Mental Disorders*. (American Psychiatric Association, 1987), which introduced a fifth axis for assessing the client's uppermost levels of functioning, and the championing efforts of a late 1990's president of the American Psychological Association, Martin Seligman, whose career trajectory shifted from an initially negative focus—namely, learned helplessness—to a positive one—learned optimism (Seligman, 1990, 1994, 1995).

This positive bent to psychology refracts much of the optimism inherent in the movement of resilience science, which allowed Garmezy (1994) to comment, "History is dotted with images of survivorship despite the most horrendous events" (p. 12). The most vanguard movement within resilience science has become more sober, perhaps we might say mature, not only in its tempering of such misleading terms as invincible or invulnerable, but even more importantly, in its recognition that resilience is more than an erratic phenomenon that "dots" the landscape, but more one that permeates it. That is, resilience is not a unique quality that only a fortunate few possess, but rather appears to be widespread, even common. Masten (2001) has described it as "ordinary magic." She writes, "The great surprise of resilience research is the ordinariness of the phenomena. Resilience appears to be a common phenomenon that results in most cases from the operation of basic human adaptational systems" (Masten, 2001, p. 227). This has capsized negative views of human functioning that overemphasize human deficits and minimize what appears to be inherent human ingenuity, elasticity, and adaptiveness.

DEFINITIONAL CONFUSION

The optimistic and even giddy flush of youth has not overtaken the sensibilities of resilience researchers, who remain true to their heritage as assiduous and critical researchers. As the field "comes of age" (Masten, 1999), researchers have begun to adopt an increasingly critical review of their own achievements and the field's future promise. Perhaps it is the field's very optimism, matched by its scientific frame of reference, that has allowed dissonant voices to rise to the surface and proclaim their skepticism. Most critics seem to display level-headed sympathy toward resilience research, even when expressing misgivings (Gordon & Wang, 1994; Kaplan, 1999; Liddle, 1994; Tarter & Vanyukov, 1999; Tolan, 1996).

An enduring difficulty in the resilience literature has been defining the concept, along with its kindred concepts—competence, vulnerability, protective factor, risk factor, and stressor. There is ample controversy and confusion regarding these terms (Glantz & Johnson, 1999; Kaufman, Cook, Arny, Jones, & Pittinsky, 1994; Windle, 1999) due, to a lesser extent, to methodological differences between studies, and, to a larger extent, to conceptual distinctions. Conceptual distinctions have included such ongoing arguments as to whether resilience is merely a behavioral pattern or whether it also (perhaps entirely) involves intrapersonal phenomena such as well-being. There also remains debate about whether resilience is a set of skills, usually attributed to the individual, or resources, which include the individual and also his or her various social, cultural, familial, and peer environments. Kaplan contributes his compelling uneasiness about the confusion between resilience understood as outcome and resilience understood as cause. He explains, "Is resilience the variation in good outcomes among individuals who are at-risk for bad outcomes, or is resilience the qualities possessed by individuals that enable them to have good outcomes?" (Kaplan, 1999, pp. 19–20). These concerns present conceptual jigsaw puzzles that current researchers are obligated to begin assembling.

In its most generic and well-established formulation, resilience has denoted "a process whereby people bounce back from adversity" (e.g., Dyer & McGuinness, 1996; Masten & Coatsworth, 1998; Rutter, 1987). Generally speaking, most agree with this overarching image. Masten (1999) notes, for example, "There does appear to be agreement about the nature of the ballpark we are in when 'resilience' is invoked" (p. 283). This is commendable, especially given the diverse disciplines that have contributed to resilience research. On the other hand, when one looks more closely at resilience within specific contexts, this very diversity has raised anxiety. Does resilience as studied in one domain carry over to other domains (Davis, 1999; Greenbaum & Auerbach, 1992; Luthar & Zigler, 1991)? Is the ability to rebound from a childhood illness (as studied by epidemiologists) the same as the ability rebound from childhood abuse (as studied by developmental psychologists)? This parallels concerns in educational psychology over the transferability of knowledge. The general finding has been that knowledge does not translate well from one domain to another (Gagne, Yekovich, & Yekovich, 1993). The transferability of resilience also parallels, to a certain degree, to questions raised within the study of psychotherapy about transferring therapeutic interventions amongst varying psychological disorders. Indeed, one might borrow Gordon Paul's (1967) ultimate clinical question from the psychotherapy literature and apply it, mutatis mutandis, to resilience: "What treatment [that is, resilience mechanism] delivered by whom, is most effective for this individual with that specific problem, under which set of circumstances, and how does it come about" (p. 111). Clearly, resilience research faces important challenges in trying to address these issues.

METHODOLOGICAL TURBULENCE

The difficulty of defining resilience directly relates to the difficulty of measuring the construct. This is complicated by the fact that resilience researchers come from such diverse fields, many employing diverse methodologies. The measurement of resilience becomes particularly elaborate, because the construct usually involves the appraisal of three main sets of constructs: measures of risks, vulnerabilities, and stressors; measures of protective processes or factors and competencies; and finally, measures of outcome. All of these pose idiosyncratic, and often knotty, difficulties. Regarding the measure of risks, vulnerabilities, and stressors, Greenbaum and Auerbach (1992) comment on the confusion that reigns, quipping that "One investigator's 'risk' is another's 'vulnerability'" (p. 18). Even where researchers do agree on definition, they often go about operationalizing their constructs in different ways. Luthar and Zigler (1991) list five different though commonly practiced ways of measuring risks: 1) using self-reported major life events; 2) using self-reported small events or hassles more characteristic of everyday life; 3) studying specific stressors such as divorce, parental schizophrenia, or natural disasters; 4) employing socioeconomic status as a global indicator of stress; and 5) using a combination of one or more of the above.

The measurement of protective factors and resilient outcomes has been no less complicated. Indeed, Greenback and Auerbach's witticism might be aptly transplanted here: that is "One researcher's 'resilient outcome' is another's 'protective factor.'" Kinard (1998) characterizes this confusion as being the conflation of "factors defining resilience and factors related to resilience" (p. 670). Lösel, Bliesener, and Köferl (1989) identify several resilience-related constructs, including "hardiness, adaptation, adjustment, mastery, plasticity, person-environment fit, or social buffering" (p. 187). There are likely many more, but the relations between these constructs have yet to be investigated.

Even in the face of these difficulties, there has been notable progress concerning methodological issues. Greenbaum and Auerbach (1992) report, for example, that there is growing agreement about how to measure certain specific risks. Luthar and Zigler (1991) suggest similar progress, though to a lesser extent, in regards to measurements of protective factors and resilient outcomes. In addition, researchers have placed definitional and methodological issues as top-tier concerns to be addressed by future research programs (Glantz & Johnson, 1999; Masten, 1999; Windle, 1999).

PUBLIC POLICY CONSIDERATIONS

Researchers and practitioners (e.g., Gitterman, 2001; Rolf, 1999) have expressed concerns about the ramifications of the study of resilience on public policy. These concerns likely grow out of the field's acute awareness of the needs of the primary population it has studied, at-risk children and youth. Describing several of the researchers we mentioned above, Cicchetti (1984) comments, "These scientists, whose work constitutes a kind of contemporary center of gravity for the discipline of developmental psychopathology, have advanced human knowledge while also helping to alleviate human suffering" (p. 5). Perhaps, too, these researchers have enough experience with policy makers to know that scientific research does not necessarily translate into effective public policy, especially when subjected to the vested, often factional interests of powerbrokers. This concern is not likely to abate. Masten (1999) reports, "There is a sense of emergency rising with the tide of child causalities of violence, drug abuse, and poverty in the United States" (p. 292); these words likely represent a broad contingent of contemporary resilience researchers. Social policy, then, clearly resides close to the heart of many resilience researchers, and that is perhaps rightly so. This trend may very well gain momentum. Romano and Hage (2000), for instance, entreat psychologists to expand their work to include the creation of public policy and other forms of activism, so that social justice receives maximum consideration within the field of prevention, and prevention science has a strong kinship and overlap with resilience science (Robinson, 2000).

FUTURE DIRECTIONS

Though concerns over public policy may influence the future trajectory of resilience research, it is not likely to eclipse the scientific agenda of the field, which is posed to tackle the literature's thorniest issues. Perhaps the first order of business is to impose some organization upon the Byzantine empire that is resilience research. Luthar, Cicchetti, and Becker take a major step in this direction, opening the current century with a thoughtful analysis of the key criticisms that have been lodged against resilience research, including its multifarious definitions, the multidimensional nature of the construct, its alleged statistical instability, and the meager theory behind much research (2000). These authors provide a helpful summary of three crucial, interrelated shifts in the literature over its brief lifespan. The first was from an early, somewhat limited focus on internal factors, such as high-self esteem and easy temperament, to an expanded focus on three levels of factors: individual, familial, and social. A second shift demarks a transition from viewing resilience (and its components) as simple *traits* or *factors* to viewing it as a complex *mechanism* or *process*. Demos (1989), as an illustration of this second shift, has gone so far as to suggest replacing the term "resilience" with the phrase "pattern of resiliency" (p. 4). He explains, that this captures the fact that "resiliency, like other complex, psychic organizations, does not function uniformly and automatically, but waxes and wanes in response to contextual variables" (Demos, 1989, p. 4). The third shift consist of the move away from conceptualizing resilience as absolute (that is, as "invulnerability"), to seeing it as environmentally or contextually circumscribed.

All three shifts highlight the field's growing conviction that resilience draws upon multiple layers of adaptational systems, ranging from the biological and genetic to the cognitive and social, these systems interacting with the individual's environment in complex ways. To a large extent, the emerging conceptualization of resilience builds upon the successes of early resilience research, which has identified several general factors that have repeatedly been correlated with resilience, including good relationships with caring adults, good cognitive skills, the capacity to self-regulate, high self-esteem or positive self-view, and a motivation to succeed (Masten, 2001). Masten (2001) confidently states, "Despite all the flaws in the early studies of resilience pointed out by early and later reviewers, recent studies continue to corroborate the importance of a relatively small set of global factors associated with resilience" (p. 234).

Having shifted "toward multifactorial, multisystem, process-oriented theories and investigations" (Masten, 1999, p. 292), researchers seem primed to address the complexity of the resilience construct. Masten (1999) optimistically concedes, "finer-grained inquiry is just beginning" (p. 291). Progress calls for the implementation of more complex and expensive research schemes that address multiple, interacting processes over time. This reflects the main agenda of the next phase of the resilience literature, which is to utilize the established short-list of resilience factors and begin putting together what some have claimed has been "lacking throughout the resilience literature," the development of an "adequate understanding of how at-risk children integrate these factors to promote resiliency" (Brown & Rhodes, 1991, p. 174).

REFERENCES

Ainsworth, M.D.S., & Wittig, B.A. (1969). Attachment and exploratory behavior of one-year-olds in a strange situation. In B.M. Foss (Ed.), *Determinants of Infant Behavior* (pp. 111–136). London: Methuen.

American Psychiatric Association. (1987). *Diagnostic and statistical manual of mental disorders* (3rd-Revised ed.).

Anthony, E.J. (1974). The syndrome of the psychologically invulnerable child. In E.J. Anthony & C. Koupernik (Eds.), *The child in his family: Children at psychiatric risk* (Vol. 3, pp. 529–544). New York: Wiley.

Bowlby, J. (1951). *Mental care and mental health*. Geneva: WHO.

Bowlby, J. (1958). The nature of the child's tie to his mother. *International Journal of Psycho-Analysis, 39*, 350–373.

Bretherton, I. (1991). The roots and growing points of attachment theory. In P. Marris (Ed.), *Attachment across the life cycle* (pp. 9–32). New York: Routledge.

Brown, W.K., & Rhodes, W.A. (1991). Factors that promote invulnerability and resiliency in at-risk children. In W.A. Rhodes & W.K. Brown (Eds.), *Why some children succeed despite the odds* (pp. 171–177). New York: Praeger.

Cicchetti, D. (1984). The emergence of developmental psychopathology. *Child Development, 55,* 1–7.

Cicchetti, D., & Garmezy, N. (1993). Milestones in the development of resilience [Special issue]. *Development and Psychopathology, 5*(4), 497–774.

Davis, N. J. (1999). Unpublished Working Paper: *Resilience: Status of the research and research-based programs.* Prepared for the Center for Mental Health Services. (301-443-2844, www.mentalhealth.org).

Demos, E.V. (1989). Resiliency in infancy. In T.F. Dugan & R. Coles (Eds.), *The Child in our times: Studies in the development of resiliency* (pp. 3–22). New York: Brunner/Mazel.

Dyer, J.G., & McGuinness, T.M. (1996). Resilience: Analysis of the concept. *Archives of Psychiatric Nursing, 10*(5), 276–282.

Gagne, E.D., Yekovich, C.W., & Yekovich, F.R. (1993). *The cognitive psychology of school learning* (2nd ed.). New York: Harper Collins.

Garmezy, N. (1971). Vulnerability research and the issue of primary prevention. *American Journal of Orthopsychiatry, 41*(1), 101–116.

Garmezy, N. (1994). Vulnerability research and the issue of primary prevention. In R.J. Haggerty, L.R. Sherrod, N. Garmezy & M. Rutter (Eds.), *Stress, risk, and resilience in children and adolescents: Procceses, mechanisms, and interventions* (pp. 1–18). New York: Cambridge University Press.

Gitterman, A. (2001). Vulnerability, resilience, and social work with groups. In T.B. Kelly, T. Berman-Rossi & S. Palombo (Eds.), *Group work: Strategies for strengthening resilience.* New York: Haworth Press.

Glantz, M.D., & Johnson, J.L. (Eds.). (1999). *Resilience and development: Positive life adaptations.* New York: Kluwer Academic/Plenum Publishers.

Gordon, E., & Wang, M.C. (1994). Epilogue: Educational resilience—Challenges and prospects. In E. Gordon (Ed.), *Educational resilience in inner-city America: Challenges and prospects* (pp. 191–194). Hillsdale, NJ: Erlbaum.

Greenbaum, C.W., & Auerbach, J.G. (1992). The conceptualization of risk, vulnerability, and resilience in psychological development. In C.W. Greenbaum & J.G. Auerbach (Eds.), *Longitudinal studies of children at psychological risk: Cross-national perspectives.* Norwood, New Jersey: Ablex.

Gullestad, S.E. (2001). Atachment theory and psychoanalysis: Controversial issues. *Scandinavian Psychoanalytic Review, 24,* 3–16.

Guttman, H.A. (1989). Children in families with emotionally disturbed parents. In L. Combrinck-Graham (Ed.), *Children in family contexts: Perspectives on treatment* (pp. 252–276). New York: Guilford Press.

Hetherington, E.M. (1980). Children and divorce. In R. Henderson (Ed.), *Parent-child interaction: Theory, research and prospect.* New York: Academic Press.

Horowitz, F.D. (1989). *The concept of risk: A re-evaluation.* Paper presented at the Society for Research in Child Development, Kansas City, MO.

Kagan, J. (1996). Three pleasing ideas. *American Psychologist, 51*(9), 901–908.

Kaplan, H.B. (1999). Toward an understanding of resilience: A critical review of definitions and models. In M.D. Glantz & J.L. Johnson (Eds.), *Resilience and development: Positive life adaptations* (pp. 17–83). New York: Kluwer Academic/Plenum Publishers.

Kaufman, J., Cook, A., Arny, L., Jones, B., & Pittinsky, T. (1994). Problems defining resilience: Illustrations from the study of maltreated children. *Development and Psychopathology, 6,* 215–229.

Kinard, E.M. (1998). Methodological issues in assessing resilience in maltreated children. *Child Abuse & Neglect, 22*(7), 669–680.

Lazarus, R.S., DeLongis, A., Folkman, S., & Gruen, R. (1985). Stress and adaptational outcomes: The problem of confounded measures. *American Psychologist, 40*(7), 770–779.

Liddle, H.A. (1994). Contextualizing resiliency. In M. Wang & E. Gordon (Eds.), *Educational resilience in inner-city America: Challenges and prospects* (pp. 167–177). Hillsdale, NJ: Erlbaum.

Lösel, F., Bliesener, T., & Köferl, P. (1989). On the concept of "invulnerability": Evaluation and first results of the Bielefeld Project. In M. Brambring, F. Lösel & H. Skowronek (Eds.), *Children at risk: Assessment, longitudinal research, and intervention* (pp. 186–219). New York: Walter de Gruyter.

Luthar, S.S., Cicchetti, D., & Becker, B. (2000). The construct of resilience: A critical evaluation and guidelines for future work. *Child Development, 71*, 543–562.

Luthar, S.S., & Zigler, E. (1991). Vulnerability and competence; A review of research on resilience in childhood. *American Journal of Orthopsychiatry, 61*(1), 6–22.

Masten, A.S. (1999). Resilience comes of age: Reflections on the past and outlook for the next generation of research. In M.D. Glantz & J.L. Johnson (Eds.), *Resilience and development: Positive life adaptations* (pp. 281–296). New York: Kluwer Academic/Plenum Publishers.

Masten, A.S. (2001). Ordinary magic: Resilience processes in development. *American Psychologist, 56*(3), 227–238.

Masten, A.S., & Coatsworth, J.D. (1998). The development of competence in favorable and unfavorable environments: Lessons from research on successful children. *American Psychologist, 53*(2), 205–220.

Murphy, L.B., & Moriarty, A.E. (1976). *Vulnerability, coping, and growth.* New Haven: Yale University.

Paul, G.L. (1967). Strategy of outcome research in psychotherapy. *Journal of Consulting Psychology, 31*(2), 109–118.

Pines, M. (1975, December). In praise of "invulnerables." *APA Monitor,* 7.

Pines, M. (1979, January). Superkids. *Psychology Today,* 53–63.

Robinson, J.L. (2000). Are there implications for prevention research from studies of resilience. *Child Development, 71*(3), 570–572.

Rolf, J.E. (1999). Resilience: An interview with Norman Garmezy. In M.D. Glantz & J.L. Johnson (Eds.), *Resilience and development: Positive life adaptations* (pp. 5–14). New York: Kluwer Academic/Plenum Publishers.

Romano, J.L., & Hage, S.M. (2000). Prevention and counseling psychology. *Counseling Psychologist, 28*(6), 733–763.

Rutter, M. (1971). Parent-child separation: Psychological effects on children. *Journal of Child Psychology & Psychiatry, 12,* 233–260.

Rutter, M. (1979). Protective factors in children's responses to stress and disadvantage. In M.W. Kent & J.E. Rolf (Eds.), *Primary prevention of psychopathology: Vol. 3. Social competence in children* (pp. 49–74).

Rutter, M. (1985). Resilience in the face of adversity: Protective factors and resistance to psychiatric disorder. *British Journal of Psychiatry, 147*(3), 598–611.

Rutter, M. (1987). Psychosocial resilience and protective mechanisms. *American Journal of Orthopsychiatry, 57*(3), 316–331.

Rutter, M. (1991, December). *Resilience: Some conceptual considerations.* Paper presented at the Institute of Mental Health Initiatives Conference on "Fostering Resilience," Washington, DC.

Rutter, M., Maughan, B., Mortimore, P., Ouston, J., & Smith, A. (1979). *Fifteen thousand hours.* Cambridge, MA: Harvard University Press.

Seligman, M.E.P. (1990). *Learned optimism: How to change your mind and your life.* New York: Simon & Schuster Trade.

Seligman, M.E.P. (1994). *What you can change and what you can't: The complete guide to successful self-improvement.* New York: Knopf.

Seligman, M.E.P. (1995). *The optimistic child.* Boston: Houghton Mifflin.

Tarter, R.E., & Vanyukov, M. (1999). Re-visiting the validity of the construct of resilience. In M.D. Glantz & J.L. Johnson (Eds.), *Resilience and development: Positive life adaptations* (pp. 85–100). New York: Kluwer Academic/Plenum Publishers.

Tolan, P.T. (1996). How resilient is the concept of resilience? *The Community Psychologist, 29,* 12–15.

Wallerstein, J.S., & Kelly, J.B. (1980). *Surviving the breakup: How children and parents cope with divorce.* New York: Basic Books.

Werner, E.E., & Smith, R.S. (1982). *Vulnerable but invincible: A longitudinal study of resilient children and youth.* New York: McGraw Hill.

Windle, M. (1999). Critical conceptual and measurement issues in the study of resilience. In M.D. Glantz & J.L. Johnson (Eds.), *Resilience and development: Positive life adaptations* (pp. 161–176). New York: Kluwer Academic/Plenum Publishers.

Wolff, S. (1995). The concept of resilience. *Australian and New Zealand Journal of Psychiatry, 29*(4), 565–574.

Chapter 3

Re-inventing Resilience
A Model of "Culturally-Focused Resilient Adaptation"

CAROLINE S. CLAUSS-EHLERS

INTRODUCTION

Traditional paradigms in counseling and clinical psychology literature have placed a tremendous emphasis on pathology-driven models. The search to classify what was wrong with the individual dates back to 1833 when Emil Kraepelin published the first classification of adult psychopathologies. Kraepelin (1833) assumed an organic etiology for each disease classification and led the way for the disease-focused zeitgeist in psychology. Pietrofesa, Hoffman, and Slete (1984), for instance, describe psychotherapy as an enterprise that deals with the more serious problems of mental illness. For Trotzer & Trotzer (1986), the goal of psychotherapy is to develop a long-term relationship focused on reconstructive change. More recently, the growing field of developmental psychopathology has attempted to understand how developmental processes contribute to the onset and formation of psychopathology throughout the life span (Wenar & Kerig, 2001). While this literature asks important questions about childrens' well being, exploration is also needed about critical issues connected to health promotion and prevention. If developmental variables such as behavior, unconscious processes, and cognition can contribute to maladaptive behaviors and poor emotional health, wouldn't we expect to see the same combination of factors contribute to positive, adaptive behaviors?

Positive psychology has moved away from a focus on disease to scientifically explore protective factors, assets, and strengths (Lopez, Prosser, Edwards, Magyar-Moe, Neufeld, & Rasmussen, 2002). Resilience is one such concept in positive psychology and has been defined as "the ability to thrive, mature, and increase competence in the face of adverse circumstances or obstacles" (Gordon, 1996, p. 63). More broadly defined, resilience has been viewed as a "process, capacity or outcome of successful adaptation despite challenges or threatening circumstances . . . good outcomes despite high risk status, sustained competence under threat and recovery from trauma" (Masten, Best, & Garmezy, 1990, p. 426). The concept of resilience is critical for youth as it means they are better equipped to cope with life circumstances. Resilience is also important in a preventive sense as it is thought that sufficient resilience will prevent children and adolescents from future problems (Arrington & Wilson, 2000; Kumpfer, 1999). Kumpfer (1999), for instance, describes how the "systematic application of methods for increasing resilience could improve child outcomes and prevent future problem behaviors and poor life adjustment, which are becoming increasingly costly to treat" (p. 180).

To date, however, there has been little research and writing that highlights cultural factors that influence resilience. As discussed below, resilience has often been defined as consisting of particular "resiliency factors" or "personality traits" (Kumpfer, 1999; Wolin & Wolin, 1993). While this research helps us understand what promotes resilience in the individual child, more recent literature has begun to examine the connection between the resilient individual and his or her surrounding environment. The focus of much of this work centers on how risk and resilience processes present themselves in the child's environmental context. According to Kumpfer (1999), family, neighborhood, school, and the peer group have an impact on the child's socialization process. In the face of stress, these environmental factors can either provide a protective buffer that supports the child or contribute to a negative impact that the child experiences.

This chapter discusses how cultural background is an additional aspect of socialization that must be explored in our understanding of resilience. Culture is defined as the transmission of shared values, beliefs, skills, and adaptive behaviors between generations and through shared participation in settings and situations (Carter, 1995; Falicov, 1995). The author defines *cultural resilience* as the way that the individual's cultural background, supports, values, and environmental experience help facilitate the process of overcoming adversity. Examining resilience through a sociocultural lens means we begin to look at individuals *in interaction* with a cultural environment that presents opportunities and challenges (Clauss-Ehlers, 2003). The purpose of this chapter is to critically explore resilience from a sociocultural perspective. For the author, this means moving away from the traditional definition of resilience as a conglomeration of character traits. Rather, readers are invited to become more culturally responsive by considering a new contextual model of resilience that the author introduces as *culturally-focused resilient adaptation* (CRA). This model attempts to explore how culture relates to resilience as it incorporates culture and diversity into resilience efforts and views successful adjustment to stress as a function of individual traits in interaction with the larger sociocultural environment.

To highlight the importance of incorporating culture and diversity into resilience processes, this chapter will first discuss the trait-based approach to resilience. It will then review current studies that include culture as an important aspect of resilience. From these reviews, the culturally-focused resilient adaptation model will be discussed as a dynamic framework that examines the individual in interaction with his/her environment in a sociocultural context.

TRAIT-BASED APPROACH TO RESILIENCE

As mentioned in Chapter Two, the construct of resilience evolved out of research conducted in the developmental psychopathology field (Cicchetti, 1990; Garmezy 1987; Rutter, 1975). Developmentalists gradually turned their interest from studying the onset of severe psychopathology, to learning about etiology and prevention for children at risk of developing problems *before* they became symptomatic. For instance, Garmezy (1987) and colleagues moved away from looking at adults with schizophrenia to study sources that support stress resistance in children of parents with schizophrenia. Following Garmezy's (1987) study, a large body of research looks at resilience in terms of different individual character traits. These studies found that individuals with greater amounts of certain characteristics were more apt to successfully negotiate negative life experiences. The inherent idea in much of this work is that if we can instill such characteristics in a child, that individual will be better equipped to cope with adverse life experiences.

The character-trait approach to resilience has looked at and identified various correlates of resilient people that include: easy temperament, secure attachment, basic trust, problem-solving abilities, an internal locus of control, an active coping style, enlisting people to help, making friends, acquiring language and reading well, realistic self-esteem, a sense of harmony, a desire to contribute to others, and faith that one's life matters (Davis, 2001). Werner and Smith (1982), for instance, found easy temperament to be a protective factor among infants. Their longitudinal study indicated that resilient children were more responsive and flexible, both of which led to more positive responses from caretakers. Gordon (1996) found five personal characteristics contributed to resilience in adolescence that included intelligence, androgyny, independence, social skills, and internal locus of control.

In her comprehensive review of resilience literature, Kumpfer (1999) organizes internal personality capabilities into five major cluster variables: 1) spiritual or motivational characteristics, 2) cognitive competence, 3) behavioral/social competencies, 4) emotional stability and emotional management, and 5) physical well-being and physical competencies. Each of Kumpfer's (1999) internal competencies is summarized below. It is suggested that her work be consulted for an excellent, in-depth description of those traits and processes that contribute to resilience.

Spiritual/Motivational Competencies

According to Kumpfer (1999), spiritual/motivational resiliency characteristics include belief systems that "serve to motivate the individual and create a direction for their efforts" (p. 197). Several studies, have shown that spirituality predicts resilience (Dunn, 1994; Masten, 1994). Variables to be included in this domain include (but are not limited to) purpose in life (Neiger, 1992), spirituality (Dunn, 1994), an internal locus of control (Werner & Smith, 1992), and hopefulness and optimism (Seligman, 1975). It appears that having a belief system helps individuals confront and cope with fears and adversities. Resilient individuals have also shown that spirituality helps them believe they can create better results for themselves and know when to give up on what they cannot control (Werner & Smith, 1992).

Cognitive Competencies

Variables that correlate with resilience in the cognitive competence category are characterized by cognitive abilities that help an individual accomplish their goals. Some of the competencies in this category include intelligence (Long & Vaillant, 1984), reading skills (Luthar & Zigler, 1992), insight (Wolin & Wolin, 1993), and self-esteem (Bandura, 1989). Intelligence has been found to correlate with children who are resilient (Werner, 1985) and acts as a protective factor that can promote school success and work achievement in later life. Reading is one such component of intelligence that fosters resilience by promoting verbal competence. Some researchers state that insight is the number one factor in resilience (Wolin & Wolin, 1993). States Kumpfer (1999): ". . . resilient children from dysfunctional parents are aware very early in life that they are different from and stronger than their sick parent. While empathetic and caring, they develop "adaptive distancing" to protect their sense of healthy separation from the parent's maladaptive coping skills and life patterns" (p. 203). Finally, positive self-esteem helps children take on challenges that can further their development and subsequent competencies.

Behavioral/Social Competencies

The behavioral/social competence domain involves the ability to carry out much of what is known in the cognitive arena. Variables include social skills, street smarts (Garmezy & Masten, 1986), communication (Wolin, 1991) and problem solving skills (Rutter & Quinton, 1994). The ability to effectively interact with people and be aware of the situation has been found to correlate with resilience (Garmezy & Masten, 1986). It is also hypothesized that those who are comfortable with the direction they plan to take are more likely to have great problem solving abilities. Trusting oneself to resolve issues is connected to self-efficacy in that it creates self-trust, initiative, and a belief in personal control (Wolin, 1993).

Emotional Stability and Emotional Management

The emotional stability and emotional management domain refers to the individual's ability to deal with and manage emotional reactions to life circumstances. Variables that fall under this competency include recognition of feelings, humor, hopefulness, and the ability to control anger and depression. A key characteristic of resilient people is their optimism and ability to recognize feelings. Recognizing feelings can subsequently lead to greater emotional management in tense situations where angry and depressive feelings might arise. Humor has been found to correlate with maintaining friendships (Masten, 1982), positive temperament (Werner, 1989) and the ability to "find the comic in the tragic" (Kumpfer, 1999, p. 208).

Physical Well-Being and Physical Competencies

Variables that correlate with resilience in the physical well-being and physical competence domain include good health (Werner & Smith, 1992), health maintenance skills, and physical attractiveness (Kaufman & Zigler, 1989). Kumpfer (1999) states that children with good physical health might internalize this as being strong and competent. Masten (1994) discusses how mastery of a physical talent such as music or sports can enhance self-esteem. Finally, physical attractiveness has been found to correlate with resilience, particularly if it also relates to charm and social skills (Kaufman & Zigler, 1989).

CROSS-CULTURAL RESEARCH ON RESILIENCE

While critical in terms of the characteristics we want to foster in children, the problem with the trait-based approach is that it leaves resilience way too much up to the individual child. To the extent that protective processes interact with stressors in the environment, resilience is actually a much more dynamic construct than first conceptualized (Rutter, 1987). Having said this, increasingly the literature has come to view resilience not as static, but as an ever-changing concept that emerges from environmental interactions. Winfield (1994) describes resilience as a dynamic construct whose processes involve the supports and stressors available to individuals as they interact with the surrounding environment. Similarly, Pianta and Walsh (1998) emphasize that "behavior cannot be understood without reference to the context(s) in which that behavior is demanded and/or supported" (p. 410). In recent work, Masten (2001) went on to define resilience as "a class of phenomenon characterized by good outcomes in spite of serious threats to adaptation or development" (p. 228).

The importance of environment is also apparent in research that indicates a child may do well in one setting, such as school, while simultaneously doing poorly in another, like home. Luthar, Doernberger, and Zigler (1993) talk about how a child may be socially competent in a high stress situation but an ineffective coper in others. These researchers define resilience as a "process that results when an individual reacts to risk factors, or vulnerabilities, that are present in their environment. As a result, resilience is an interactional process consisting of individual characteristics and the environment. The process of resilience can be fostered by . . . protective processes" (Arrington & Wilson, 2000, p. 225; Winfield, 1994).

While this working definition reflects the dynamic complexity at the root of resilience and moves beyond a trait-based model, research is just beginning to look at how resilience manifests itself in different cultural contexts. Much of the research that explores positive psychology constructs such as resilience has focused on predominantly White samples (Lopez et al., 2002). As a result, little is known about how resilience plays out in non-White cultural groups. Some writing has begun to move towards an understanding of resilience that incorporates culture and diversity. The following section reviews current work that looks at how culture and diversity influence resilience processes, or "what works for different people" (Lopez et al., 2002).

Cohler, Scott, and Musick (1995) discuss how culture can interact with stressors and development so that risk has a different impact and manifestation on different individuals. This is evidenced in the cultural formulation of illness section in the American Psychiatric Association (1994) *Diagnostic and Statistical Manual of Mental Disorders (4th ed.) (DSM-IV)* where the meaning of symptoms are viewed in relation to the norms of the cultural reference group. *Ataques de nervios* is one widely recognized culture bound syndrome in Latin America. An *ataque de nervios* might initially look like Panic Disorder as symptoms include being out of control, trembling, heat in the chest rising to the head, crying, and uncontrollable shouting. However, because *ataques* are associated with a precipitating event such as the loss of a family member, a separation from a spouse, or witnessing an accident, coupled with the individual's fairly quick return to normal functioning, they are not related to Panic Disorder. Rather, *ataques* can be seen as a culturally acceptable way to express emotional distress.

Belgrave, Chase-Vaughn, Gray, Addison, and Cherry (2000) conducted a study on the effectiveness of a cultural and gender specific intervention program designed to increase resiliency among African American preadolescent females. These researchers decided to implement a resilience-based intervention for adolescents who faced contextual risk factors such as drugs, criminal activity, and violence. The intervention incorporated two strategies: resource enhancement (e.g., gives access to new resources) and process orientation (e.g., supports relationships needed for successful development). The first strategy consisted of providing after-school activities while the second involved a focus on developing positive relationships with others. A third intervention strategy focused on strengthening Africentric values and traditions found among individuals of African descent (Akbar, 1996; Azibo, 1991) such as spirituality; harmony; collective responsibility; oral tradition; sensitivity to emotional cues; authenticity; balance; concurrent time orientation to past, present and future; and interpersonal/communal orientation (Belgrave et al., 2000).

Results of the study indicated that after participating in the intervention, participants scored significantly higher on 1) Africentric values; 2) ethnic identity; and 3) physical appearance self-concept than those who did not engage in the exercises designed to increase feelings of self-worth, Africentric values, and ethnic/gender identity. The researchers hypothesized that their study contributed to an understanding about how to promote resiliency as a protective factor in African American girls. They concluded that this gender and ethnically congruent intervention was responsive to the group as it promoted self-esteem, ethnic identity, and cultural values.

Researchers have also found that relational and environmental support promotes academic resilience among different cultural groups. Gonzalez and Padilla (1997) conducted a study that identified factors that contributed to the academic resilience and achievement among Mexican American high school students. They administered a 314-item questionnaire to three high schools in California. Students who identified themselves as Mexican were included in the subject pool that consisted of 2,169 participants.

Demographic data allowed the researchers to distinguish between resilient (students who reported getting "mostly A's") vs. nonresilient students (students who reported getting "mostly D's"). The demographic portion of the study found that resilient students were more likely to be female, have immigrant parents, have been born outside the United States, have had foreign schooling, and be more likely to live with both parents in comparison to nonresilient students. In contrast, nonresilient students were more likely than resilient students to live with their mothers, and have parents with lower education levels in comparison to resilient students.

The researchers conducted a factor analysis of the questionnaire and found it reflected three variables: support (a variable that included family and peer support, parental monitoring, and teacher feedback); sense of belonging in school (a variable that reflected the students' sense of acceptance); and cultural loyalty (a variable that consisted of familism, nonassimilation, and cultural pride/awareness). Gonzalez and Padilla (1997) found that a supportive academic environment and a sense of belonging to school predicted greater resilience among Mexican American students. Family and peer support were also significant with regard to the participant's grade point average (GPA).

The study also found that, although cultural loyalty did not predict resilience, *t* tests indicated that the familism subscale showed significant differences between resilient and nonresilient students. These investigators concluded that "students' sense of belonging to school and their supportive environments can have important effects on academic achievement" (Gonzalez & Padilla, 1997, p. 315). With regard to looking at resilience as something that is trait-based vs. environmentally driven, the authors state that their study reinforces the idea that resilience is not a trait, but rather "a capacity that develops over time in the context of environmental support" (Egeland, Carlson, & Sroufe, 1993, p. 19).

In another study, Brodsky (1999) suggests that African American single mothers consider resilience as the ability to find a balance between risk and protective factors in eight domains: neighborhood, parenting, family, friends, men, personal characteristics/activities, and spirituality. Her qualitative analysis was conducted on 10 single African American mothers living in risky neighborhoods. Brodsky (1999) found that, for the women, "making it" involved balancing stressors and resources in these eight domains. In addition, the study found that each woman achieved this balance in her own way, thus finding a unique person-environment fit. There were, however, three skills that fostered resilience in all the women. These skills included the ability to "1) appreciate resources and success and reframe some stressors to allow for contentment in one's current situation; 2) reframe stressors in ways that are motivating; and 3) locate, recognize, and utilize resources from supportive domains to deal with the demands of stressful domains—and to set and strive for new goals" (Brodsky, 1999, p. 157).

Some studies have supported the hypothesis that culture can influence how one understands and copes with an event (Lopez et al., 2002). Strong's (1984) study compared coping behaviors between Native American and White families who took care of elderly relatives. Strong (1984) found differences between the two groups in terms of their sense of control and expression of anger. Specifically, White families felt more in control and experienced a greater sense of coping than Native American families. Strong (1984) concluded that perhaps Native Americans were more apt to accept their situation since they felt less control, a dynamic that corresponds with the traditional Native American value of noninterference.

Again, moving beyond a trait-based focus, other research looks at how support systems can be critical to coping. De la Rosa (1988) found Puerto Rican adolescents with strong support systems were more equipped to deal with stressful situations and less likely to get ill. Similarly, Colomba, Santiago, and Rossello (1999) found that the more Puerto Rican adolescents seek out family and social support, the less likely they will become depressed when faced with a stressful situation.

Spencer and Dupree (1996) incorporate culture and diversity in their perspective of resilience. Their identity-focused ecological model states that ecology and culture have an impact on how children adjust to the environment. They discuss the concept of an *ecocultural character* that involves cultural values and practices that have an impact on social interactions and development. For them, the identity-focused cultural ecological model takes a dynamic approach to looking at risk, coping, resilience, and outcomes. Keogh and Weisner (1993) also discuss how both vulnerability and resilience must be understood within the individual's ecological and cultural context. They state that an assessment of supports and risk factors must go beyond the individual and the family to look at the community and culture as they are experienced by the child.

A NEW MODEL: CULTURALLY-FOCUSED RESILIENT ADAPTATION

This review of resilience literature within a multicultural context suggests that resilience processes lie in the environmental context in addition to individual traits. The previously cited investigations take a culturally contextual systems perspective in their understanding of the development of problems and stress (Belgrave et al., 2000; Brodsky, 1999; Colomba et al., 1999; Gonzalez & Padilla, 1997; Kumpfer, 1999; Strong, 1984). Central to this approach is the idea that behavior must be understood within the contexts in which that behavior is demanded or supported. Lopez et al. (2002) state that the multicultural coping literature, such as that mentioned above, indicates similarities and differences between coping behaviors of Whites and other groups. They conclude that, because of these differences, current models of stress and coping may not sufficiently address the unique coping styles of diverse groups.

Similarly, Pianta and Walsh (1998) state that too often, researchers and theorists follow the single characteristic approach to resilience by looking at only one system as the location of success or failure. This "single-location discourse" (Pianta & Walsh, 1996) looks only at the child, school, or home environment to determine what either fostered competence or failed development. Pianta and Walsh (1998) caution against looking at the impact of only one system on development and instead state that resilience consists of the "characteristics of a process involving the interactions of systems" (p. 411). A developmental systems approach to resilience argues that resilience is complex (Pianta & Walsh, 1998; 1996) and involves the interaction of many factors over time which, occasionally, initiate success in a particular domain. What deserves closer scrutiny is the child's embeddedness in a context that can either mobilize resources that lead to positive outcomes or introduce stressors that initiate risk. Here resilience is conceptualized as the positive result of interactions among child, school, family, peers, and community. The more these interactions are child-focused, the more resilience-resources the child will bring to key developmental tasks and experiences.

A paradigmatic shift from disease to health must be central to new objectives in the field of psychology. Prevention, early intervention, and integrating sociocultural support are integral tasks to emerge from a move toward health. Sociocultural contexts reflect resources and stressors relevant to a particular child's experience (Johnson, 1990). It is the larger sociocultural system that is thought to influence a superordinate cultural framework through which behavior, language, and communication patterns are understood. Looking at the sociocultural environment allows us to explore ways in which normative and non-normative experiences influence resilience or stress among diverse groups of children. For instance, sociocultural experiences like socioeconomic and cultural differences are increasingly thought to have an impact on development (Dryfoos, 1996).

To this end, *cultural resilience* is a term that considers those aspects of one's cultural background such as cultural values, norms, supports, language, and customs that promote resilience for individuals and communities. Because culture is all around us, because children operate within different cultural mindsets, and because there are inherent values built into these frameworks, we can no longer talk about resilience without incorporating culture and diversity. Resilience as it is defined and practiced, must be relevant to a wide spectrum of culturally diverse youth. The author's perspective, the *culturally-focused resilient adaptation (CRA) model*, asserts that culture and the sociocultural context influence resilient adaptation. Here resilience is not defined as a conglomeration of individual characteristic traits alone. Culturally-focused resilient adaptation in the face of adversity is defined as a dynamic, interactive process in which the individual negotiates stress through a combination of character traits, cultural background, cultural values, and facilitating factors in the sociocultural environment.

Cultural values are those beliefs about what is important to one's cultural background. Cultural values are posited to enhance resilience since they build support and protective processes into communities. For instance, Clauss-Ehlers and Lopez-Levi (2002a; 2002b) talk about cultural values in the Latino community such as *familismo, respeto*, and *personalismo. Familismo* means that family needs come before individual desires and include family obligation, view of family as a social support, and looking to family members as role models. *Respeto* compliments familismo as it "acknowledges the authority of elder family members and senior people in positions of power" (Clauss-Ehlers & Lopez-Levi, 2002a, p. 8). *Personalismo* refers to valuing relationships in and of themselves and not as a means to an end (Clauss, 1998).

The intersection of these cultural values creates what the author introduces as the *child's cultural script for resilience*. Latino cultural values, for instance, allow children to look to extended family for ongoing support, seek out older, experienced role models, and be encouraged to develop positive relationships with which they can identify and develop healthy attachments. Such influences help define contexts of resilience for Latino children who benefit from an extended family support network. Certainly this hypothesis has been supported by empirical studies such as those conducted by De La Rosa (1988) and Colomba et al. (1999).

Conversely, this literature also provides information about stressors. For children whose families immigrate to the United States, for instance, vulnerability might be the sudden loss of extended family support from members in the country of origin. The sociocultural context that arises out of Latino cultural values illustrates a key concept in the CRA model that the author calls *facilitating developmental environments*. A facilitating developmental environment is an environment that supports optimal development, mastery, and health, and is *culturally syntonic* with the individual's objectives and needs. In the Colomba et al. (1999) study, for instance, the fact that family support prevented depressive symptoms provides an example of a facilitating developmental environment.

In contrast, an *interfering developmental environment* is one that fails to promote resilience and optimal development. The interfering developmental environment is the context that does not respond to the individual, does not support mastery and competence, is *culturally dystonic*, and creates a barrier in development. Interfering developmental environments can be active or passive. The passive interfering developmental environment fails to support the child simply because it lacks key resources. Such an environment might be experienced by the family that immigrates to the United States and experiences cultural value conflicts, loss of extended family support, and language barriers. The active interfering developmental environment is the context where intentional behaviors and actions exist such that they create an adversity potential that undermines the child.

The interaction between contexts and the individual, cultural values, and interpersonal dynamics create a response to the facilitating or interfering environment. The process is one of culturally-focused resilient adaptation since the child brings multiple aspects of self and culture to confront and manage environmental adversity. Out of this process, it is hoped that children develop competent responses to the various sociocultural environments where they live.

CONCLUSION

The purpose of this chapter has been to promote a shift from disease to health by putting resilience in a multicultural context. Resilience research has made extraordinary contributions to the positive psychology literature (Cicchetti & Garmezy, 1993; Conrad & Hammond, 1993; Dunn, 1994; Gordon, 1996). Incorporating culture and diversity into these efforts means that we build on scientific findings to determine how they correspond to and reflect the needs of diverse communities.

It is thought that by understanding the sociocultural contexts in which children function, we can provide culturally relevant interventions. By looking at resilience as a culturally-adaptive competency, the author's hope is that we will also look at clinical interventions that are responsive to the backgrounds of children, families, and the communities we serve. A Latino child who adheres to the cultural value of *familismo*, for instance, might feel she's betraying her parents if she has to share family secrets in individual therapy. This same child, however, might be an active participant in family therapy since the modality doesn't raise the conflict of talking to a stranger, i.e., the therapist, outside the family. Similarly, the value of *personalismo* (Clauss, 1998) suggests that personal, informal treatment settings may be more germane to treatment than sterile impersonal medical settings. Through discussing the history and current status of resilience, the author's goal has been to place resilience in a sociocultural framework. To this end, aspects of the CRA model include:

- Building on the trait-based literature by looking at environmental factors that promote resilience
- Recognizing that coping and resilience processes might differ for different cultural groups
- Considering how interaction with the sociocultural context can promote the development of resilience
- Exploring the Culturally Resilient Adaptation model that seeks to incorporate culture and diversity with resilience processes
- Conducting empirical research on resilience with diverse groups to explore what works for different people

Re-visiting resilience as a function of culture means that protective factors and subsequent interventions are viewed as culturally syntonic for African American, Asian and Asian American, Latino, American Indian, and White American children. To accomplish this fundamental task, readers are invited to consider three paradigmatic shifts in psychology: a change from a *pathology-driven* to a *health-promotion* model of mental health; a change from an exclusively trait-based approach to one that incorporates a socioculturally-focused understanding of resilience; and last, a move towards culturally relevant interventions at individual, family, and community levels. Through concerted efforts in all these areas, we will truly be in a position to build on solid research foundations and together, re-invent resilience.

REFERENCES

Akbar, N. (1996). African metapsychology of human personality. In D.A. Azibo (Ed.), *African psychology in historical perspective and related commentary* (pp. 29–46). Trenton, NJ: Africa World Press.

American Psychiatric Association. (1994). *Diagnostic and statistical manual of mental disorders* (4th ed.). Washington, DC: Author.

Arrington, M.A., & Wilson, M.N. (2000). A re-examination of risk and resilience during adolescence: Incorporating culture and diversity. *Journal of Child and Family Studies, 9*(2), 221–230.

Azibo, D. (1991). African-centered theses on mental health and nosology of Black/African personality disorders. *Journal of Black Psychology, 15*, 173–214.

Bandura, A. (1989). Human agency in social cognitive theory. *American Psychologist, 44*(9), 1175–1184.

Belgrave, F.Z., Chase-Vaughn, G., Gray, F., Addison, J.D., & Cherry, V.R. (2000). The effectiveness of a culture-and gender-specific intervention for increasing resiliency among African American preadolescent females. *Journal of Black Psychology, 26*(2), 133–147.

Brodsky, A.E. (1999). "MAKING IT": The components and process of resilience among urban, African American, single mothers. *American Journal of Orthopsychiatry, 69*(2), 148–169.

Carter, R.T. (1995). *The influence of race and racial identity in psychotherapy: Toward a racially inclusive model*. New York: John Wiley & Sons.

Cicchetti, D. (1990). A historical perspective on the discipline of developmental psychopathology. In J. Rolf, A. Masten, D. Cicchetti, K. Nuechterlein, & S. Weinbtraub (Eds.), Risk and protective factors in the development of spychopathology (pp. 2–28). New York: Cambridge University Press.

Cicchetti, D., & Garmezy, N. (1993). *Prospects and promises in the study of resilience. Development and Psychopathology, 5*, 497–502.

Clauss, C.S. (1998). Language: The unspoken variable in psychotherapy practice. *Journal of Psychotherapy, 35*(2), 188–196.

Clauss-Ehlers, C.S. (2003). Promoting ecological health resilience for minority youth: Enhancing health care access through the school health center. *Psychology in the Schools, 40(3)*, 265–278.

Clauss-Ehlers, C.S., & Lopez Levi, L. (2002a). Violence and community, terms in conflict: An ecological approach to resilience. *Journal of Social Distress and the Homeless, 11*(4), 265–278.

Clauss-Ehlers, C.S., & Lopez Levi, L. (2002b). Working to promote resilience with Latino youth in schools: Perspectives from the U.S. and Mexico. *The International Journal of Mental Health Promotion, 4*(4), 14–20.

Cohler, B.J., Scott, F.M., & Musick, J.S. (1995). Adversity, vulnerability, and resilience: Cultural and developmental perspectives. In D. Cicchetti & D.J. Cohen (Eds.), *Developmental psychopathology, Vol. 2: Risk, disorder, and adaptation* (pp. 753–800). NY: John Wiley.

Colomba, M.V., Santiago, E.S., & Rossello, J. (1999). Coping strategies and depression in Puerto Rican adolescents: An exploratory study. *Cultural Diversity and Ethnic Minority Psychology, 5*, 65–75.

Conrad, M., & Hammond, C. (1993). Protective and resource factors in high and low-risk children: A comparison of children with unipolar, bipolar, medically ill, and normal mothers. *Development and Psychopathology, 5*, 593–607.

Davis, N.J. (2001). *Resilience in childhood and adolescence*. Panel presentation delivered at George Washington University, Media Conference, Washington, DC, April.

De La Rosa, M. (1988). Natural support systems of Puerto Ricans: A key dimension for well-being. *Health and Social Work, 13*, 181–190.

Dryfoos, J.G. (1996). Adolescents at risk: Shaping programs to fit the need. *Journal of Negro Education, 65*, 5–18.

Dunn, D. (1994). Resilient reintegration of married women with dependent children: Employed and un employed. (Doctoral Dissertation, Department of Health Education, University of Utah, Salt Lake City, Utah).

Egeland, B., Carlson, E., & Sroufe, L.A. (1993). Resilience as process. *Development and Psychopathology, 5*(4), 517–528.

Falicov, C.J. (1995). Training to think culturally: A multidimensional comparative framework. *Family Process, 34*, 373–387.

Garmezy, N. (1987). Stress, competence, and development: Continuities in the study of schizophrenic adults, children vulnerable to psychopathology, and the search for stress-resistant children. *American Journal of Orthopsychiatry (57)* 2, 159–174.

Garmezy, N., & Masten, A.S. (1986). Stress, competence, and resilience: Common frontiers for therapist and psychopathologist. *Behavior Therapy, 57*(2), 159–174.

Gonzalez, R., & Padilla, A.M. (1997). The academic resilience of Mexican American high school students. *Hispanic Journal of Behavioral Sciences, 19*(3), 301–317.

Gordon, K.A. (1996). Resilient Hispanic youths, self-concept and motivational patterns. *Hispanic Journal of Behavioral Sciences, 18,* 63–73.

Johnson, S.D. (1990). Toward clarifying culture, race, and ethnicity in the context of multicultural counseling. *Journal of Multicultural Counseling and Development, 18*(1), 41–50.

Kaufman, J., & Zigler, E. (1989). The intergenerational transmission of child abuse. In D. Cicchetti & V. Carlson (Eds.), *Child Maltreatment: Theory and research on the causes and consequences of child abuse and neglect* (pp. 129–150). Cambridge: Cambridge University Press.

Keogh, B.K., & Weisner, T. (1993). An ecocultural perspective on risk and protective factors in children's development: Implications for learning disabilities. *Learning Disabilities Research and Practice, 8,* 3–10.

Kraepelin, E. (1883). *Compendium der psychiatire.* Liepzig: Abel.

Kumpfer, K.L. (1999). Factors and processes contributing to resilience: The resilience framework. In M.D. Glantz & J.L. Johnson (Eds.), *Resilience and development: Positive life adaptations* (pp. 179–224). New York: Kluwer Academic/Plenum Publishers.

Long, J.V.F., & Vaillanta, G.E. (1984). Natural history of male psychological health XI: Escape from the underclass. *American Journal of Psychiatry, 141,* 341–346.

Lopez, S.J., Prosser, E.C., Edwards, L.M., Magyar-Moe, J.L., Neufeld, J.E., & Rasmussen, H.N. (2002). Putting positive psychology in a multicultural context. In C.R. Snyder & S.J. Lopez (Eds.), *Handbook of positive psychology.* (pp. 700–714). New York: Oxford University Press.

Luthar, S.S., Doernberger, C.H., & Zigler, E. (1993). Resilience is not a unidimensional construct: Insights from a perspective study of inner-city adolescents, *Development and Psychopathology, 5,* 703–717.

Luthar, S.S., & Zigler, E. (1992). Intelligence and social competence among high-risk adolescents. *Development and Psychopathology, 4,* 287–299.

Masten, A.S. (1982). *Humor and creative thinking in stress resistant children.* Unpublished doctoral dissertation, University of Minnesota.

Masten, A.S. (2001). Ordinary magic: Resilience processes in development. *American Psychologist, 56*(3), 227–238.

Masten, A.S. (1994). Resilience in individual development: Successful adaptation despite risk and adversity. In M.C. Wang & E.W. Gordon (Eds.), *Educational resilience in inner-city America* (pp. 3–25). Hillsdale, NJ: Erlbaum.

Masten, A.S., Best, K.M., & Garmezy, N. (1990). Resilience and development: Contributions from the study of children who overcome adversity. *Development and Psychopathology, 2,* 425–222.

Neiger, B. (1991). *Resilient reintegration: Use of structural equations modeling.* Doctoral dissertation, University of Utah, Salt Lake City.

Pianta, R.C., & Walsh, D.J. (1998). Applying the construct of resilience in schools: Cautions form a developmental systems perspective. *School Psychology Review, 27*(3), 407–417.

Pianta, R.C., & Walsh, D. (1996). *High-risk children in the schools: Creating sustaining relationships.* New York: Routledge.

Pietrofesa, J.J., Hoffman, A., & Splete, H.H. (1984). *Counseling: An introduction* (2nd Ed.), Boston: Houghton Mifflin.

Rutter, M. (1987). Psychosocial resilience and protective mechanisms. *American Journal of Orthopsychiatry, 52,* 316–331.

Rutter, M., & Quinton, D. (1994). Long-term follow-up of women institutionalized in childhood: Factors promoting good functioning in adult life. *British Journal of Developmental Psychology, 18*, 225–234.

Seligman, M. (1975). *Helplessness: On depression, development, and death.* San Francisco: Freeman.

Spencer, M.B., & Dupree, D. (1996). African-American youths' ecocultural challenges and psychosocial opportunities: An alternative analysis of problem behavior outcomes. In D. Cicchetti & S.L. Toth (Eds.) *Adolescence: Opportunities and challenges* (pp. 259–282). Rochester, NY: University of Rochester Press.

Strong, C. (1984). Stress and caring for the elderly relatives: Interpretation and coping strategies in an American Indian and White sample. *The Gerontologist, 24*, 251–256.

Trotzer, J.P., & Trotzer, T.B. (1986). *Marriage and family.* Muncie, IN: Accelerated Development.

Wenar, C., & Kerig, P. (2001). *Developmental psychopathology: From infancy through adolescence. (4th Ed.)*, Boston: McGraw Hill.

Werner, E.E. (1985). Stress and protective factors in children's lives. In A.R. Nicol (Ed.), *Longitudinal studies in child psychology and psychiatry* (pp. 335–355). New York: John Wiley and Sons.

Werner, E.E. (1989). High-risk children in young adulthood: A longitudinal study from birth to 32 years. *American Journal of Orthopsychiatry, 59*, 72–81.

Werner, E.E., & Smith, R.S. (1992). *Overcoming the odds: High risk children from birth to adulthood.* Ithaca, New York: Cornell University Press.

Winfield, L.F. (1994). Developing resilience in urban youth, NCREL Monograph, Oak Park, IL: North Central Regional Educational Laboratory.

Wolin, S.J. (1991). Paper presented at the Protecting Vulnerable Children Project, Children of Alcoholics Foundation, Inc. Princeton University, Princeton, NJ, November, 1991.

Wolin, S.J., & Wolin, S. (1993). *Bound and determined: Growing up resilient in a troubled family.* New York: Villard Press.

Part 2

Promoting Resilience in Diverse Communities

Chapter 4

Sacred Spaces
The Role of Context in American Indian Youth Development

TERESA LAFROMBOISE AND LISA MEDOFF

For many decades attempts have been made to assimilate American Indians[1] into the dominant culture. Many have been removed from their homes as children and placed in boarding schools intended to erase all aspects of their traditional culture; others have been relocated from the reservation to large urban areas with the promise of housing and jobs, only to find themselves alone in the city with little assistance and limited contact with extended family or fellow tribal members. Institutional and systemic problems, such as discrimination and poverty, which increase the effects of potential risk factors, may obscure the underlying strengths of Native cultures and hinder the efforts of Native communities in fostering resilience. However, much of the traditional practices and beliefs still live on today, demonstrating the strength of cultural identity within Native individuals and the resilience of Native cultures as a whole.

Currently, there are 558 federally recognized American Indian tribes, many of which practice their own customs, maintain particular social organizations, and speak different tribal languages. It is important to bear in mind that while many tribes share similar traditions and a common basis for beliefs, as with any group of individuals, complete homogeneity in those beliefs cannot be assumed. Approximately 2.5 million people identify themselves solely as American Indian and Alaska Native, but when including those who consider themselves part American

---

[1] The name "American Indian" is used to refer to all Native American individuals, including Alaska Natives, Aleuts, Eskimos, and those of mixed blood. The terms American Indian, Native American, and Native are used interchangeably in this chapter, but it should be noted that these words represent diverse people from distinct tribes.

Indian or part Alaska Native, the number grows to 4.1 million (Ogunwole, 2002). Currently, American Indians are a young population, with approximately 840,300 individuals under the age of eighteen and a median age of twenty-eight years (U.S. Bureau of the Census, 2002a), in comparison with the national average of thirty-five years (U.S. Bureau of the Census, 2002b).

Due to outside interference, such as the boarding school and relocation movements, many tribes have encountered difficulty in sustaining intact family relations and preserving traditional ways of life. In many Native communities these factors have served to impair healthy functioning, impacting social, economic, and educational arenas. Native American women are less likely to marry and are more likely to be divorced than U.S. women in general. According to Sandefur and Liebler (1996), Indian women and children are in more precarious economic and social situations than those of other groups in the United States. Willeto (2002) confirms this negative conception, noting that poverty rates for American Indian and Alaska Native children are nearly three times higher than that of the general population. She also points out that American Indians have the lowest educational attainment. Estimations of high school dropout range from 30 to 60%. However, in some cases the urban Indian high school dropout rate has been reported to be as high as 85% (E. Webster, personal communication, July 15, 2003), underscoring the importance of taking into account the distinctiveness of different tribes and regions.

Despite difficulties, many aspects of American Indian culture have enabled it to survive great obstacles, particularly the strength of extended family support and the sense of belongingness enhanced by enculturation (an involvement in traditional cultural activities[2]). In American Indian communities still living the traditions, there is a very close link between the family and the community, creating a sacred space for youth development. Extended family members and other individuals there often serve as active mentors and supportive role models. These adults take a special interest in youth, through both personal contact and by promoting involvement in traditional cultural activities, such as ceremonies, powwows, feasts, and preparing Native foods. According to socialization theory (Maccoby, 1992), children learn the values, attitudes, and norms of behavior that are most valued by their social group from socializing agents such as the family, teachers, and other community members. These individuals function as role models who help contour the perceptions and goals of youth in relation to what roles and ways of living they are likely to adopt. In evaluating communities with both high and low rates of healthy youth within mainstream society, Blyth and Leffert (1995)

---

[2] Rogoff (2003) points out that because cultural practices fit together and are connected, it is important to bear in mind that cultural processes involve patterned relations that cannot be reduced to independent variables. A practice that is undertaken in one community may serve a different purpose than the same practice in another community.

found that the factors distinguishing the two were associated less with how the young people perceived their families and more with how they were linked to other socializing agents, such as schools, neighborhoods, and youth organizations. Werner and Smith's (1993) longitudinal study of multi-ethnic Hawaiian children showed that those who were the most resilient as adults had the strongest support network, consisting of both related and non-related members of older generations, as they were growing up. As young children, resilient adults tended to have more contact with caring others such as teachers, neighbors, and spiritual leaders.

Both the concern of extended family members and the involvement in traditional activities serve to reinforce feelings of connectedness, emphasizing not only the responsibility of the community to care for individuals, but the obligation of those individuals to be productive members of the community. A major source of many youth problems is the experience of feeling that one has no significant and meaningful role in the larger community (Nightingale & Wolverton, 1993). Bowlby (1969) has suggested that the need to belong is one of the strongest motivational needs. Thus, individuals act as if they are eager to become part of a larger social group, which often involves adopting the norms, values, and behaviors of the group. The longer the person is exposed to the activities of the group, the stronger the identification with the group becomes and the more likely the individual is to internalize the group values and norms. The behaviors that an individual exhibits are likely to be predicated upon such ideas, which highlights the importance of youth belonging to a group that advocates healthy, pro-social values and norms. Eccles and Gootman (2002), in their review of eight positive features of developmental settings, point out the importance of opportunities that give rise to a sense of belonging, noting that no matter what ethnic or racial background one comes from, it is often difficult to figure out how and where one fits in the diverse sphere of cultural identity. This may be difficult for Native youth who often must learn to function biculturally (in both American Indian and European American cultures), especially if they do not live on the reservation. However, bicultural competence, the ability to function effectively in diverse cultural settings, may be a protective factor for adolescent well-being (LaFromboise, Coleman, & Gerton, 1993).

Goodluck (2002) believes that the future is optimistic for American Indians. She notes a current trend toward increased tribal sovereignty, population growth, and an increasing economic base, which undoubtedly strengthens the community context. According to Blum, Potthoff, and Resnick (1997), over 80% of Indian youth feel that their parents care about them. Indian youth are increasingly able to emulate nationally known role models such as Notah Begay, the professional golfer; actress Irene Bedard; Ben NightHorse Campbell, the first American Indian United States Senator (R-Colorado); folk singer Buffy Sainte-Marie; and the hip-hop group, Haida. Thirty-five tribal colleges currently exist, allowing both youth and adults to advance their education and engage in lifelong learning within a comfortable and familiar environment. American Indians are constantly engaging in a process of cultural renewal and revitalization. James Clairmount, a Lakota spiritual elder, expresses how the concept of resilience is inherent in the Native culture: "The closest translation of 'resilience' is a sacred word that means 'resistance' . . . resisting bad thoughts, bad behaviors. We accept what life gives us, good and bad, as gifts from the Creator. We try to get through hard times, stressful times, with a good heart. The gift [of adversity] is the lesson we learn from overcoming it." (Graham, 2001, p. 1)

SPIRITUALITY

Some protective factors that assist children in coping with times of difficulty are having a sense of hope, a sense of meaning, and a sense of purpose (Benson, 1997). In addition to being an internal factor that fosters resilience, spirituality can also be viewed as an external factor, as adult members of a society transmit spiritual and religious beliefs through daily interactions and sacred rituals that increase the opportunity for promoting connectedness. It is important to take into consideration the interaction between internal and external protective factors. Werner and Smith (1993) noted a continuity over the life course of individuals who successfully overcame a variety of childhood adversities. The individual dispositions of each person directed him or her to select or construct environments that reinforced a positive disposition and rewarded competencies.

A theme that is frequently noted in American Indian spiritual belief systems is that of interconnectedness of all things, both living and non-living. Human beings are seen as a small part of the larger structure of the universe. They are morally intertwined with the natural world such that the past of one's family and community is linked to the present and teaches valuable lessons about proper and harmonious behavior. All creatures are an integral part of the sacred life force. Spirituality integrates American Indian society, giving rise to collective consciousness and social cohesion. Natural locations can also figure prominently in American Indian spirituality. Sacred mountains, such as Bear Butte in South Dakota, rocks, lakes, and rivers often serve as an anchor for spiritual practice. According to Hungry Wolf and Hungry Wolf (1987), for American Indians, spiritual life and tribal life cannot be separated. Spirituality pervades all aspects of American Indian culture. Religion is not generally seen as a separate institution from tribal life. Spirituality is the preferred term, as the spiritual aspect of humans is perceived to be an integral part of daily life.

The Native American Church acts as a resource for many American Indian youth (Office for Substance Abuse Prevention, 1990). The Church promotes abstinence from alcohol use, in addition to other ideals that promote health, wellness, and the preservation of cultural values. Members are encouraged to develop a strong social support network, and group meetings provide a safe environment in which members are able to express their emotions. It should be noted that many American Indians also belong to Christian churches and are able to draw strength, support, and a sense of belonging from these institutions in the same manner as other individuals. There is mounting evidence that American Indian people do not see Christianity and traditional practices as incompatible (Csordas, 1999).

Goodluck (2002) identified a list of 42 strengths in a sample of 22 American Indian documents (such as newspapers, dissertations, and book chapters) from a variety of specific tribal groups. Spirituality appeared quite frequently, second only to extended family. Goodluck defines three domains of well-being indicators that are specific to tribal groups: helping each other, group belonging, and spiritual belief systems and practices. In the spiritual domain behaviors include: knowing traditional Native American songs and dances, practicing traditional religion, participating in sweat lodge ceremonies/fasting/vision quests, and learning languages, songs, and traditions from a traditional person. Goodluck's findings coincide with those of other researchers. Jagers (1996) determined that cultural orientations of spirituality were associated with a lower number of aggressive and delinquent behaviors in inner-city adolescents. Resnick, Harris, and Blum (1993) found that a sense of spirituality served as a protective factor against high-risk behaviors for adolescents. Other studies have found a connection between spirituality and decreased self-report of depressive symptoms (Wright, Frost, & Wisecarver, 1993), decreased risk of suicide (Stein, Witzum, & Brom, 1992), and decreased involvement in substance abuse (Benson, 1992).

FAMILY

One of the most devastating policies of the US government was the boarding school experiment that began in the early 1700's and continued through the 1960's. As a result of the boarding school movement, traditional American Indian parenting practices have been severely compromised.[3] It was believed that American Indian children would learn to be self-sufficient participants in the larger society if they were reared away from their families in boarding schools. These schools were designed to destroy the family unit. Children as young as five years old were forcibly separated from their homes and sent far away to school, often across the country, for many years, ostensibly for the purposes of spiritual conversion, education, and other forms of "civilization." They were often severely punished for speaking their language or practicing any of their tribal customs. Since children

---

[3] The authors recognize that the practices of contemporary schooling with Indian children vary considerably in the extent to which they connect to Native cultures. For a more comprehensive treatment of this issue, see Demmert (2001); McCarty (2002); and Peshkin (1997).

had minimal interactions with their families, many lost their community identity and adapted to routine, institutional practices.

Not only were these children denied the opportunity to be taught traditional ways and practices, they were denied ongoing contact with their loved ones and the opportunity to be nurtured through traditional American Indian childrearing methods. When they returned to their communities after lengthy separations, they were often welcomed by family members who did not know how to relate to them. Unfortunately, the children were often deemed to be culturally incompetent. These disruptions in family living have produced generations of American Indian parents with a sense of uncertainty about how children should be raised. However, in recent years, there has been an attempt to rekindle traditional childrearing practices in order to strengthen the quality of life in Indian communities (National Indian Child Welfare Association, 1986). One example of this revival can be seen in the Minnesota "Cherish the Children" manual (Buffalohead, 1988). This manual includes lessons about the traditional Ojibwa way of parenting, as well as incorporating corresponding new ways of parenting.

Traditional Parenting Practices

In traditional times children were highly valued in most North American tribes and were often seen as sacred beings because they had the most recent contact with the spirit world (Gfellnert, 1990; Riley, 1993). All children were fully accepted as members of the family, clan, and tribe, whether they came from natural birth, were adopted, or were stepchildren (Babcock, 1991; Hungry Wolf & Hungry Wolf, 1987). They were considered to be beloved gifts from the Creator, the pathways through which the ancestors could offer help to the tribe. As with the Lakota, from conception onward the transmission of unconditional love to children was the primary role of American Indian parents (Atkinson & Locke, 1995). Like the Lakota, Ojibwa and Kickapoo parents made special efforts to protect their children's spirits (Cross, 1987), believing that children could be taken back to the spirit world if they were not treated well (Hill Witt, 1979; Morey & Gilliam, 1972).

Many childrearing processes that modern developmental psychologists have recommended for raising healthy and productive children have their counterparts in traditional American Indian ways of parenting still practiced by some American Indians today (K. Alvy, personal communication, May 16, 1995). The learning processes of modeling and behavioral demonstration of skills are widely practiced among caregivers. American Indian adults and older children often demonstrate the strategy of cognitive structuring, which includes giving children reasons for learning a new behavior or treating others with respect. Long before psychologists determined the positive effects of parental acceptance and warmth, native people understood its importance and practiced it regularly through praise, affection, and devotion to children. They allowed their children to learn from natural and logical consequences, despite outside judgments that they were laissez-faire in their approach (Gray & Cosgrove, 1985). Many behavioral modification programs teach parents and teachers about the positive impact of systematically ignoring child misbehaviors. When American Indian children misbehave, many Indian families still practice collective inattention until the child displays remorse or makes restitution for the behavior.

In the traditional extended family system everyone shares responsibility for meeting the needs of children. No one person has sole responsibility for child rearing. Thus, when parents cannot raise their own children, members of the extended family take them in and treat them well. In many tribes grandparents eagerly raise a child in a separate home and train them in particular skills and traditional teachings (MacPhee, Fritz, & Miller-Heyl, 1996; Ward, Henckley, & Sawyer, 1995). Among the Navajo, this alliance between grandparent and grandchild is considered to be the strongest bond in their culture. Grandparents recognize that age and life experiences are essential for child rearing. They readily offer assistance to parents, as young parents are not considered to have the years of experience necessary to raise children alone (Joe & Malach, 2000). Elders even adopt children when they lack strong family ties (Swinomish Tribal Mental Health Project, 1989). Currently, middle-aged adults are taking on increasing responsibilities for running the tribe, thus placing more childrearing responsibility upon elders who remain at home (Gray & Cosgrove, 1985).

In traditional practices American Indian children learn early on about the complex relationships between family and clan members. A prevalent expectation is the utmost display of respect for elders, as they hold the most honored positions in the community. Many children are encouraged to visit older people on an ongoing basis, especially their namesake (Buffalohead, 1988). Both children and adults often refer to elder men and women as "grandfather" and "grandmother," and the men and women of their parents' generation as "uncle" and "aunt" (Morey & Gilliam, 1972), highlighting the concept of extended family within the tribe.

Many of the methods of influencing appropriate behavior are based on the values that underlie traditional life. These include respect, bravery, generosity, and harmony (Eastman, 1924; Franzen, 1992). Respect is the foundation for discipline and authority. Many tribes believe that respect is situated at the very center of a person's relationship with all others. This begins with the child's relationship with the family. Children learn early to show respect, especially to elders. In years past they were told to stand or sit quietly by them, to obey them, and to learn from them by watching their daily activities. In turn, adults showed respect for children by being polite to them and using punishment sparingly, only when necessary (Morey & Gilliam, 1972). After misbehaving, a child might be ignored, or else quickly experience disapproving looks, words, or "tsk-tsk" sounds from adults.

Erickson (1963) noted that members of the Oglala communities he studied often modeled disdain for ownership and the importance of generosity in a variety of ways, such as giving away objects admired by others and always displaying hospitality by sharing food and drink with visitors. Adults still readily share resources, such as clothes and tools, with other members in the community, perpetuating the values of generosity and community responsibility.

The concept of harmony refers to balance between all living things. This value involves people co-existing cooperatively with the forces around them. Among the Cherokee, the harmony ethos provides regulatory norms for children. Avoidance and tolerance seem to be the most important methods of operationalizing this value (French, 1987). Children are encouraged not to insult or offend anyone. Within traditional families, adults demonstrate the importance of this value by using diffuse communication patterns that go to great length to avoid direct confrontation or conflict. For example, information about a child's misbehavior might be passed from the child's mother to an aunt or uncle who has been designated as responsible for guiding the child's character development (Morey & Gilliam, 1972). This indirect line of communication serves to keep the bond between parents and child harmonious and reinforces the extended family involvement in maintaining standards of behavior. Brendtro, Brokenleg, and Van Bockern (1990) describe the Circle of Courage, an incorporation of traditional practices that focuses on harmony and balance in the education and empowerment of children, which is believed to promote self-esteem through child-rearing practices. Cross (1998) points out that a relational worldview that stresses harmony and balance is conducive to resilience.

Contemporary Families

In many contemporary American Indian families, relational values and their behavioral manifestations have remained intact. Extended family networks still provide extensive psychological support despite the fact that families have been transformed over time due to geographic movements and intertribal marriages (Mohatt, 1988). Indian families that live in urban areas tend to have nuclear households, whereas families that live on the reservation tend to include extended family members (Joe & Malach, 2000; Lobo & Peters, 2001). In contrast to the European model of an extended family that is defined as three generations within a single household, Red Horse and colleagues (1978) describe a traditional American Indian extended family as structurally open with a village-like characteristic, including several households and relatives along both vertical and horizontal lines. Currently, many American Indian families operate biculturally by maintaining some of the traditional ways of the tribe and blending them with conventional American practices (National Indian Child Welfare Association, 1986). Families may shift along the continuum, becoming more traditional at times and less so at others.

A key feature of contemporary American Indian families is the growing proportion of children within them who reside with only one parent. Women head 45% of American Indian households (Sandefur & Liebler, 1996). According to Jacobson (1995), 54% of American Indian women had never married, compared to 39% of all American women. The extent of single parenthood, never marrying, and divorce appears to be higher on reservations with high unemployment and poverty rates. However, it is important to bear in mind that what may appear to be a negative life event to an outside assessor may, in fact, foster more successful adaptation. For example, an early pregnancy by an unwed mother is not necessarily a risk factor for American Indian women. They do not experience the stigma that is seen in other communities; in fact, the pregnancy may be seen as anchoring them. Being a mother is viewed as sacred, and as such, one's status in the community is elevated. In a similar fashion, limited employment or school drop-out may indicate that the individual is helping elders and/or the community through the provision of services and labor (Goodluck, 2002).

Although oftentimes there is only one parent in the family, there are often other adults in the household, including grandparents, aunts, uncles, and live-in partners, who continue the informal practice of caregiving that has gone on within the extended family for centuries. Most extended family members, especially females, readily work together to help children develop a sense of personal worth and well-being. Furthermore, grandparents often willingly assume child-rearing responsibilities, especially while parents of young children are employed. Parents frequently seek the much-valued advice and assistance of older family members and elders, recognizing the worth of counsel from those with a great deal of life experience when making major decisions (Joe & Malach, 2000). Following the tradition of story telling, elders often relate tales of abuse that has been directed at American Indian families, highlighting the powerful resources that allow individuals and communities to be resilient and survive (Red Horse et al., 1978).

Two major external factors that contribute to resiliency are a caring adult and family support (Eccles & Gootman, 2002). Parental support has been found to be one of the most powerful predictors of reduced delinquency and drug use in American Indian youth (King, Beals, Manson, & Trimble, 1992). Although Cowan and Cowan (1990) found that a warm, involved, supportive husband and caring authoritative father can promote the well-being and positive adjustment of children, especially sons, Cross (1998) indicated that though American Indian fathers provide part of the balance within a family, fathers do not need to be present in the household in order to contribute strength to the family system. LaFromboise, Oliver, and Hoyt (in press) found no significant relationship between American Indian resiliency and the presence of a male caregiver in the household. When an American Indian family is unable to instill moral values and provide guidance and support for children, the community is obligated to take responsibility for ensuring that children receive optimal levels of care. Although there are exceptions, for the most part Indian communities, both on and off the reservation, help to reinforce a protective sense of self-worth, identity, safety, and environmental mastery (Kipke, 1999). As one American Indian woman stated, "our children have dozens of parents if we allow it, if we utilize that. That helps us to bounce back from problems" (Goodluck & Willeto, in press).

Rolf and Johnson (1999) describe a mentoring relationship as one of the few key factors in promoting resilience. Mentors provide a modeling of useful skills and the rewards that are associated with those skills. The mentoring relationship allows for a practical, hands-on fostering of competencies through on-going communication and social interaction. Werner and Smith (1993) found that resilient children who succeeded against many odds overwhelmingly and exclusively gave credit to members of their extended family, neighbors, teachers, and mentors. This informal type of support was sought out more often and was more highly valued than professional and bureaucratic social services. Mentoring by members of the extended family is prevalent in many American Indian communities. For example, in the Navajo kinship system, mentoring is a birthright (Waller, 2002). In one such mentoring relationship, it is expected that the maternal uncle will mentor his sisters' children, particularly guiding them through their education. Within this kinship system, individual standing in the community is related to the extent to which a person fulfills his or her responsibilities to relatives.

A sense of mutual obligation is prevalent in the extended family system. Individuals are expected to fulfill cultural obligations to family members, thus heightening the sense of connectedness and belonging that help to foster resilience. Obligations can include caring for a young family member for an extended period of time or giving family members financial support without expectation of repayment. Cheshire and Kawamoto (2003) discuss the idea that mutual obligation produces collateral relationships that create a system of family support that is consistently maintained and secure; being a responsible individual in a collateral relationship fosters a sense of approval and self-worth. Whitehorse (1988) describes a giveaway as an event that exemplifies mutual obligation and collateral relationships. A giveaway is usually held in conjunction with a special occasion such as a graduation, a return home from active duty in the military, or a marriage. During this ritual, a friend may speak for the family of the individual being honored and call forth family and friends to receive gifts, while discussing the role these individuals have played in the life of the honored person. In this way, the community acknowledges the individual as a part of the community, as well as displays gratitude to the community for supporting the individual. This practice points out the importance of the extended family and community in taking responsibility for rearing children, as well as illustrating the obligation of the individual to continue the ways of the community.

TRADITIONAL INVOLVEMENT

Individuals are not passive receptors of the culture in which they happen to be raised. Rogoff (2003) conceptualizes human development as "a process in which people transform through their ongoing participation in cultural activities, which in turn contribute to changes in their cultural communities across generations" (p. 37). Enculturation involves gaining knowledge of and identifying with one's traditional culture. Zimmerman, Ramirez, Washienko, Walter, and Dyer (1998) view enculturation as the extent to which one identifies with his or her cultural heritage, takes pride in it, and participates in cultural activities. Although these authors suggest that a strong cultural identity and participation in traditional practices are related to resilience and can buffer negative influences, leading to decreased problem behaviors, it should be noted that others disagree with this perspective. Researchers such as Gil, Vega, and Dimas (1994) and Vega and Gil (1998) argue that enculturation may serve to increase the stress experienced by young minorities. Strong identification with traditional cultures may serve to create contradicting demands and value conflicts between minority and majority cultures, as well as an increase in perceived discrimination. LaFromboise, Oliver, and Hoyt (in press) point out this duality, noting that a traditional practice such as living on the reservation allows for more social interactions, exposure to traditional culture, and community support, but may also bring negative consequences such as geographical isolation, high unemployment, and low income. However, living on the reservation is not a necessary component of enculturation, as cultural involvement and community support often occurs regardless of where a Native person lives (Snipp, 1992).

Evidence for the positive aspect of enculturation is emerging, despite its possible negative features. Beauvais (2000) contends that devotion to traditional values and pride in one's culture provides a foundation for American Indian adolescents as they attempt to combine the strengths of their people with the opportunities that are available in the larger society. Oetting and Beauvais (1990) found that enculturation is associated with lower amounts of substance use. This result is supported by LaFromboise, Oliver, and Hoyt (in press), who found a significant relationship between enculturation and American Indian adolescent resiliency. However, this relationship may not be a simple one. Whitbeck, Hoyt, Stubben, McMorris, and LaFromboise (in press) found that the effects of enculturation on early substance use among American Indian adolescents are indirect, via two distinct pathways. One pathway indicates that enculturation decreases use through enhancing school compentency, while the other suggests that enculturation increases the likelihood of perceived discrimination, which, in turn, increases risk for early substance use.

Phinney (1992) identified a connection between enculturation and higher self-esteem, and Parham and Helms (1985) noted a relationship between enculturation and lower levels of anxiety. LaFromboise and BigFoot (1988) found that successful Native American adolescents tend to possess characteristics that embody traditional tribal values, such as a sense of spirituality, remembering ancestors, patience, comparing oneself with others who are less fortunate, endurance, and self-talk. Supporting these findings is research with Lakota people by Han et al. (1994). They found that healthier Lakota females demonstrated values that are consistent with traditional Lakota female gender roles, such as cultural isolationism, altruism, personal control, and devaluation of wealth and occupation.

From the time of birth, traditional American Indians mark their children's developmental milestones with great ritual. Most tribes have ceremonies to welcome a newborn into the world. As soon as an Ojibwa child can walk, traditional parents prepare a great feast. However, if the walk takes place at a neighbor's home, the neighbors give the honoring feast (Buffalohead, 1988). Among the Crow, the grandmother immediately makes a pudding to feed the parents and other relatives who happen to be present in honor of a child's first step. Wishes are then made for the child to take many more steps in the future (Morey & Gilliam, 1972). Children are recognized for their achievement throughout their lives. Rights of passage into adolescence, such as the first successful hunt, are marked with ceremony. Parents sometimes share children's achievement with others at powwows or ceremonial encampments by imparting relevant information to a "camp crier" who visits among the participants to broadcast information about the child's accomplishments. All of these traditional activities serve to cement a child's sense of belonging to the community, as well as instill a sense of obligation to fulfill one's duty as a tribal member.

Beavais and Oetting (1999) agree that cultural identification can be a resilience factor, noting that when a family has a high level of cultural identification, this indicates that the family is successfully functioning in a cultural context where the members are meeting appropriate cultural demands and being reinforced in a way that is personally and culturally meaningful. Applying this framework to American Indians, an enculturated child has access to cultural resources, such as a network of social support and rituals that increase a sense of belonging. Most American Indian families consist of members with differing levels of cultural involvement and adherence to traditional teachings.[4] For example, the grandparents of an extended family may live on the reservation, yet speak only English. Some of their grandchildren may be becoming bilingual, whereas some of their grandchildren who live in the city may predominantly speak English. However, all of the members of this extended family may be involved in enculturation activities such

---

[4] Although the role of the Indian youth as embedded within the family as the primary context is emphasized in this chapter, it is necessary to acknowledge the important influences of peers upon children and adolescents. For a general discussion of peer influence, see Cotterrell (1996) and Harris (1999).

as beading, attending or participating in powwows, hunting, fishing, and cooking Native foods. Because of the family structure, girls tend to be more involved in traditional activities (Whitbeck, Hoyt, Stubben, McMorris, & LaFromboise, in press). Male-oriented traditional activities require leadership and involvement with older men, but with current conditions, men are not as active in the traditional or ongoing activities of the tribe, and thus are not as available for this type of mentoring. It should not be assumed that every child has an equal opportunity to be involved in traditional activities; in attempting to determine the extent of involvement, opportunity must be taken into account.

Two examples of common traditional activities frequently engaged in by Native Americans across the life span are the sweat lodge ceremony and the talking circle. "Sweats" are often conducted among American Indian groups for the purpose of purification and prevention. Participation in the sweat lodge involves preparatory fasting, prayers, and offerings throughout serial purification sessions, known as "rounds." Participants make offerings for health and balance in life during a ceremony that lasts for several hours. Garret and Osborne (1995) point out that a sweat lodge ceremony can help to integrate a recovering individual back into the larger community. In the talking circle, sage or sweet grass is burned to produce purifying smoke and provide direction for group conversation. The leader begins by sharing feelings or thoughts about the group. Each participant is free to speak and interruptions are not allowed. A sacred object such as an eagle feather or talking stick is often circulated, and the ceremony concludes with the joining of hands in prayer (Manson, Walker, & Kivlahan, 1987). Both of these practices foster a sense of belonging and connection that affirms identity and acceptance by the community.

Another potential protective factor is the use of humor. Humor is a vital component of American Indian life, and is often used as a method of social control. Joe and Malach (1997) describe one such instance at a sacred dance, where clown dancers entertain the crowd, and in doing so, may single out a community member to reprimand through teasing and humorous demonstrations. This reprimand often serves to point out behaviors that are offensive to the rest of the community and directs the individual back to a healthier, more harmonious path.

Cheshire and Kawamoto (2003) describe more modern community efforts to enhance American Indian connectedness, particularly for urban youth who may not have direct access to the resources that are available on the reservation. Lorie Lee, a radio personality in Window Rock, Arizona, hosts a program called, "Navajo Nights," which features American Indian talent such as Casper, a Hopi reggae band, and Indigenous, an American Indian blues band. Litefoot, another American Indian entertainer, recently worked to organize a gathering of American Indian youth intended to recognize the talent of these youth and to help them see how they can function effectively in a bicultural manner. Cheshire and Kawamoto see these initiatives as filling the essential role of integrating urban and reservation concerns with traditional values and practices. Another example of this integration is the White Bison Wellbriety Movement that promotes maintaining sobriety from addictions and aids in recovery from the harmful effects of drugs and alcohol on individuals, families and communities. White Bison encourages going beyond sobriety and recovery, and committing to a life of wellness and healing every day. Included in the Wellbriety for Youth activities are youth talking circles and caring adult Wellbriety mentor/friends to whom young people can turn (White Bison, 2003).

CONTEMPORARY ECONOMIC DEVELOPMENT

The passage of the Indian Gaming Regulatory Act of 1988 can be viewed as a source of native empowerment, as revenues allow for employment training and investment in solutions to social and economic problems. On the other hand, some worry that reservation gaming enhances exposure to negative influences such as gambling and alcohol, and increases contact with non-natives, which may lead to further erosion of traditional values. Cozzetto (1995) in discussing the case of American Indian gaming in Minnesota, finds that although compulsive gambling seems to be on the rise among American Indians in Minnesota, tribal gaming has created jobs and increased education and training opportunities. Many of the tribes in Minnesota have invested in social programs such as establishing college scholarship funds, building childcare centers, and creating comprehensive health plans. The Mille Lacs Chippewa constructed a new school and health center and the Fond du Lac Chippewa were able to implement youth drug treatment programs with gaming revenue.

The Harvard Project on American Indian Economic Development (Spilde, Taylor, & Grant, 2002) explored the impact of gaming on tribes in Oklahoma. They found because of gaming, tribal nations were becoming more self-sufficient and were able to raise revenues for social programs and economic development, thus decreasing the insidious effects of welfare status on tribal members. Tribal governments spend a significant percent of the profits in efforts to revitalize native communities. Indian nations in Oklahoma and elsewhere have invested in community needs, such as highway infrastructure and health care. Contrary to the Minnesota findings, the Harvard Project concluded that the growth of tribal gaming is not likely to be associated with significant changes in the prevalence of pathological gambling.

The Harvard Project also found that gaming monies have been used to support cultural preservation programs such as tribal history courses and native language immersion programs. Many Cherokee and Choctaw tribal members are able to discover their history and language for the first time because of educational programs funded by gaming. Miami tribal members have implemented a tribal library that includes historical documents and an archive of over 16,000 items. The Citizen

Potawatomi Nation uses gaming revenue to host powwows and other traditional events, which strengthen connectedness and increase a sense of community. Charmaign Benz, publications specialist of the Ziibiwing Cultural Society, notes that the Saginaw Chippewa tribe from Michigan bought back some of their historic land. They also housed a museum, *Diba Jimooyung* ("Our Story" in the Ojibwa language) near their casino to share their history with visitors as well as tribal members (personal communication, March 24, 1998). Perhaps most importantly, tribes are able to use their new capital to become major lobbyists at the state and federal level, advocating for programs that will be serve their people.

SUMMARY AND CONCLUSIONS

According to Masten and Coatsworth (1998), the term resilience denotes patterns of positive adaptation in the context of significant risk or adversity. Native Americans have faced a great deal of adversity in economic, social, and health matters. Impediments, such as governmental removal policies and the devastating poverty facing some reservations, served to chip away at many aspects of Native American culture by separating families and communities, either by force or by necessity. However, the current prevalence of traditional beliefs and practices, together with the on-going revitalization of Native culture across the country, testifies to the incredible resilience that is inherent in the Native way of life. The major areas of importance in Native American culture, extended family, participation in traditional activities, and the role of spirituality, all function as protective factors. These factors increase a sense of belongingness and connectedness, reminding the individual of his or her place in the community and the natural world, including one's obligation to be a contributing member of both the family and the community. We hope that this overview of select external factors will shed light upon the processes that contribute to resilience for Native Americans. Undoubtedly, the external influence of the mass media, tribal governments, contemporary schooling practices, relationships between reservations and their bordering towns, local employment settings, and relationships with peers also influence the dynamic nature of Indian youth development, and should be explored in future research undertakings. Understanding resilience within a Native American context can lead to better outcomes not only for Native youth, but for all families and communities that would be able to blend positive Native strategies with their own.

REFERENCES

Atkinson, R., & Locke, P. (1995). The Lakota view of the child. *The Maine Scholar, 8*, 207–220.
Babcock, B.A. Ed. (1991). *Pueblo mothers and children: Essays by Elsie Clews Parsons 1915–1924.* Santa Fe: Ancient City Press.

Beauvais, F. (2000). Indian adolescence: Opportunity and challenge. In R. Montmeyer, G. Adams, & T. Gullota (Eds.), *Adolescent diversity in ethnic, economic, and cultural contexts* (pp. 110–140). Thousand Oaks, CA: Sage.

Beauvais, F., & Oetting, E.R. (1999). Drug use, resilience, and the myth of the golden child. In M.D. Glantz & J.L. Johnson (Eds.), *Resilience and development* (pp. 229–249). New York: Kluwer Academic/Plenum Publishers.

Benson, P.L. (1992). Religion and substance use. In J.F. Schumaker (Ed.), *Religion and mental health* (pp. 211–220). New York, NY: Oxford University Press.

Benson, P.L. (1997). Spirituality and the adolescent journey. *Reclaiming Children and Youth, 5(4),* 190–193.

Blum, R.W., Potthoff, S.J., & Resnick, M.D. (1997). The impact of chronic conditions on Native American adolescents. *Families, Systems, and Health, 15(3),* 275–282.

Blyth, D.A., & Leffert, N. (1995). Communities as contexts for adolescent development: An empirical analysis. *Journal of Adolescent Research, 10,* 64–87.

Bowlby, J. (1969). *Attachment.* New York: Basic Books.

Brendtro, L.K., Brokenleg., M., & Van Bockern, S. (1990). *Reclaiming youth at risk: Our hope for the future.* Bloomington, IN: National Educational Service, Inc.

Buffalohead, P. (1988). *Cherish the children: Parenting skills for Indian mothers with young children.* Minneapolis: Minnesota Indian Women's Resource Center.

Cheshire, T.C., & Kawamoto, W.T. (2003). Positive youth development in urban American Indian adolescents. In F.A. Villarruel, D.F. Perkins, L.M. Borden, & J.G. Keith (Eds.), *Community youth development: Programs, policies, and practices* (pp. 79–89). Thousand Oaks, CA: Sage.

Cotterrell, J. (1996). *Social networks and social influences in adolescence.* London: Routledge.

Cowan, P.A., & Cowan, C.P. (1990). Becoming a family: Research and intervention. In I.E. Siegel & G.H. Brody (Eds.), *Methods of family research: Biographies of research projects: Volume I: Normal families* (pp. 1–51). Hillsdale, NJ: Lawrence Erlbaum.

Cozzetto, D.A. (1995). The economic and social implications of Indian gaming: The case of Minnesota. *American Indian Culture and Research Journal, 19(1),* 119–131.

Cross, T.L. (1987). Positive Indian parenting: Honoring our children by honoring our traditions. In *Conference Proceedings of the 5th Annual National American Indian Conference on Child Abuse and Neglect* (pp. 5–18). Norman, OK: American Indian Institute, University of Oklahoma.

Cross, T.L. (1998). Understanding family resiliency from a relational world view. In H.I. McCubbin, E.A. Thompson, A.I. Thompson, & J.E. Fromer (Eds.), *Resiliency in Native American and immigrant families* (pp. 143–157). Thousand Oaks, CA: Sage.

Csordas, T.J. (1999). Ritual healing and the politics of identity in comtemporary Navajo society. *American Ethnologist, 26,* 3–23.

Demmert, W.G. (2001). *Improving academic performance among Native American students: A review of the research literature.* Charleston, WV: ERIC Clearinghouse on Rural Education and Small Schools.

Eastman, C. (1924). *Indian boyhood.* Boston: Little, Brown.

Eccles, J., & Gootman, J. (2002). *Community programs to promote youth development.* Washington, DC: National Academy Press.

Erikson, E. (1950, reprinted 1963). *Childhood and society. (2nd ed.).* New York: Norton.

Franzen, L.L. (1992). *The spirit within: Encouraging harmony and health in American Indian children.* Minneapolis, MN: Minnesota Indian Women's Resource Center.

French, L. (1987). *Psychocultural change and the American Indian: A ethnohistorical analysis.* New York: Garland Publishing, Inc.

Garrett, M.T., & Osborne, W.L. (1995). The Native American sweat lodge as metaphor for group work. *Journal for Specialists in Group Work, 20,* 33–39.

Gfellnert, B.M. (1990). Culture and consistency in ideal and actual child-rearing practices: A study of Canadian Indian and White parents. *Journal of Comparative Family Studies, 21(3)*, 413–423.

Gil, A.G., Vega, W.A., & Dimas, J.M. (1994). Acculturative stress and personal adjustment among Hispanic adolescent boys. *Journal of Community Psychology, 21*, 43–54.

Goodluck, C. (2002). *Native American children and youth well-being indicators: A strengths perspective*. Seattle, WA: Casey Family Programs.

Goodluck, C., & Willeto, A.A.A. (in press). *American Indian and Alaskan Native family resiliency*. Seattle, WA: Casey Family Programs.

Graham, B.L. (2001). *Resilience among American Indian youth: First Nations' youth resilience study* (Doctoral dissertation, University of Minnesota, 2001).

Gray, E., & Cosgrove, J. (1985). Ethnocentric perception of childrearing practices in protective services. *Child Abuse and Neglect, 9*, 389–396.

Han, P., Hagel, J., Welty, T., Ross, R., Leonardson, G., & Keckler, A. (1994). Cultural factors associated with health-risk behavior among the Cheyenne River Sioux. *American Indian and Alaska Native Mental Health Research, 5(3)*, 15–29.

Harris, J.R. (1999). *The nuture assumption*. New York: Touchstone.

Hill Witt, S. (1979, August). *Pressure points in growing up Indian*. Paper presented at the 87th annual meeting of the American Psychological Association, New York, NY.

Hungry Wolf, A., & Hungry Wolf, B. (1987). *Children of the sun: Stories by and about Indian kids*. New York, NY: William Morrow.

Jacobson, C.K. (1995). An analysis of Native American fertility in the public use microdata samples of the 1990 census. In C.K. Jacobson (Ed.), *American families: Issues in race and ethnicity* (pp. 119–130). New York: Garland Publishers.

Jagers, R.J. (1996). Culture and problem behaviors among inner-city African-American youth: Further explorations. *Journal of Adolescence, 19*, 371–381.

Joe, J.R., & Malach, R.S. (2002). Families with Native American roots. In E.W. Lynch & M.J. Hanson (Eds.), *A guide for working with children and their families: Developing cross cultural competence* (pp. 127–164). Baltimore, OH: Paul H. Brookes Publishing Co.

King, J., Beals, J., Manson, S.M., & Trimble, J.E. (1992). A structural equation model of factors related to substance abuse among American Indian adolescents. In J.E. Trimble, C.S. Bolek, & S.J. Niemcryck (Eds.), *Ethnic and multicultural drug abuse: Perspectives on current research* (pp. 253–268). Binghamton, NY: Haworth Press.

Kipke, M.D. (Ed.) (1999). *Risks and opportunities: Synthesis of studies on adolescence*. Washington, D.C.: National Academy Press.

LaFromboise, T., & BigFoot, D.S. (1988). Cultural and cognitive considerations in the prevention of American Indian adolescent suicide. *Journal of Adolescence, 11(2)*, 139.

LaFromboise, T., Coleman, H., & Gerton, J. (1993). Psychological aspects of bicultural compentence: Evidence and theory. *Psychological Bulletin, 114*, 395–412.

LaFromboise, T., Oliver, L., & Hoyt, D.R. (in press). Strengths and resilience of American Indian adolescents. In L. Whitbeck (Ed.), *This is not our way: Traditional culture and substance use prevention in American Indian adolescents and their families* Tucson: University of Arizona Press.

Lobo, S., & Peters, K. (Eds.). (2001). *American Indians and the urban experience*. Walnut Creek, CA: AltaMira Press.

Maccoby, E.E. (1992). The role of parents in the socialization of children: An historical overview. *Developmental Psychology, 28*, 1006–1017.

MacPhee, D., Fritz, J., & Miller-Heyl, J. (1996). Ethnic variation in personal social networks and parenting. *Child Development, 67*, 3278–3295.

Manson, S.M., Walker, R.D., & Kivlahan, D.R. (1987). Psychiatric assessment and treatment of American Indians and Alaska Natives. *Hospital and Community Psychiatry, 38*, 165–173.

Masten, A.S., & Coatsworth, J.D. (1998). The development of competence in favorable and unfavorable environments: Lessons from successful children. *American Psychologist, 53*, 205–220.

McCarty, T.L. (2002). *A place to be Navajo: Rough Rock and the struggle for self-determination in indigenous schooling.* Mahwah, NJ: Lawrence Erlbaum Associates.

Mohatt, G.V., McDiarmid, G.W. & Montoya, V. (1988). Societies, families and change: The Alaskan example. *American Indians and Alaska Native Mental Health Research, 1, Monograph No. 1,* 325–369.

Morey, S.M., & Gilliam, O.J. (Eds.) (1972). *Respect for life: The traditional upbringing of American Indian children.* New York, NY: Myrin Institute.

National Indian Child Welfare Association. (1986). *Positive Indian parenting: honoring our children by honoring our traditions.* Portland, OR: Author.

Nightingale, E.O., & Wolverton, L. (1993). Adolescent rolelessness in modern society. In R. Takanishi (Ed.), *Adolescence in the 1990's: Risk and opportunity* (pp. 14–28). New York: Teachers College Press.

Oetting, E., & Beauvais, F. (1990). Adolescent drug use: Findings of national and local surveys. *Journal of Consulting and Clinical Psychology, 58*, 385–394.

Office for Substance Abuse Prevention. (1990). *Breaking new ground for American Indian and Alaska Native youth at risk: Program summaries.* U.S. Department of Health and Human Services.

Ogunwole, S. (2002). *The American Indian and Alaska Native population: 2000.* Washington, D.C.: U.S. Bureau of the Census, U.S. Department of Commerce.

Parham, T., & Helms, J. (1985). Relation of racial identity attitudes to self-actualization and affective states of Black students. *Journal of Counseling Psychology, 32*, 431–440.

Peshkin, A. (1997). *Places of memory: Whiteman's schools and Native American communities.* Mahwah, NJ: Lawrence Erlbaum Associates.

Phinney, J. (1992). *Ethnic identity in adolescents and adults: Review of the research. Psychological Bulletin, 108*, 499–514.

Red Horse, J., Lewis, R.G., Feit, M., & Decker, J. (1978). Family behavior of urban American Indians. *Social Casework, 59*, 67–72.

Resnick, M., Harris, L., & Blum, R. (1993). The impact of caring and connectedness on adolescent health and well-being. *Journal of Pediatrics and Child Health, 29(1)*, 53–59.

Riley, P. (Ed.) (1993). *Growing up Native American: An anthology.* New York: Morrow.

Rogoff, B. (2003). *The cultural nature of human development.* Oxford: Oxford University Press.

Rolf, J.E., & Johnson, J.L. (1999). Opening doors to resilience intervention for prevention research. In M.D. Glantz & J.L. Johnson (Eds.), *Resilience and development* (pp. 229–249). New York: Kluwer Academic/Plenum Publishers.

Sandefur, G.D., & Liebler, C.A. (1996). The demography of American Indian families. In G.D. Sandefur, R.R. Rindfuss, & B. Cohen (Eds.), *Changing numbers, changing needs: American Indian demography and public health* (pp. 196–217). Washington, D.C.: National Academy Press.

Snipp, C.M. (1992). Sociological perspectives on American Indians. *Annual Review of Sociology, 18*, 351–371.

Spilde, K.A, Taylor, J.B., & Grant, K.W. (2002). *Social and economic analysis of tribal government gaming in Oklahoma.* Cambridge, MA: Harvard Project on American Indian Economic Development.

Stein, D., Witzum, E., & Brom, D. (1992). The association between adolescents' attitudes toward suicide and their psychosocial background and suicidal tendencies. *Adolescence, 27*, 949–959.

Swinomish Tribal Mental Health Project. (1989). *Cultural considerations for tribal mental health* (Booklet II). LaConner, WA: Author.

U.S. Bureau of the Census. (2002a). *American Indian and Alaska Native population, by age and sex for the United States: 2000.* Washington, D.C.: U.S. Department of Commerce.

U.S. Bureau of the Census. (2002b). *Total population, by age and sex for the United States: 2000.* Washington, D.C.: U.S. Department of Commerce.

Vega, W.A., & Gil, A.G. (1998). *Drug use and ethnicity in early adolescence.* New York: Plenum Press.

Waller, M. (2002). Family mentors and educational resilience among Native students. The *Prevention Researcher, 9(1),* 14–15.

Ward, C., Hinckley, G., & Sawyer, K. (1995). The intersection of ethnic and gender identities: Northern Cheyenne women's roles in cultural recovery. In C.K. Jacobson (Ed.), *American families: Issues in race and ethnicity* (pp. 201–227). New York: Garland Publishing.

Werner, E.E., & Smith, R.S. (1993). *Overcoming the odds: High risk children from birth to adulthood.* Ithaca, NY: Cornell University Press.

Whitbeck, L., Hoyt, D., Stubben, J., McMorris, B., & LaFromboise, T. (in press). Enculturation and early substance abuse among American Indian Adolescents. In L. Whitbeck (Ed.), *This is not our way: Traditional culture and substance use prevention in American Indian adolescents and their families.*

White Bison. (2003). *The Center for Wellbriety Movement.* Retrieved July 29, 2003, from http://www. whitebison.org/youth/index.html.

Whitehorse, D. (1988). *POW-WOW: The contemporary Pan-Indian celebration.* San Diego, CA: San Diego State University.

Willeto, A.A.A. (2002). *Native American kids 2002: Indian children's well-being indicators data book for 13 states.* Seattle, WA: Casey Family Programs.

Wright, L., Frost, C., & Wisecarver, S. (1993). Church attendance, meaningfulness of religion on, and depressive symptamology among adolescents. *Journal of Youth and Adolescence, 22(5),* 559–568.

Zimmerman, M., Ramirez, J., Washienko, K., Walter, B., & Dyer, S. (1998). Enculturation hypothesis: exploring effects among Native American youth. In McCubbin, E.A. Thompson, A.I. Thompson, & J.E. Fromer (Eds.), *Resiliency in Native American and immigrant families* (pp. 143–157). Thousand Oaks, CA: Sage.

Chapter 5

Risk and Resilience in Latino Youth

RAFAEL ART. JAVIER AND ALINA CAMACHO-GINGERICH

Discussing the issue of risk factors and resilience in the Latino population is a monumental task because we are not dealing with a monolithic population with the same experience but rather with individuals who, although may have a great deal of communality, also have a great deal of diversity in their experiences (Javier & Yussef, 1995). Understanding what factors are involved in making possible for an individual to excel even in the face of challenges and for another to flounder in the face of stress has been of great interest to behavioral scientists (Eccles et al., 1993; Garbarino, 2001; Jessor, 1993; Masten, Best & Garmezy, 1990; Quadrel, Fischoff & Davis, 1993). With regard to understanding of resilience and vulnerability in Latino individuals, different considerations need to be made depending upon whether we look at the Latino individuals in their country of origin or in the context of their immigration experience. With regard to Latinos in the United States, the fact that Latino individuals come from different countries; that they may have spent their formative years in their country of origin or in the United States; that there is an immigration experience that is different for the different Latino communities; that the sociopolitical and socioeconomic realities for these individuals prior to and following the immigration experience may be different; that the nature and quality of their environmental and ecological context while in the United States may have different impact; that the extent of acculturation may be different and hence may become a factor on the ability of the less acculturated to adjust to the demands of the host country; that their linguistic abilities, level of education, nature of employment, extent of family support may be different, add additional challenges to behavioral scientists interested in understanding the nature of resilience and vulnerability in individuals where these experiences are central.

There is a wealth of literature (Piaget, 1972; Sullivan, 1953) that focuses on the description of the general developmental pathways that the individual goes through, in the context of which, achievement of specific competences are acquired at critical developmental stages. It is in the context of this development that cognitive and emotional schemata are developed. These function as the necessary structure that allows the individual to handle the different challenges in his or her environment. In the case of Latino individuals, factors specific to Latino individuals' experiences that are likely to have a differential impact on their cognitive and emotional development and general function should also be included in this conceptual matrix. It would be helpful, in this context, to understand the nature of their resilience, what contributes to its development and in what areas are they most vulnerable and in what context. Identifying the specific factors associated with resilience and vulnerability in the Latino context will allow us to create more targeted interventions for this group.

That this is important is seen in a recent study on depression among Mexican women. The level of depression experienced by these women was found to be significantly different depending on whether they were born in Mexico or the United States and was greater if born in the United States (Heilemann, Lee & Kury, 2002). Mexican Americans born in Mexico also reported significantly lower suicide thoughts and attempts than Mexican Americans born in the United States (Sorenson & Golding, 1988). These findings suggest that the closer to the cultural of origin these women were, the more they were protected from emotional difficulties. The farther removed the women were (i.e., being born in the United States) the least they were protected by whatever their parents' culture could offer to handle difficult situations and hence more despair and hopelessness became evident. Acculturation has been implicated in many deleterious health effects (Vega, Kology, Aguilar-Gaxiola, Alderete, Catalano, Caraveo-Anduaga, 1998).

We have divided the chapter into five major components to address the relevant issues related to the definition and assessment of resilience and risk factors when dealing with Latino youth. The first section will deal with the problem defining the Latino individual, followed by sections dealing with issues of resilience in general and specifically with Latinos, protective factors in the Latino context, and general recommendations.

ON DEFINING THE LATINO INDIVIDUAL

As indicated earlier, the difficulty in studying and understanding resilience in the Latino population has to do with how are we to define the Latino or Hispanic individual. In the United States 'Latino' and 'Hispanic' are terms frequently used to identify an individual whose place of origin, either by birth or inherited culture, is a Latin American country or Spain. Many have attempted to group such a diverse people under a single term or 'ethnic' category. Until recently many government agencies, educational and business institutions were using the term 'Hispanic' as a racial category. Some still do. They do not take into consideration the historical, geographical, racial, socio-economic, educational, linguistic, religious and other cultural factors that differentiate these groups of individuals not only from one country of origin to another but within the same country. How much does a nahuatl-speaking Mexican or a quechua-speaking Peruvian have in common with their Spanish-speaking countrymen, descendants of Europeans? In terms of educational and economic achievement, how similar are the first waves of Cuban exiles, mostly from the upper and middle classes, to the majority of 'Marielitos' who arrived in 1980? How similar is La Paz, with its rich Indian traditions (Inca, Aymara, Guarani) co-existing with descendants of Europeans, with Buenos Aires, made up of mostly European immigrants and their descendants?

Furthermore, the Latino individual living in the United States is not the same as the one living in the country of origin. Once in the United States, the individual's culture, traditions and values, which may have served as sources of identity and personal meaning, begin to change gradually in the process of contact with the new culture. Conflicts are likely to emerge which then result in some degree of accommodation to the demands of the host country if the immigrant is to adjust to the new reality (Baca & Javier, 1995; Camacho-Gingerich, 2002; Salgado de Snyder, 1987). The nature and degree of that conflict and the necessary accommodation should be assessed in the context of each individual's immigration experience, including the reason (s) for immigration, educational level, professional preparation, and other personal resources. That is, whether we are dealing with an 'immigrant in progress' (or an immigrant who has already reached a high level of integration into new culture although still maintains a close contact with the culture of origin), an 'immigrant in conflict'(or an immigrant who is unhappy about being in the new country and long for the time when he/she can return to the country of origin), or 'a progressive immigrant' (an immigrant who has reached great integration in the new country and has decided to establish completely into the new culture) (Baca & Javier, 1995; Javier, 2002). In the case of the Latino youth, we also need to ascertain how the normal developmental issues will play out in the context of the immigration experience.

Another difficulty with the definition has to do with the fact that Latino individuals are different in various ways—we can see these differences by just walking around the different Latino communities who migrated to the United States and now live in many metropolitan cities. This is particularly important with regard to the youth who are in the midst of consolidation of self-definition and are dealing with identity issues. What cultural value will be used as a point of reference for identity development, self-reference and self-esteem? Problems in self-esteem have been associated with serious academic, behavioral problem and affective disorders (National Advisory Mental Health Council, 1996). Thus, the Latino adolescent not only has to negotiate the general Latino identity in the context of the host culture but also has to navigate among the other Latino individuals' distinctive differences.

One can easily observe the distinctive differences among Latinos by looking at the more or less predominant Indian features and African and Spanish influences in the skin color, hair quality and other physical characteristics, as well as in the unique flavor of the food, music, clothing, speech styles and voice inflexion (Javier & Yussef, 1995; Preble, 1979). This is the case because most Latin American countries were under the control of the Spaniards for centuries that resulted in different degrees of mixing with the native Indian population and later with the African slaves (Gutierrez, 1991). An important component of this influence is the Catholic Church with all of what that represents with regard to the development of morality and code of conduct, although other religious influences are now competing for the souls of Latino individuals (Javier & Yussef, 1995). As in their countries of origin, Latinos today, although still predominantly Catholic, practice almost every religion and creed.

Certain cultural, racial and linguistic traits help distinguish Latinos from Mexico, the Caribbean, Central and South America, and from one another. For instance, in the Andean music enjoyed by the people from Bolivia, Peru and Ecuador you can hear the influence of pre-Colombian civilizations like the Incas, while African influence is more evident in Cuban, Dominican and Puerto Rican music (Padilla, 1998). Thus, Merengue becomes unique to the Dominican Republic; Salsa becomes more identified with Puerto Rico; Mambo, Guaguanco y Chachacha more to Cuba; Cumbia to Colombia, and Mariachis and Las Rancheras to Mexico. With regard to religious influence, in addition to the strong Catholic presence, Mexicans are more likely to also include the use of 'Curanderos' as part of their religious practice in dealing with the supernatural and difficult situations, while some Cubans may resort to the work of 'Santeros' and Puerto Rican to the work of 'Espiritistas' (Argueta-Bernal, 1990; Tejada, Sanchez, & Mella, 1993). Dominicans may also rely on voodoo tradition as part of their religious practice in dealing with the supernatural and difficult situations (Tejada, Sanchez, & Mella, 1993).

We can also see how the different ecologies, geographies and climates have a palpable impact on the diet, dress, and other personal habits or through their preferences for the different fruits, produce, and crafts specific to the regions from which they came. This is epitomized in the legendary Cuban tobacco, the Chilean and Argentinian wines, Argentinian and Brazilian beef, and Colombian coffee. Indeed, there is a great deal of pride connected to these different countries' unique experiences with their history and ecology, and how each evolved as people.

Thus, using 'Hispanic' or 'Latino' to refer to individuals coming from Spanish speaking countries rather than the adjective referring to the specific country (such as Dominican, Cuban, Puerto Rican) or one that makes closer reference to their uniqueness (such as Central American, Caribbean, or South American) can create a great deal of tension and conflict, in addition to not providing a clear enough specification about the individual. Part of the specific characteristics of the different countries in most of Latin America include a unique history of struggle for independence from Spain (in the case of Brazil, from Portugal) with the resulting creation of country-specific symbols (country-specific national flags) and patriotic anthems (national anthems) which become part of each country's folklore and literary tradition (such as Jose Marti for Cuba, Ruben Dario for Nicaragua, Eugenio Maria de Hostos for the Dominican Republic and Puerto Rico). All of these different country-specific influences offer the Latino individual the opportunity to develop a unique sense of self closely connected to these influences. Again, this is particularly important during adolescence.

However, these differences notwithstanding, there are fundamental threads that connect and characterize the psychological and emotional make-up of all individuals coming from Spanish speaking countries and that, paradoxically, grew mostly out of the colonial experience. It is the love for Spanish as a romance language, spoken by the great majority of Latin Americans, including those whose native language might be other; the strong influence of the Catholic religion in the lives of most Latinos; the view of family and family structure, including the extended family; the codes of conduct that guide the relationship between woman and man (machismo and marianismo), between children and parents, with the authorities and with oneself (Camacho-Gingerich, 2002; Gil & Vazquez, 1996). Thus, the essence of Latino individuals should be defined in the context of the similarity of their cultural influences as well as the uniqueness that the country of origin and the individual's own personal background provide. Only then we will be able to develop more sophisticated ways of studying and understanding issues affecting the Latino population, including the issue of resilience and risks in adolescence. This lack of refinement as to the differential uniqueness of the Latino experience is, indeed, a major problem in the current literature that makes it difficult to fully appreciate the relevance of its findings when applied to this population. For instance, a study discussed by Gutierrez (2003), Vega, Gil, Zimmerman and Warheit (1993) found that acculturation stress was a co-factor along with drug use for increased vulnerability to suicide attempts for Hispanic adolescents. What is not clear in this study is where these adolescents are from and where they are in terms of the acculturation dimension.

DEVELOPMENT OF RESILIENCE IN THE LATINO CONTEXT

A number of theories about human development have attempted to describe the complex evolution of the individual as he or she develops as a person in his or her context. Since the brevity of this chapter will not allow us to discuss these contributions in detail, the reader is referred to the seminal works of Piaget (1969, 1972) in terms of cognitive development, and Freud (1965), Sullivan (1953, 1973), Mahler (1975), Erickson (1963), and Offer (1979) with regard to the emotional and social development. According to these authors, there are important stages where the individual has to achieve specific competencies, and these competencies change in nature as the individual progresses from an early stage of development to a more advanced stage. Early achievements focus on the acquisition of basic skills having to do with the ability to recognize the environment, crawling and finally walking; they also focus on the ability to develop attachment and then to separate and individuate; and the development of internal representation of the experience. Language skills also become progressively more sophisticated, from the acquisition of the ability to make and recognize the proper phonemes, to the acquisition of the individual's ability to understand and communicate more complex thoughts; to making his or her behavior become more regulated by more sophisticated cognitive and linguistic processes (Piaget, 1972; Vygotsky, 1978). More complex cognitive operation allows the individual to develop functional schemata that are then used to organize and respond to future experiences and challenges.

Emotionally, the individual learns to understand and regulate his or her reactions to the environment and develops emotional schemata in this regard. The individual learns to identify situations of anxiety and frustration and those likely to produce anger and other emotions. The initial stage of the development of these competencies occur in the context of the family, making the quality of the family environment, the quality of the mother interaction fundamental for the development of basic competencies. It is in the context of the development of these competencies that the individual develops a sense of self as competent or incompetent. The nature of the self-esteem is fostered and crystallized in this development and so the view of the world. Serious psychopathology can develop, as described by Sullivan (1973), Winnicott (1974), and Kernberg (1975), when the child is forced to create malevolent transformations to respond to a toxic family environment and other trauma, when his or her sense of self is compromised, when the individual does not learn to regulate his or her affect, and when the basic internal system becomes disorganized. In fact, the presence of psychopathology, especially affective disorders, and conflict in the family are strong predictors to suicide ideation and attempts in adolescence (Brent et al., 1993).

A developmental model of competence suggests that the extent of success and strength of future competencies are based on the extent to which the individual successfully accomplishes early competencies. Thus, for adolescents, although the issue may center on school demands, peer relations, athletic competence and academic achievements, early successes may soften the impact of the tremendous emotional upheaval normally expected during this time (Offer, 1979). Adolescence

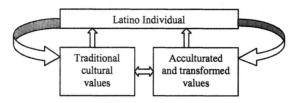

Figure 1. Latino Individuals and the Process of Culture

is the time when the individual strives for separation from parents, and peer and friends of the opposite sex become more important for their emotional life. He or she tries to disengage from parental influence and there is a profound reorganization of emotional life. In this context, there is an undoing of previous personality and the crystallization of the adult personality and the restructuring of his or her character (Offer, 1979). This is the time in which tremendous changes occur to their bodies and fashionable clothing and music acquire a self-defining role. The extent to which these developmental challenges have a permanent impact on adolescents will be a function of early developmental successes and care that the adolescent may have experienced (Garbarino, 2001; Garmezy & Maten, 1986; Losel & Bliesener, 1990).

It is against this backdrop that we need to understand the development of resilience in Latino youth along with the influences associated with specific conditions in the Latino individual's experience referred to earlier. We can say that the developmental challenges and the final definition of Latino youth has to be seen along a continuum, that includes, on the one end, the influence of traditional cultural values on the Latino development and the ways the influence of these values change over time in the individual as a result of the immigration experience and contact with the host culture, on the other end (Fig. 1) (Javier, 2002). In the more traditional Latino experience, development occurs in the context of an extended family system that may include parents, grandparents, aunts and uncles, cousins, in-laws, second-uncles and aunts, 'padrinos' (godparents), 'compadres' (co-parents), and 'vecinos' (neighbors). All major institutions, such as schools and churches, are expected to be part of this large system of influence and to function as an extension of the parental influence. 'Respeto' (refers to the deference and special consideration given to adults and other people) and the importance to protect the family "honra" (Canino & Canino, 1980; Lauria, 1964) are the backbone of cultural-based disciplinary techniques used by the family and other institutions to instill and transmit behavioral expectations. In this context, being concerned with "el que diran" (what neighbors would think or say) and that God is always looking or present, are important components of this technique.

Religious beliefs are also used to give the Latino individual a 'protective shield' against desperation and hopelessness in the face of adversity. That God, the

Guardian Angel, the Virgin Mary, and specific saints are there to assist in difficult times are strong beliefs usually found in Latino individuals to derive strength and resilience. We can witness this phenomenon by going to any of the houses of worship frequented by Latino individuals and hear the tremendous reliance on these beliefs or devotions and strong feelings that, at the end, things will be o.k. It will be "lo que Dios quiera" (God's willing) or what their patron saint's will is (i.e., 'Lo que quiera mi Virgencita del Cobre,' de La Altagracia, de Guadalupe).

In the more assimilated context, some of these influences become less obvious, such as the extended family structure; the degree of influence of traditional cultural values is related to factors such as education, socioeconomic status, the extent of affiliation with the Latino community, among others. It is in the context of these influences that the Latino youth's view of the world, sense of himself/herself, sense of hope and hopelessness, frustration, tolerance, strengths and weaknesses, and personal determination, are developed and incorporated into the self-definition and coping mechanism. It is also in this context that the Latino individual's sense of resoluteness and determination in the face of difficulties are forged and so his/her sense of fatalism and vulnerability.

A LOOK AT RESILIENCE AND VULNERABILITY IN LATINO YOUTH

Resilience refers to an ability to maintain a good level of function and emotional stability in the midst of or in spite of tremendous challenges and obstacles. According to Masten and Coatsworth (1998), it refers to "manifested competence in the context of significant challenges to adaptation or development" (p. 207). Thus, resilience can only be defined in the context of the individual's competence in reference to specific domains. It refers to good outcomes despite high-risk status; to sustained competence under threat; and to the ability to recover from trauma (Masten, et al., 1990) (see fig 2). That is, resilience includes the individual's capacity to respond effectively to environmental and internal challenges and to maintain an adequate level of competence in important areas in his/her life. It requires the necessary flexibility to adjust to new situations and to maintain effective coping or sustained competent functioning in spite of severely challenging circumstances (Masten et al., 1990).

According to Masten and Coatsworth (1998), competence refers to

A pattern of effective adaptation in the environment, either broadly defined in terms of reasonable success with major developmental tasks expected for a person of a given age and gender in life context of his or her culture, society and time, or more narrowly defined in terms of specific domains of achievement, such as academics, peer acceptance, or athletics (p. 206).

The crucial areas of concern for competence change depending on the tasks demanded of the individual for his or her emotional/professional/scholastic survival and the developmental stage. That is, the infant is concerned with different issues than adolescents and adults and vis-a-versa. With regard to adolescents, domains pertaining to school, friends and athletics become most crucial in assessing competences (National Advisory Mental Health Council, 1996).

There are a number of factors that have been identified in the literature to contribute to the development of resilience and dysfunctionality in adolescents (Jessor, 1993; Masten et al., 1990; Masten & Coastworth, 1998; National Advisory Mental Health Council, 1996). For instance, children coming from a divorced family, from a single parent home, with a history of abuse, experiencing homelessness and poverty, are at high risk for the development of a number of problems (Masten, 1992). Poverty, low maternal education, low socioeconomic status, low birth-weight, family instability, presence of psychopathology in the mother have been associated with lower academic and work achievements, more emotional or behavioral problems and/or trouble with the law (Masten et al., 1990).

Thus, we can identify different clusters of risks for the individual that could have a deleterious effect in the development of adequate competences:

- *Individual characteristics*: Neurological and perinatal complications have been associated with reading disability and behavioral disorders (Pasamanick & Knobloch, 1961; Masten et al., 1990). Low birth rate, questionable early attachment, difficult temperament and low intelligence have also been associated with bad outcomes in at risk children and youth (National Advisory Mental Health Council, 1996). Gender characteristics have been associated with at risk rate. For instance, under condition of stress, boys have been found to exhibit more disruptive or aggressive behavior than girls, while girls are more prone to anxiety and depression. Autism and conduct disorder are more prevalent in boys while eating disorder more prevalent in girls (Rutter, 1989 as cited by Masten et al., 1990).

  In a series of studies discussed by Masten and Coatsworth (1998), children with problems in self-regulation of attention and negative emotions have been associated with a variety of academic and emotional difficulties. For instance, difficulties in regulation of attention have been linked to attention-deficit hyperactivity disorder, antisocial behavior and academic problems. By contrast, good attention regulation has been linked to pro-social behavior and peer popularity. Negative emotions, such as irritability or difficult temperament, have been linked to aggressive and disruptive behaviors (Rothbart & Bates, 1998). These, in turn, affect school performance, resulting in academic placement, and make it more likely for the individual to be rejected by teachers and peers.

- *Parental/family characteristics*: Low maternal education, rigid and un-
democratic parenting style, absent father, history of criminal behavior,
history of serious emotional problems (i.e., depression and schizophrenia), history of substance abuse, physical and domestic abuse, family
instability, and divorce have all been associated with high risk children
and youth (Garbarino, 2001; Masten et al., 1990; 1998). The extent to
which problems with parents will have a deleterious impact of the children depends on the age and the gender of the children. For instance, in the
case of divorce, preschoolers appear to be more negatively affected in the
short-tem while the effect in adolescents may be more enduring (Emery,
1988; Wallerstein, Corbin, & Lewis, 1988 cited by Masten et al., 1990).

In looking at these risk factors, it is important to consider that it is the cumulative effect of risks that tends to be most damaging and that there are specific
protective factors that tend to mitigate the impact of these risks in the individual
(Garbarino, 2001). For instance, for a group of Salvadorian immigrants, English
language skills, a positive and hard-working attitude, use of social supports, and
religious faith were found to be useful adoptive coping strategies in dealing with
stress (Pante, Manuel, Menendez & Marcotte, 1995). Moreover, the extent of impact of risk factors on the individual is a function of whether one is dealing with
proximal versus distal risks. According to Masten et al. (1990), citing the work of
Baldwin, Baldwin and Cole (1990), proximal-risk factors (such as inadequate nutrition, discord between parents, or antisocial behaviors in a parent) are more likely
to impinge directly on the child. On the other hand, the effects of distal-risk factors
(such as poverty or economic hardship, community violence, political instability)
are mediated by proximal variables. For instance, if the child or adolescent comes
from an unstable family environment, unfavorable school environment and has
poor intellectual skills, the effect of these distal risk factors increases.

With regard to the Latino youth, how are we to assess the extent to which
the risk factors delineated above will apply in the same manner? If our focus
is academic achievement, mental health, and coping skills as compared with the
performance of individuals from the larger population it is likely that we will
be missing the point. As indicated earlier, a more comprehensive assessment of
resilience and risks factors should include the specific characteristics of those who
may be coming from a recently immigrated family; whose life's conditions may
be characterized by poverty and low socioeconomic status but without the despair
and the lack of hope that may characterize others in poverty; whose parents have
to spend long hours working in order to support the family and hence may not be
able to attend school meetings, without the children necessarily feeling abandoned
and unattended; and those who live in rundown neighborhoods but in the context
of a determination to improve their lots. How are we to assess resilience and risks
in those whose capacity to communicate is inadequate and whose knowledge of

this society is limited but who have learned to survive in a neighborhood where violence and drug addiction behavior may be the norm? What about for those where part of the family is still in the country of origin and do not have much family support in the host society and yet continue to struggle to improve their lots?

To assume that stressful conditions in the lives of Latino families are enough to cause serious emotional damage is to overlook the fact that a great number of Latinos and youth in general are not affected in the same manner and many flourish in the midst of adversity (Masten & Coastworth, 1998). Additionally, we have a serious problem with how competence is assessed. The same child may be judged to be competent in one context and incompetent in another, depending on what areas of competence are being considered in the measure and the context of reference. This issue has been raised repeatedly by a number of authors (Armour-Thomas & Gopaul-McNicol, 1997; Flanagan, McGrew, & Ortiz, 2000; Sternberg, 1985) who put the blame for this problem partly on the assessment instruments utilized for evaluation. They criticize the traditional assessment instruments as contributing to our inability to accurately determine issues such as cognitive ability, level of affective function and the like. For instance, Latino individuals and other minorities are more likely to be judged as having a learning disability and other cognitive deficiencies and behavioral problems when the assessment instruments utilized are linguistically and culturally inappropriate or the instrument utilized is unable to assess other competencies that may be more relevant to the individuals by virtue of their specific reality (Armour-Thomas & Gopaul-McNicol, 1997; Flanagan, McGrew, & Ortiz, 2000). According to these authors, the inclusion of all relevant information about the individual's true cognitive and emotional ability in the assessment process can only occur if a more comprehensive system of assessment, such as the *'Bio-Ecological Assessment System,' 'Bio-Cultural Model of Cognitive Functioning,' or 'Hypothesis-based Model of Assessment,'* is systematically utilized. A description of this system is found in Armour-Thomas and Gopaul-McNicol (1997) and Flanagan, McGrew and Ortiz (2000).

With regard to understanding the differential manner in which stress affects the Latino youth in this country, we need to take a closer look at the specific factors contributing to the phenomenon in this population. Take, for instance, the increase in suicide ideation and attempts found among Latino adolescents (Razin, O'Doud, Nathan, Rodriguez, & Goldfield, 1991; Tortolero & Roberts, 2001); socioeconomic factors were found to be insufficient to explain the rate of suicide ideations among a sample of Mexican American adolescents when compared to European American adolescents (Tortolero & Roberts, 2001). Ethnicity did appear to be involved in the difference. This same finding was reported by Olvera (2001) who assessed suicide ideation, depressive symptomatology, acculturation and coping strategies in a middle school sample of Hispanic, non-Hispanic White and mixed ancestry adolescents. Mexican American and mixed ancestry adolescents exhibited the highest risks of suicide ideation even when socioeconomic status, gender and age were controlled for. In studies discussed earlier, the level of depression was also found to be greater among Mexican American women born in the USA when compared with Mexican American women born in Mexico (Heilemann et al., 2002). Mexican Americans born in Mexico also reported significantly lower suicide thoughts and attempts than Mexican Americans born in the United States (Sorenson & Golding, 1988).

It is clear that more research is needed to identify the specific factors that may be more relevant to Latino youth with regard to the experience of resilience and vulnerability. For instance, we would like to encourage those interested in this phenomenon to make sure to consider issues of hope, and areas of success in the family and immediate community environment, improvement in linguistic ability and school performance in the context of limited English proficiency and difficult economic conditions, and the performance and general function in the country of origin as important components in reaching a more comprehensive view of these individuals' true level of skills and vulnerabilities. In this context, it would also be important to identify the specific risk factors in order of importance for Latino youth and what series of risk factors (i.e., breaking point) have to be present for the individual beyond which problems are likely to emerge. For instance, in a study discussed by Gutierrez (2003), cultural gender role prescriptions, poverty, migrational generationality, family structure and dynamics, mother's personality structure and suicide behavior, and sexuality were found to predispose and precipitate suicide attempts (Razin et al., 1991). What would be important is to determine the relative sequential impact relevant to each of these factors with regard to resilience, risks and similar phenomena.

In this context, the *"Vulnerable Populations Conceptual Model"* could be useful in assessing the effect of cumulative risks in the Latino youth. This model suggests that exposure to more stressful life events is related to an increase in risk factors. Increased exposure to risk factors lead to increased morbidity, psychopathological changes, or disease states (Flaskerud & Winslow, 1998; Heilemann et al., 2002). This model suggests that gender and ethnicity contribute to the intensity of the effect of risks factors.

A VIEW OF PROTECTIVE FACTORS IN THE LATINO CONTEXT

There are a number of protective factors that have been found to facilitate and promote good functioning in children and youth in general that may be applicable to the Latino youth (see Fig. 2). For instance, children who experience chronic adversity fare better or recover more successfully when they received good and stable care from someone (Masten et al., 1990). As indicated earlier, familism

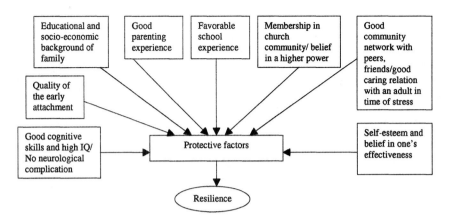

Figure 2. Protective Factors and Latino Youth

and extended family are important aspects of the Latino experience and members of the immediate family, the compadres (co-parents), neighbors, clergy and the community at large may function as a protective shield against feeling that one is alone. The extent to which there is a lessening of this protective shield as a result of the immigration experience, should be part of the assessment of the Latino youth experience.

Similarly, favorable school experiences were found to mitigate the effects of stressful home environment (Werner, 1990). Higher childhood IQ scores predicted low delinquency rate in adolescent boys and girls for all risk groups (White, Moffitt, & Silva, 1989). Finally, good cognitive skills predict academic achievement and other aspects of competence, such as rule-abiding behavior (Masten & Coatsworth, 1998). Again, as discussed earlier, in assessing these skills we need to consider instruments and methods that are more appropriate for the Latino youth population.

Solid self-esteem and sense of self-efficacy are important factors in helping the individual deal better with difficult situations. Self-esteem in adolescence gets reinforcement from a number of avenues, including good family relations, favorable school experiences, good peer relations, good relation with members of the opposite gender, achievement in sports, and music or other similar activities, among others. (Masten & Coatsworth, 1998; National Advisory Mental Health Council, 1996). For the Latino individual, the sense of self-efficacy may also be reinforced by his or her ability to assist family members in dealing with difficult situations or the extent to which he or she is able to help the family still in the country of origin and the extent to which he or she is able to negotiate his or her surroundings.

In a series of studies discussed by Masten et al. (1990), church membership and faith in a higher power were found to function as protective factors in diverse high-risk situations. These authors suggested that "religion may influence appraisals of stressful situations or fears of death, availability of social resources, or choices of coping behavior" (p. 430). Similarly, having someone to rely on in a time of stress greatly reduced the impact of the stressful experience in children dealing with disasters and war or in children living in a home with severe marital conflict. Finally, trusting that things will be o.k. and believing in one's self-efficacy have been found to help the individual to enter into a situation more prepared for effective action. This is particularly important for the Latino individual whose life is likely to be influenced by strong beliefs, including the traditional religious beliefs and beliefs in the power of other supernatural practices (such as Espiritistas, Santeria, voodoo, among others). Again, the extent to which there is a lessening of this protective shield as a result of the immigration experience should be part of the assessment for Latino youth.

Another important culturally-based mechanism to deal with stress and emotionally-laden situation is what is known as "ataque" among Latinos (similar mechanisms exist in other cultures). An ataque is an epileptic-like attack that is exhibited mostly by females that includes psychomotor agitation, palpitation, screaming, and throwing themselves on the floor, and finally a partial loss of consciousness (Ghali, 1982; Javier, 1996). This is a transitory state that leaves no clear residual effect. It is likely for the individual, in a short time, to be able to sit up and resume the activity that she was engaged in prior to the episode. It is believed that this culturally-syntonic discharge offers a unique relief of the tension and contributes to better coping.

CONCLUSIONS

In this chapter we attempted to elucidate a series of important factors that should be considered when dealing with Latino youth. We put particular emphasis on the cultural and ethnic influences that tend to color the developmental progression traversed by Latino youth. This includes culturally-based codes of conduct, religious beliefs, the importance of the family and extended family structure, the specific geopolitical, socioeconomic and ecological influences that contribute to the Latino youth's self definition and identity. We made emphasis in this regard on the need to consider both the distinctiveness and similarities of different Latino individuals in terms of the definition of resilience and vulnerability.

We indicated in this chapter that the current literature does not offer enough specificity to help us understand the different Latino individuals with regard to the specific factors that contribute to resilience and those that contribute to dysfunctionality. Thus, the complex relations that exist among the different coping strategies, ethnicity and culture or the different coping strategies and immigration experience, level of linguistic proficiency or acculturation are still in need of systematic research. An important issue in this regard is the need to ascertain how and the extent to which the emotional state and self-esteem of Latino youth could be affected by the above factors. As also suggested by the National Advisory Mental Health Council in its report on vulnerability and resilience (1996), future investigations need to clarify the different cultural orientations and levels of acculturation as well as to identify and define those cultural strengths that help maintain a solid sense of self among Latino youths, collectively and individually. This is particularly important since self-esteem has been found to play a role in depression, eating disorders, achievements, self-destructive actions and antisocial behaviors.

REFERENCES

Argueta-Bernal, G.A. (1990). Stress and stress-related disorders in Hispanics: Biobehavioral approaches to treatment. In F.C., Serafia, A.I. Sheweber, R.K. Russell, P.D. Issac, & L.B. Myers (eds.), *Mental health of ethnic minorities* (pp. 202–21). New York: Praeger.

Armour-Thomas, E., & Gopaul-McNicol, S. (1997). In search of correlates of learning underlying "Learning Disability" using a Bio-Ecological Assessment System. *Journal of Social Distress and the Homeless,* 6(2), 143–159.

Baca, E., & Javier, R.A. (July, 1995). *El role de los objectos transicionales en el proceso de la separation de la tierra madre: Un estudio realizado con mujeres emigrantes latinas.* Presented at the XXV Interamerican Congress of Psychology, San Juan Puerto Rico.

Baldwin, A., L., Baldwin, C., & Cole, R.E. (1990). Stress-resistant families and stress-resistant children. In J. Rolf, A.S. Masten, D. Cicchetti, K. H. Nuechterlein & S. Weintraum (Eds.). *Risk and protective factors in the development of psychopathology* (pp. 257–280). New York: Cambridge University Press.

Brent, D.A., Perper, J.A., Moritz, G., Allman, C., Friend, A., & Roth, C. (1993). Psychiatric risk factors for adolescent suicide: A case control study. *Journal of the American Academy of Chidren and Adolescents, 32,* 521–529.

Camacho-Gingerich, A. (Ed.) (2002). *Coping in America: The Case of Caribbean East Indians.* New York: The Guyanese East Indian Civic Association.

Canino, I.A., & Canino, G. (1980). Impact of stress on the Puerto Rican family: Treatment considerations, *American Journal of Orthopsychiatry,* 50(3), 232–238.

Delgado, R., & Stefancic, J. (Eds.) (1998). *The Latino/a Condition: A Critical Reader.* New York: New York University Press.

Eccles, J., Midgley, C. Wigfield, A. Buchanan, C.M., Reuman, D., & Flanagan, C. (1993). Development during adolescence: The impact of Stage-Environment Fit on young adolescents' experience in school and in families. *American Psychologist, 48* (2): 90–101.

Emery, R.E. (1988). *Marriage, divorce, and children's adjustment (vol. 14).* Newbury Park, CA: Sage.

Erickson, E. (1963). *Childhood and society.* W.W. Norton & Company, Inc., New York.

Flanagan, D.P., McGrew, K.S., & Ortiz, S.O. (2000). *The Wechsler Intelligence Scales and Gf-Gc theory: A contemporary approach to interpretation. Boston:* Allyn and Bacon.

Flaskerud, J.H., & Winslow, B.J. (1998). Conceptualizing vulnerable populations health-related research. *Nursing Research, 47* (2), 69–78.

Freud, A. (1965). *Normality and pathology in childhood.* New York: International University Press.

Garbarino, J. (2001). An ecological perspective on the effects of violence on children. *Journal of Community Psychology, 29* (3), 361–378.

Garmezy, N., & Masten, A. (1986). Stress, competence, and resilience: Common frontiers for therapist and psychotherapist. *Behavior Therapy, 17,* 500–607.

Ghali, S.B. (1982), Understanding Puerto Rican tradition. *Social Work* January, 98–102.

Gil, R.M., & Vazquez, C.I. (1996). *The Maria paradox: How Latinas can merge old world traditions with new world self-esteem.* New York: G.P. Putnam & Sons.

Gutierrez, M. (2003). *Attitude toward suicide among Hispanic adolescents.* Unpublished doctoral dissertation, St. John's University.

Gutierrez, R.A. (1991). *When Jesus came, the Corn Mothers went away: Marriage, sexuality, and power in New Mexico, 1500–1845,* Stanford, CA: Stanford University Press.

Heilemann, M.V., Lee, K., & Kury, F.S. (2002). Strengths and vulnerabilities of women of Mexican descent in relation to depressive symptoms. *Official Journal of the Eastern Nursing Research Society and the Western Institute of Nursing,* 51(3), 175–182.

Javier, R.A. (1996). Psychodynamic treatment with the urban poor. In R.P. Foster, M. Moskowitz, R.A. Javier (Eds.) *Reaching across boundaries of culture and class: Widening the scope of psychotherapy* (pp. 93–113). Northvale, New Jersey, London: Jason Aronson, Inc.

Javier, R.A. (2002). Coping in America: A psychological journey. In A. Camacho-Gingerich (Ed.). *Coping in America: The Case of Caribbean East Indians* (pp. 135–139). New York: The Guyanese East Indian Civic Association.

Javier, R.A., & Yussef, M.B. (1995). A Latino perspective on the role of ethnicity in the development of moral values: Implications for psychoanalytic theory and practice. *Journal of the American Academy of Psychoanalysis, 23, 79–97.*

Jessor, R. (1993). Successful adolescent development among youth in high-risk Setting. *American Psychologist,* 48(2), 117–126.

Kernberg, O. (1975). *Borderline conditions and pathological narcissism.* New York: Jason Aronson, Inc.

Lauria, A. (1964). "Respeto," "relajo" and interpersonal relations in Puerto Rico. *Antropological Quarterly, 38,* 53–66.

Losel, F., & Bliesener, T. (1990). Resilience in adolescence: A study on the generalizability of protective factors. In K. Hurrelmann & F. Losel (Eds.) *Health hazards in adolescence* (pp. 104–135). New York: Walter de Gruyter.

Mahler, M.S., Pine, F., & Bergman, A. (1975). *The psychological birth of the human infant.* New York: Basic Books.

Masten, A.S. (1992). Homeless children in the United States: Mark of a nation at risk. *Current Directions in Psychological Science, 1,* 41–44.

Masten, A.S., Best, K.M., & Garmezy, N. (1990). Resilience and development: Contributions from the study of children who overcome adversity. *Development and Psychopathology, 2,* 425–444.

Masten, A.S., & Coatsworth, J.D. (1998). Development of competence in favorable and unfavorable environments. Lessons from research on successful children. *American Psychologist,* 53(2), 205–220.

National Advisory Mental Health Council (1996). Basic behavioral science research for mental health-vulnerability and resilience. *American Psychologist, 51* (1), 22–28.

Offer, D. (1979). Adolescent turmoil. In A.H. Esman (Ed.), *The Psychology of Adolescence, Essential Readings* (pp. 141–154), New York: International Universities Press, Inc.

Olvera, R. (2001). Suicide ideation in Hispanics and mixed ancestry adolescents. *Suicide and Life Threatening Behavior, 31,* 416–427.

Padilla, F. (1998). Salsa: Puerto Rican and Latino music. *Journal of Popular Culture, 24, 87–104.*

Pasamanick, B., & Knobloch, H. (1961). Epidemiological studies on the complications of pregnancy and the birth process. In G. Caplan (Ed.), *Prevention of Mental Disorders in Children: Initial Explorations* (pp. 74–94). New York: Basic Books.

Piaget, J. (1969). The intellectual development of the adolescent. In A.H. Esman (Ed.) *The psychology of adolescence: Essential readings* (pp. 104–108). New York: International University Press.

Piaget, J. (1972). *The psychology of intelligence.* Totowa, NJ: Littlefield Adams.

Plante, T.G., Manuel, G.M., Mendendez, A., & Marcotte, D. (1995). Coping with stress among Salvatorian immigrants. *Hispanic Journal of Behavioral Sciences, 17* (4), 471–479.

Preble, E. (1979). The Puerto Rican-American teen-ager in New York City. In A.H. Esman (Ed.). The *Psychology of Adolescence, Essential Readings* (pp. 52–71). New York: International Universities Press, Inc.

Quadrel, M.J., Fischoff, B., & Davis, W. (1993). Adolescent (in)vulnerability. *American Psychologist, 48 (2),* 102–116.

Razin, A.M., O'Doud, M.A., Nathan, A., Rodriguez, I, Goldfield, A., & Martin, C. (1991). Suicide behavior among Inner-city Hispanic adolescent females. *General Hospital Psychiatry, 13,* 45–58.

Rothbart, M.T., & Bates, J.E. (1998). Temperament. In W. Damon (Series Ed.) & N. Eisenberg (Vol. Ed), *Handbook of child psychology: Vol.3 Social, emotional, and personality development* (5th ed. pp. 105–176). New York: Wiley.

Rutter, M. (1989). Temperment: Conceptual issues and clinical implications. In G.A. Kohnstamn, J.E. Bates, & M.K. Rothbart (Eds.), *Temperment in childhood* (pp. 463–479). New York: Wiley.

Salgado de Snyder, V. Nelly (1987). Factors associated with acculturative stress and depressive symptomatology among married Mexican women. *Psychology of Women Quarterly,* 11, 475–488.

Sorenson, S.B., & Golding, J.M. (1988). Prevalence of suicide attempts in a Mexican-American population: Prevention implications of immigrant and cultural issues. *Suicide and Life-Threatening Behavior, 18,* 322–333.

Sternberg, R.J. (1985). Beyond IQ: A *triarchic theory of human intelligence.* New York: Cambridge University Press.

Suarez-Orozco, C., & Suarez-Orozco, M. (2001). *Children of Immigration.* Cambridge: Harvard University Press.

Sullivan, H.S. (1953). *The interpersonal theory of psychiatry.* New York: Norton.

Sullivan, H.S. (1973). *Clinical Studies in Psychiatry.* New York: W.W. Norton & Company, Inc.

Tejada, D., Sanchez, F., & Mella, C. (1993). *Religiosidad popular dominicana y Psiquiatra.* Santo Domingo, D.R.: Corripio.

Tortolero, S.R., & Roberts, R.E. (2001). Differences in nonfatal suicide behaviors among Mexican and European American middle school children. *Suicide and Life Threatening Behavior, 31,* 214–223.

Vega, W.A. Gil, A., G., Zimmerman, R.S., & Warheit, G. (1993). Risk factors for suicide behavior among Hispanic, African American, and non-Hispanic White boys in early adolescence. *Ethnicity and Disease, 3,* 229–241.

Vega, W.A., Kolody, B. Aguilar-Gaxiola, S., Alderet, E., Catalano, R., & Caraveo-Anduaga, J. (1998). Life time prevalence of DSM-R psychiatric disorders among urban and rural Mexican Americans in California. *Archives of General Psychiatry, 55,* 771–778.

Vygotsky, L.S. (1978). *Mind in society: The development of higher psychological processes.* Cambridge, MA: Harvard University Press.

Wallerstein, J.S., Corbin, S.B., & Lewis, J.S. (1988). Children of divorce: A two-year study. In M. Hetherington & J.D. Arasteh (Eds.). *Impact of divorce, single parenting, and stepparenting on children* (pp. 197–214). Hillsdale, N.J.: Earbaum.

Werner, E.E. (1990). Protective factors and individual resilience. In S.J. Meisels & M. Shonkoff (Eds.), *Handbook of early intervention.* New York: Cambridge University Press.

White, J.L., Moffitt, T.E., & Silva, P.A. (1989). A prospective replication of the protective effects of IQ in subjects at high risk for juvenile delinquency. *Journal of Consulting and Clinical Psychology, 57,* 719–724.

Winnicott, D.W. (1974). *The maturational processes and the facilitating environment.* New York: International University Press.

Chapter 6

Building Strengths in Inner City African-American Children
The Task and Promise of Schools

R. DWAYNE LAGRANGE

For several years now, researchers have attempted to better conceptualize the lives of children who are exposed to a variety of risks, and develop interventions that foster resilience and create better life opportunities (Garmezy, 1987, 1991; Masten, 1994; Rutter, 1987). While problems of some sort exist for almost all children, few have garnered as much attention in the literature as inner city African-American youth. The fact that this focus is so well justified is a disturbing reality. Studies indicate that children from the typical American inner city neighborhood are exposed to a wider range of negative influences than those experienced by their suburban and rural peers (Barbarin, 1993; Hellison & Cutforth, 1997; Myers, 1989).

African-American children reared in our nation's inner cities often suffer from a "double jeopardy" that exposes them to even greater risks and fewer resilience-promoting conditions (Borman & Rachuba, 2001). The child poverty rate in the United States is highest for African-American children (30%), most of whom live in large, urban areas (National Center for Children in Poverty [NCCP], 2003)[1]. Children reared in these communities commonly face obstacles to their development that include poverty, violence, single parent families, teenage motherhood, disorderly and stressful environments, lack of employment opportunities,

---

[1] The child poverty rate is 29% for Latino-American and 13% for White American children (NCCP, 2003).

institutionalized racism, poor health care, and highly fragmented patterns of service (Safyer, 1994; Wang, Haertel, & Walberg, 1994). In a report on mental health and race in America, the U.S. Surgeon General reported that minorities have less access to mental health services and are less likely to receive needed mental health care (U.S. Department of Health and Human Services [DHHS], 2001). The emotional and behavioral problems disadvantaged children endure are likely to reduce their quality of life and future opportunities. Children with these challenges are at much greater risk for dropping out of school and of not being fully functioning members of society when they reach adulthood (DHHS, 2000). As a result, many inner city African-American children do not have an opportunity to grow in an environment that is conducive to their cognitive, emotional, and social development (Myers, 1989; Taylor, 1994).

In spite of their exposure to extraordinary environmental stressors and the lack of available protective mechanisms, many inner city African-American children excel. In the early 1980s, investigators seeking to understand how resiliency develops in disadvantaged children focused on identifying their deficits and pathologies (Werner, 1995). Child developmentalists, psychologists, and educators have played a leading role since that time in the introduction of new methods for studying resilience and have contributed to the knowledge base on African-American youth who overcome adversity.

Several findings have consistently identified a small number of factors that help protect children against stressful environmental conditions (Garmezy, 1991; Smokowski, Reynolds, & Bezruczko, 2000; Werner, 2000). The most important *protective mechanism* seems to be a strong relationship with a competent, caring, positive adult—preferably a parent, while the most important *personal attributes* are average or above-average intellectual development with good attention and interpersonal skills (Osofsky & Thompson, 2000). Given the disproportionately high level of stress faced by poor, African-American parents living in urban areas, children from these families can easily be deprived of the very agents that are so critical to their survival and prosperity. Therefore, resilience promoting interventions that protect inner city African-American children against stressful life circumstances must be culturally competent and designed to meet their unique educational and social needs.

African-Americans have traditionally viewed education as a mechanism for overcoming societal obstacles (Clark, 1983; Winfield, 1995). It represents a potentially powerful construct for fostering resilience and success among children who are enduring stressful life circumstances (Wang, Haertel, & Walberg, 1997a). Schools may be in the ideal position to provide a place of refuge and hope for inner city African-American children. To a degree, some do; others put forth a valiant effort; but sadly, many inner city schools miss the opportunity to significantly alter the negative trajectories of their African-American students. Especially for children living in disadvantaged communities, the conditions for learning, both in school and out, are established in their families and in their communities (Taylor, 1994). Resilience in inner city African-American children is facilitated when available school, family, and community resources are complementary, coordinated, and devoted to promoting healthy development and academic success (Wang et al., 1994; Winfield, 1995).

Thus, school-based solutions designed to help build strengths in inner city African-American children should be wide-ranging enough to embrace elements of the family and community. In order to earnestly prepare these youth for the future, schools must assume a more proactive role in fostering their healthy development. This will entail integrating more comprehensive prevention efforts that are dedicated to increasing resilience, helping avert adjustment problems, and promoting adaptive functioning. The remainder of this chapter will describe how inner-city schools can play an integral role in helping to develop resilient African-American children. Included will be a discussion of the construct of resilience and its cultural context, the role that environmental factors such as parenting have in fostering resilience, and a solution for schools to become a more prominent developmental agent in the lives of its students.

RESILIENCE IN CONTEXT

Regardless of race, ethnicity, class, or geographic boundaries, resilient children make use of environmental support systems more effectively than their less resilient peers (Werner, 2000). The relational bonds of resilient children are often credited for buffering risks and facilitating adaptive development (Garmezy, 1983; Werner & Smith, 1982) as well as encouraging important personal attributes like trust, autonomy, and initiative (Werner, 1995). These protective factors appear to make a more profound impact on the life course of children growing up in adversity than do specific risk factors or stressful life events (Werner, 1995). Evidence suggests that the need to strengthen environmental support systems is especially relevant to disadvantaged African-American children and can enable them to cope under adverse conditions (Nettles & Pleck, 1994; Zimmerman, Ramirez-Valles, & Maton, 1999).

Focusing on environmental resources rather than the individual characteristics of resilient children accurately emphasizes the importance of social conditions in fostering success. Research pursuits that concentrate on the small proportion of youth who surmount adverse circumstances create the misperception that individual fortitude develops without outside influences and undermines the support needed to initiate social interventions (Garmezy, 1987; Nettles & Pleck, 1994). Investigations on the resilience of African-American children have often suffered shortcomings by failing to differentiate between such within-group variables as social class, region, country of origin, recency of immigration, language or other characteristics (Nettles & Pleck, 1994). Treating African-American children as a homogeneous group ignores important distinctions. Too often, studies have confounded the demographic categories of ethnicity and social class, thereby ignoring the interaction of these two variables and obscuring subsequent findings (McKenry, Everett, Ramseur, & Carter, 1989; Slaughter-DeFoe, Nakagawa, Takanishi, & Johnson, 1990). The information presented in this chapter is intended to focus on the issues most relevant to a discussion of resilience among *inner city* African-American youth. The chapter does not mean to suggest that all African American youth live in inner cities. In contrast, there is a range of diversity within African American youth in terms of socioeconomic status and geographical region, whether it be urban, suburban, or rural. The decision to focus on inner city African American youth was made to address some of the specific stressors that poverty presents.

RESILIENCY IN INNER CITY AFRICAN-AMERICAN CHILDREN

The rising number of children at risk for poor developmental outcomes due to poverty and associated stressors emphasizes the need to determine both those factors that promote resilience and those that are alterable (NCCP, 2003; Reynolds, 1998). This need is especially significant for African-American children who are disproportionately raised in poor communities. Low-income, urban African-American youth must negotiate the stressors associated with economic deprivation and disadvantage, institutionalized racism, unemployment, poor educational opportunities, violence, high death rates and similar obstacles as they traverse the normal trials and tribulations associated with childhood (Rosella & Albrecht, 1993; Taylor, 1994; Zimmerman et al., 1999). Seligman and Peterson (1986) argue that inner city African-American youth often perceive their environments as unalterable and as a result, may be prone to feelings of helplessness and negative expectations. Studies link these emotional responses to future psychological problems such as depression, anxiety, and low self-esteem (Lloyd, 1980; Seligman & Peterson, 1986; Zimmerman et al., 1999).

Despite extraordinary stressors, however, many inner city African-American youth can and do grow up to be well-adapted and productive adults (Anderson, Eaddy, & Williams, 1990). Most of the early research on resilient African-American children endeavored to categorize pathology, risk factors, problem behaviors, or social class traits (McKenry et al., 1989; Zimmerman et al., 1999). Fortunately, contemporary investigators have veered from this path and accelerated efforts to determine the social and cultural mechanisms that underlie resilience in the face of adversity (Cicchetti & Garmezy, 1993; Nettles & Pleck, 1994). This approach broadens the understanding of how environmental factors affect resiliency in African-American children beyond the scope of individual characteristics.

During the 1990s, several researchers increased their efforts to determine the factors that are most important to promoting the healthy development and resilience of poor, urban African-American youth (Barbarin, 1993; Luthar, Doernberger, & Zigler, 1993; Garmezy, 1991; Miller & MacIntosh, 1999; Myers & Taylor, 1998; Spencer, Cole, DuPree, Glymph, & Pierre, 1993). Competent African-American children living in highly stressed urban areas exhibit protective factors that include a wider array of social skills, positive peer and adult interactions, and a higher degree of social responsiveness and sensitivity (Garmezy, 1983).

Reynolds (1998) sought to better understand the process through which African-American children use existing protective mechanisms to achieve resilience. His investigation analyzed data from a longitudinal study of the adjustment of 1,120 low-income African-American 12-year-olds living in an inner-city environment. Results indicated that the most salient and alterable factors contributing to resilience could be categorized as either academic influences (i.e., achievement in early childhood, perceived competence, and classroom adjustment) or parental influences (i.e., parental expectations and early childhood interventions). A strong argument is made from these findings for the need to further explore the influences of both parenting and education on resiliency in inner city African-American children.

THE INFLUENCE OF PARENTING ON RESILIENCE

Parenting is largely determined by the environmental context in which families live (Osofsky & Thompson, 2000). Although African-American children are directly influenced by a series of ongoing interpersonal interactions (e.g., with peers, teachers, family members, etc.), societal factors impact how their parents rear them in a more indirect manner. Elder, Nguyen, and Caspi (1985) outlined this tendency in poverty-stricken families through their work on the effects of parental income and job loss during the Great Depression of the 1930's. The negative psychological outcomes suffered by children in this research were not necessarily associated with their family's socioeconomic status. Instead, the emotional functioning of children who lived through the Depression was more correlated with their parents' psychological functioning. Fathers who sustained heavy financial losses, for example, became more irritable, tense and explosive. They subsequently became more punitive, arbitrary, and inconsistent in disciplining their children (Elder et al., 1985). These types of parental behaviors predict a series of resilience inhibiting and emotional responses in children, ranging from irritability and moodiness in boys to hypersensitivity and feelings of inadequacy in girls (McLoyd, 1998). Similar processes likely affect inner city African-American children considering that so many of their parents deal with poverty as well as institutionalized racism, violence and other societal obstacles on a daily basis.

Bronfenbrenner (1989) describes parent-child interactions as existing within the context of multiple relationships. A child's environment can encompass interpersonal relationships outside the family that can have a significant influence and help shape the child's overall development (Osofsky & Thompson, 2000). These extra-familial relationships play a critical role in fostering resilience when other resources are depleted or non-existent. Many African-Americans living in urban areas require additional support to help overcome the challenges of parenting with limited means. Fortunately, studies of the African-American family have documented that extended family support systems can protect children against a hostile or racist societal environment (Winfield, 1995).

Parenting Challenges in the Inner City

The linkage between poor parenting practices and negative developmental outcomes in impoverished children has been a part of both educational and developmental literature for several years (Slaughter-Defoe et al., 1990). African-American children from poor, inner city communities are at increased risk for negative outcomes not so much because of what their parents cannot afford to buy, but because of what living with limited financial resources represents (McLoyd, 1998). The connection between parental expectations and resiliency in African-American children has recently garnered more interest in the research literature (Nettles & Pleck, 1994; Reynolds, 1998; Slaughter & Epps, 1987; Wang et al., 1994). Family protective factors have typically included socioeconomic status, child behavior management, and parenting styles (Werner & Smith, 1992). Reynolds (1998) extends earlier models of educational performance that suggested parent expectations alone contributed to the scholastic development of students. Instead, he maintains that parental expectations significantly affect all resilience constructs above and beyond the influence of risk status, early childhood adjustment, and intervention experience (Reynolds, 1998).

Some individuals who are struggling to develop effective parenting styles tend to utilize inconsistent behaviors (e.g., punishing and rewarding based on parents' current mood) or over-controlling behaviors (e.g., parental overprotection, superfluous use of rewards) (Gardner, 1989; Sansbury & Whaler, 1992). However, ineffective parenting is not necessarily the result of parental neglect or lack of parental skills. Some research suggests that respondents from poor families frequently attributed their maladaptive parenting behaviors to a lack of faith in the educational system and their extraordinarily stress-filled lives. Parents negotiating their own personal, social, or financial challenges may be unresponsive, or react ambiguously to their child's defiant activities (McLoyd, 1998). In contrast, parenting that is structured and highly directive (e.g., well-defined rules at home, clear and consistent consequences for breaking rules, close supervision), when combined with high levels of warmth, helps disadvantaged children overcome obstacles in their environment that ordinarily increase their risk for negative outcomes (Baldwin, Baldwin, & Cole, 1990; McLoyd, 1998). Adaptive parenting behaviors, much like high parental expectations, distinguish disadvantaged yet resilient children from their less successful peers. Based on these findings, a strong argument can be made for providing inner city African-American families with a system that can offer support to parents.

The Role of Extended Social Networks in Adaptive Parenting

There are many ways that social networks can assist those parents whose environmental conditions make them susceptible to maladaptive parenting styles (Osofsky & Thompson, 2000). Organized and extended social networks help to reduce stress by providing a buffer against threatening events, improving the coping strategies of parents, and providing needed emotional support (Cochran, Lerner, Riley, Gunnarsson, & Henderson, 1990). Collaborative social environments improve parents' general dispositions, assist them in feeling less overwhelmed by parenting tasks, and allow them to have additional tangible and intangible resources from which to draw information (McLoyd, 1995). Additionally, extended social networks can offer parents who are struggling with child-rearing much needed advice and information regarding community resources (Osofsky & Thompson, 2000).

Reports indicate that African-Americans often have larger social networks that they rely on more frequently than other cultural groups (Cross, 1990; Kohn & Wilson, 1995; Taylor, Chatters, Tucker, & Lewis, 1990). High levels of community support in African-American families has been linked to greater levels of social interaction in children, higher levels of academic achievement, and overall enhanced social and emotional well-being (Gonzalez, Cauce, Friedman, & Mason, 1996; Taylor, 1997). Overly punitive, cruel, or controlling parenting styles are less likely in families where there is an effective and supportive network, even in the presence of extraordinarily harsh environmental stressors (Hashima & Amato, 1994). Families with access to extended social networks also tend to have a lower incidence of child abuse and violence (Crockenberg, 1987). These systems are so critical to child rearing in disadvantaged families that its absence greatly increases conditions that foster maladaptive parenting. When compared with nonabusive parents, abusive parents were more likely to be isolated from both formal and informal social networks (McLoyd, 1995). Moreover, abusive parents report having less access to external sources of support and being dissatisfied with the resources that are readily available to them (MacPhee, Fritz, & Miller-Heyl, 1996).

Since educational systems have the most sustained contact with inner city African-American students, schools can engage families through extended social networks and play an integral role in helping parents foster their children's adaptive development. Research on resilient African-American children has consistently shown that if a parent is incapacitated, unavailable, or prone to maladaptive parenting styles, other significant people in a child's life can compensate for what may be lacking (Osofsky & Thompson, 2000; Smokowski et al., 2000; Werner, 1995). Werner (2000) argues that in many situations, it makes better sense and is more cost efficient to strengthen existing resources (e.g., schools, communities) than to introduce additional layers of bureaucracy into the delivery of services. Parents who have positive relationships with effective school systems that provide organization and support in their neighborhoods are more likely to produce resilient children than those who lack these significant relationships (Osofsky & Thompson, 2000). Schools can help build resilient strengths in inner city African-American children by implementing programs that link the resources that exist in their communities and the relationships that are nurtured within them.

THE INFLUENCE OF SCHOOLS ON RESILIENCE

Several of the protective factors that promote academic success (i.e., caring and supportive school staff; safe and orderly school environment; high expectations for all students; improved partnerships between home and school) (Wang et al., 1997a) parallel the individual factors that are characteristic of resilient children (i.e., caring parents; stable and structured home environment; clear sense of one's purpose and future; well-developed interpersonal skills) (Smokowski et al., 2000; Werner, 2000). Although there is little evidence that high academic achievement alone promotes more effective coping, most studies report that intelligence (especially communication and problem solving skills) assists considerably in providing children with the ability to overcome adversity (Werner, 2000). Furthermore, the positive relationships inner city African-American students are able to establish with school staff can mitigate the effect of both individual and familial stressors (Rutter, 1987). It then stands to reason that schools can represent a strong agent of change in the lives of disadvantaged African-American students when they integrate evidence-based resilience promoting strategies within their academic framework. It is recommended that universal policy initiatives in schools be directed at enhancing the interpersonal contexts, emotional well-being, and engagement of all disadvantaged youth in educational settings (Connell, Spencer, & Aber, 1994).

Whether at home or school, children from responsive, nurturing, organized and predictable environments develop a greater degree of adaptive behavior (Hetherington, Stanley-Ragan, & Anderson, 1989). However, it is widely acknowledged that schools cannot overcome the multi-layered risks of their disadvantaged children when acting alone. In this light, a growing school reform effort has developed strategies that can be used to address the interconnected needs of disadvantaged students and their families (Kirst, Koppich, & Kelley, 1994; Rigsby,

Reynolds, & Wang, 1995; U.S. Department of Education & American Educational Research Association, 1995). The goal of this movement is for schools to harness the resources of the family and community to create an educational environment that supports student success by meeting their physical and social-wellness needs.

Building Strengths Through Schools

The Community for Learning Program (CFL) in Philadelphia demonstrates how schools can successfully alter the environmental context of its inner city African-American students and better support their overall development. CFL is based on investigations conducted at the Temple University Center for Research in Human Development and Education and builds upon findings from the Adaptive Learning Environments Model (Wang, 1992) and the Comer (1985) School Development Model. The CFL program design represents an effort to foster educational resilience through connections among school, family, and the community (Wang, 1996). It seeks to impact student outcomes in three major areas: a) increased positive attitudes by students and the school staff toward their school learning environment, b) improved student achievement for all students, especially those at the lowest end of the academic spectrum, and c) enhanced patterns of active learning and teaching processes that are consistent with the research base on effective classroom practices (Wang, 1996).

In just the first two years of CFL implementation, several notable findings became apparent that showed an improvement along program goals (Wang, Haertel, & Walberg, 1997b; Wang & Oates, 1996). For instance, students in CFL schools reported perceiving their learning environments in a profoundly more encouraging manner (e.g., more constructive feedback from teachers about their work and behavior, a higher level of aspiration for academic learning, better academic self-concept, and clearer rules for behaviors and school operations). Data also revealed CFL students increased their math and reading scores both school-wide, and in comparison to students in similar schools. A noteworthy, yet unexpected finding included the observation that student families and the community, two groups that had been a challenge to engage, became increasingly active in a wide range of school activities and in the school decision-making process (Wang & Oates, 1996). The success attained by CFL has contributed to the emergence of a variety of innovative programs that seek to improve the life circumstances of inner city African-American youth around the country (Oates et al., 1997; Wang & Oates, 1996). Nearly all of these initiatives strive to develop feasible ways to transform fragmented, inefficient systems of service delivery into a network of coordinated partnerships that cross programmatic and agency borders by placing schools at the front line of the battle.

Expanded School Mental Health (ESMH)

Through partnerships between schools and community programs and agencies, expanded school mental health (ESMH) programs provide a full range of mental health promotion and intervention that can foster resilience in inner city African-American children (Weist, 1997; Weist & Christodulu, 2000). Rutter (1987) identified four main protective processes that can be used to demonstrate how ESMH can promote the development of resilience in disadvantaged African-American children. They include: a) reducing the impact of risk exposure, b) reducing the negative chain reaction following risk exposure, c) establishing and maintaining self-esteem and self-efficacy, and d) opening up new opportunities.

Reducing Impact of Risk Exposure

Rutter (1987) suggests that reducing the impact of a child's risk exposure is a crucial protective mechanism. For those African-American children who grow up in communities where poverty, violence and other environmental stressors are commonplace, ESMH programs present valuable opportunities to improve the overall environment in inner city schools through joined efforts between health and educational staff (Knitzer, Steinberg, & Fleisch, 1991). In a study of inner city minority students, for instance, Armbruster and Lichtman (1999) reported that school administrators noted improvements in academic performance, behavior, and attendance in those receiving ESMH services.

Academic success is promoted for African-American students when they feel safe and are engaged (Fowler & Walberg, 1991; Wang et al., 1997a). Through a proactive approach to prevent problems and assist youth and families in need, ESMH programs can enhance this sense of connectedness for African-American youth. ESMH programs can offer African-American parents with a reliable, supportive network that encourages and promotes positive parenting, and assists in connecting families to needed and available community resources (e.g., tutoring, job training, GED classes, social services; see Osofsky & Thompson, 2000).

Reducing Negative Chain Reactions

The sequence of events that transpire following risk exposure perpetuates the long-term adverse effects that children suffer (Rutter, 1985). African-American students who become involved in gangs, engage in crime, or become pregnant typically fall into a downward spiral that is too difficult for them to overcome without additional support. ESMH staff can help identify and provide interventions for such common student occurrences as excessive absences, classroom disciplinary problems, and unexpected family disruptions. Interventions for these situations may range from additional student monitoring, to individual, group, or family counseling, to referral to outside social service agencies.

Establishing and Maintaining Self-Esteem

A large body of literature attests to the protective role that a strong sense of self-worth has for children (Cicchetti & Garmezy, 1993; Masten, 1994; Smokowski et al., 2000; Werner, 2000). Weist, Paskewitz, Warner, and Flaherty (1996) found that inner city adolescents receiving psychological services showed significant declines in depression and improvements in self-concept. Specific strategies that ESMH staff can employ to provide for the emotional support of African-American students include establishing clearly defined personal goals for students being seen in treatment, improving oral and interpersonal skills through structured group interactions, developing a peer mentoring system, and teaching assertiveness skills.

Opening Opportunities

This final protective mechanism involves what Rutter (1987) describes as turning points, critical junctions in the lives of children. Most of these turning points will occur for youth while they are in school when decisions are made regarding their future and their available options. Educational systems that integrate ESMH are able to maintain strong school-community collaborations and move toward providing a more comprehensive system of care. The merging of community resources reduces the likelihood that disadvantaged African-American youth will fall through the cracks of a pourous social service network. Effective ESMH programs emphasize building upon individual and community strengths and assist disadvantaged youth in making positive life choices (see Winfield, 1995).

CONCLUSION

Because resilience is not fostered in a vacuum, the co-occurring risk factors and other obstacles faced by many inner city African-American children cannot be addressed by interventions that focus solely on the child, family, school, or community. Instead, all available resources must be organized and channeled. This can help compensate for existing deficiencies and provide solutions for the educational, health, and social problems facing children in need. Since inner city African-American children are often exposed to greater risk with fewer resilience-promoting conditions, they can benefit significantly from school-led efforts that create strong, mutual partnerships between the school, family, and community to shield them from risk and stress and to promote internal and external protective factors (Borman & Rachuba, 2001; Vondra, 1999). Ultimately, leaders of urban schools confront a choice point of being complicit in closing gateways of opportunity, or accepting the responsibility of being agents of change for the youth they serve. Although schools are in the business of education, they cannot ignore student concerns that extend beyond their doors when these barriers impede learning and healthy development. For inner city schools, this junction represents both their most daunting challenge and their greatest potential. My hope is that this chapter will provide more stimulus for action towards the latter.

REFERENCES

Anderson, L., Eaddy, C.L., & Williams, E.A. (1990). Psychological competence: Toward a theory of understanding positive mental health among Black Americans. In D. Ruiz (Ed.), *Handbook of mental health and mental disorders among Black Americans* (pp. 255–271). Westport, CT: Greenwood Press.

Armbruster, P., & Lichtman, J. (1999). Are school based mental health services effective?: Evidence from 36 inner city schools. *Community Mental Health Journal, 35(6)*, 493–504.

Baldwin, A.L., Baldwin, C., & Cole, R.E. (1990). Stress-resistant families and stress-resistant children. In J. Rolf, A.S. Masten, D. Cicchetti, K., Nuechterlein, & S. Weintraub (Eds.), *Risk and protective factors in the development of psychopathology* (pp. 257–280). Cambridge, England: Cambridge University Press.

Barbarin, O.A. (1993). Coping and resilience: Exploring the inner lives of African-American children. *Journal of Black Psychology, 19*, 478–492.

Borman, G.D., & Rachuba, L.T. (2001, Feb.). *Academic success among poor and minority students: An analysis of competing models of school effects* (Report No. 52). Baltimore, MD: Johns Hopkins University, Center for Research on the Education of Students Placed at Risk. (ERIC Document Reproduction Service No. ED451281)

Broffenbrenner, U. (1989). Ecological systems theory. In R. Vasta (Ed.), *Annals of childhood development* (Vol. 6, pp. 187–249). Greenwich, CT: Jason Aaronson Press.

Cicchetti, D., & Garmezy, N. (1993). Prospects and promises in the study of resilience. *Development and psychopathology, 5*, 497–502.

Clark, R. (1983). *Family life and school achievement. Why poor Black children succeed and fail.* Chicago: University of Chicago Press.

Cochran, M., Lerner, M., Riley, D., Gunnarsson, L., & Henderson, C.R., Jr. (1990). *Extended families: The social networks of parents and their children.* New York: Cambridge University Press.

Comer, J.P. (1985, September). *The school development program: A nine-step guide to school improvement [paper].* New Haven, CT: Yale Child Study Center.

Connell, J.P., Spencer, M.B., & Aber, J.L. (1994). Educational Risk and Resilience in African-American youth: Context, self, action, and outcomes in school. *Child Development, 65*, 493–506.

Crockenberg, S. (1987). Support for adolescent mothers during the postnatal period: Theory and research. In C.F.Z. Boukydis (Ed.), *Research on support for parents and infants in the postnatal period* (pp. 3–24). Hillsdale, NJ: Erlbaum.

Cross, W.E. (1990). Race and ethnicity: Effects on social networks. In M. Cochran, M. Lerner, D. Riley, I. Gunnarson, & C. Henderson (Eds.), *Extending families: The social networks of parents and their children* (pp. 67–85). New York: Cambridge University Press.

Elder, G., Nguyen, T., & Caspi, A. (1985). Linking family hardship to children's lives. *Child Development, 56*, 361–375.

Fowler, W.J., & Walberg, H.J. (1991). School size, characteristics, and outcomes. *Educational Evaluation and Policy Analysis, 13(2)*, 189–202.

Gardner, F.E. (1989). Inconsistent parenting: Is there evidence for a link with children's conduct problems? *Journal of Abnormal Psychology, 17*, 223–233.

Garmezy, N. (1983). Stressors in childhood. In N. Garmezy & M. Rutter (Eds.), *Stress, coping, and development in children* (pp. 34–89). New York: McGraw-Hill.

Garmezy, N. (1987). Stress, competence, and development: Continuities in the study of schizophrenic adults, children vulnerable to psychopathology, and the search for stress-resistant children. *American Journal of Orthopsychiatry, 57(2)*, 159–174.

Garmezy, N. (1991). Resilience and vulnerability to adverse developmental outcomes associated with poverty. *American Behavioral Scientist, 34(4)*, 416–430.

Gonzalez, N.A., Cauce, A.M., Friedman, R.J., & Mason, C.A. (1996). Family, peer, and neighborhood influences on academic achievement among African-American adolescents: One-year prospective effects. *American Journal of Community Psychology, 24*, 82–91.

Hashima, P.Y., & Amato, P.R. (1994). Poverty, social support, and parental behavior. *Child Development, 65*, 394–403.

Hellison, D.R. & Cutforth, N.J. (1997). Extended day programs for urban children and youth: From theory to practice. In H.J. Walberg, O. Reyes, & R.P. Weissberg (Eds.), *Children and youth: Interdisciplinary perspectives* (pp. 223–249). Thousand Oaks, CA: SAGE Publications.

Hetherington, E.M., Stanley-Ragan, M., & Anderson, E.R. (1989). Marital transitions: A child's perspective. *American Psychologist, 44*, 303–212.

Kirst, M.W., Koppich, J.E., & Kelley, C. (1994). School-linked services: A new approach to improving outcomes for children. In K. Wong & M.C. Wang (Eds.), *Rethinking policy for at-risk students* (pp. 197–220). Berkeley, CA: McCutchan.

Knitzer, J., Steinberg, Z., & Fleisch, B. (1991). Schools, children's mental health, and the advocacy challenge. *Journal of Clinical Child Psychology, 20(1)*, 102–111.

Kohn, M., & Wilson, M.N. (1995). Social support networks in the African American family: Utility for culturally compatible intervention. In M.N. Wilson (Ed.), *New directions for child development: Vol 68. African American family life: Its structural and ecological aspects* (pp. 5–21). San Francisco: Jossey-Bass Publishers.

Lloyd, C. (1980). Life events and depressive disorder reviewed. *Archives of General Psychiatry, 37*, 529–548.

Luther, S.S., Doernberger, C., & Zigler, E. (1993). Resilience is not a unidimensional construct: Insights from a prospective study of inner-city adolescents. *Development and Psychopathology, 5*, 703–717.

MacPhee, D., Fritz, J., & Miller-Heyl, J. (1996). Ethnic variations in personal social networks and parenting. *Child Development, 67*, 3278–3295.

Masten, A.S. (1994). Resilience in individual development: Successful adaptation despite risk and adversity. In M.C. Wang & E.W. Gordon (Eds.), *Educational resilience in inner-city America: Challenges and prospects* (pp. 3–25). Hillside, NJ: Erlbaum.

McKenry, C.P., Everett, J.E., Ramseur, H.P., & Carter, C.J. (1989). Research on Black adolescents: A legacy of cultural bias. *Journal of Adolescent Research, 4(2)*, 254–264.

McLoyd, V.C. (1995). Poverty, parenting, and policy: Meeting the support needs of poor parents. In H. Fitzgerald, B. Lester, & B. Zuckerman (Eds.), *Children of poverty: Research health, and policy issues* (pp. 269–303). New York: Garland Press.

McLoyd, V.C. (1998). Socioeconomic disadvantage and child development. *American Psychologist, 53(2)*, 185–204.

Miller, D.B., & MacIntosh, R. (1999). Promoting resilience in urban African American adolescents: Racial socialization and identity as protective factors. *Social Work Research, 23(3)*, 159–170.

Myers, H.F. (1989). Urban stress and mental health in Black youth: An epidemiologic and conceptual update. In R. Jones (Ed.), *Black adolescents* (pp. 123–152). Berkeley, CA: Cobb & Henry.

Myers, H.F. & Taylor, S. (1998). Family contributions to risk and resilience in African American children. *Journal of Comparative Family Studies, 29,* 215–229.

National Center for Children in Poverty. (2003). *Low-income children in the United States: A brief demographic profile.* Retrieved April 21, 2003 from www.nccp.org/pub_cpf03.html

Nettles, S.M., & Pleck, J.H. (1994). Risk, resilience, and development: The multiple ecologies of Black adolescents in the United States. In R.J. Haggerty, L.R. Sherrod, N. Garmezy, & M. Rutter (Eds.), *Stress, risk, and resilience in children and adolescents: Processes, mechanisms, and interventions* (pp. 147–181). New York: Cambridge University Press.

Oates, J., Weishew, N., and Flores, R. (1997). *Achieving student success in inner-city schools is possible, provided... [paper]* Philadelphia, PA: Laboratory for Student Success, the Mid-Atlantic Regional Educational Laboratory at Temple University Center for Research in Human Development and Education.

Osofsky, J.D., & Thompson, M.D. (2000). Adaptive and maladaptive parenting: Perspectives on risk and protective factors. In J.P. Shonkoff & S.J. Meisels (Eds.), *Handbook of early childhood intervention* (2nd ed., pp. 54–75). New York: Cambridge University Press.

Reynolds, A.J. (1998). Resilience among black urban youth: Prevalence, intervention effects, and mechanisms of influence. *American Journal of Orthopsychiatry, 68(1),* 84–100.

Rosella, J.D., & Albrecht, S.A. (1993). Toward an understanding of the health status of Black adolescents: An application of the stress-coping framework. *Issues in Comprehensive Pediatric Nursing, 16,* 193–205.

Rutter, M. (1987). Psychosocial resilience and protective mechanisms. *American Journal of Orthopsychiatry, 37(3),* 317–331.

Sansbury, L.L., & Whaler, R.G. (1992). Pathways to maladaptive parenting with mothers and their conduct disordered children. *Behavior Modification, 16,* 574–592.

Safyer, A.W. (1994). The impact of inner-city life on adolescent development: Implications for social work. *Smith College Studies in Social Work, 64,* 153–167.

Seligman, M., & Peterson, C. (1986). A learned helplessness perspective on childhood depression: Theory and research. In M. Rutter, C. Izard, & P. Read (Eds.), *Depression in young people: Development and clinical Perspectives* (223–249). New York: Guilford.

Slaughter, D.T., & Epps, E.G. (1987). The home environment and academic achievement of Black American children and youth: An overview. *Journal of Negro Education, 56,* 3–20.

Slaughter-Defoe, D., Nakagawa, K., Takanishi, R., & Johnson, D. (1990). Toward cultural/ecological perspectives on schooling and achievement in African-American and Asian-American children. *Child Development, 65(2),* 562–589.

Smokowski, P.R., Reynolds, A.J., & Bezruczko, N. (2000). Resilience and protective factors in adolescence: An autobiographical perspective from disadvantaged youth. *Journal of School Psychology, 47(4),* 425–448.

Spencer, M.B., Cole, S.P., DuPree, D., Glymph, A., & Pierre, P. (1993). Self-efficacy among urban African-American early adolescents: Exploring issues of risk, vulnerability, and resilience. *Development and Psychopathology, 5,* 719–739.

Taylor, R.D. (1994). Risk and resilience: Contextual influences on the development of African-American adolescents. In M.C. Wang & E.W. Gordon (Eds.), *Educational resilience in inner-city America: Challenges and prospects* (pp. 119–130). Hillside, NJ: Erlbaum.

Taylor, R.D., Chatters, L.M., Tucker, M.B., & Lewis, E. (1990). Developments in research on Black families: A decade review. Journal of Marriage and the Family, 52, 993–1014.

U.S. Department of Education & American Educational Research Association (1995). *School-linked comprehensive services for children and families: What we know and what we do now know.* Washington, D.C.: U.S. Department of Education.

U.S. Department of Health and Human Services (2000). *Report of the Surgeon General's conference on children's mental health: A national action agenda.* Rockville, MD: U.S. Department of Health and Human Services Administration, Center for Mental Health Services, National Institute of Health, National Institute of Mental Health.

U.S. Department of Health and Human Services (2001). *Mental health: Culture, race, and ethnicity.* Rockville, MD: U.S. Department of Health and Human Services Administration, Center for Mental Health Services, National Institute of Health, National Institute of Mental Health.

Vondra, J.I. (1999). Commentary for "Schooling and high-risk populations: The Chicago Longitudinal Study". *Journal of School Psychology, 37(4),* 471–479.

Wang, M.C. (Ed.) (1992). *Adaptive education strategies.* Baltimore: Paul H. Brookes.

Wang, M.C. (1996). The community for learning program: A call for a coordinated approach to achieve student success. Philadelphia, PA: Laboratory for Student Success, the Mid-Atlantic Regional Educational Laboratory at Temple University Center for Research in Human Development and Education.

Wang, M.C., Haertel, G.D., & Walberg, H.J. (1994). Educational resilience in inner cities. In M.C. Wang & E.W. Gordon (Eds.)., *Educational resilience in inner-city America: Challenges and prospects* (pp. 45–72). Hillsdale, NJ: Lawrence Erlbaum.

Wang, M.C., Haertel, G.D., & Walberg, H.J. (1997a). Fostering educational resilience in inner-city schools. In H.J. Walberg, O. Reyes, & R.P. Weissberg (Eds.), *Children and youth: Interdisciplinary perspectives* (pp. 119–140). Thousand Oaks, CA: SAGE Publications.

Wang, M.C., Haertel, G.D., & Walberg, H.J. (1997b). Fostering educational resilience in inner-city schools. *Laboratory for Student Success Publication Series, No. 4.* Retrieved November 14, 2003 from www.temple.edu/lss/htmlpublications/ publications/pubs97-4.htm

Wang, M.C., & Oates, J. (1996). Fostering resilience and learning success in schools: The community for learning program. *Spotlight on Student Success, Laboratory for Student Success 104.* Retrieved November 14, 2003 from www.temple.edu/lss/htmlpublications/spotlights/100/spot103.htm

Weist, M.D. (1997). Expanded school mental health services: A national movement in progress. *Advances in Clinical Child Psychology, 19,* 319–351.

Weist, M. D., & Christodulu, K.V. (2000). Expanded school mental health programs: Advancing reform and closing the gap between research and practice. *Journal of School Health, 70,* 195–2000.

Weist, M.D., Paskewitz, D.A., Warner, B.S., & Flaherty, L.T. (1996). Treatment outcomes of school-based mental health services for urban teenagers. *Community Mental Health Journal, Vol., 32(2),* 149–157.

Werner, E. (1995). Resilience in development. *Current Directions in Psychological Science, 4(3),* 81–85.

Werner, E. (2000). Protective factors and individual resilience. In J.P. Shonkoff & S.J. Meisels (Eds.), *Handbook of early childhood intervention* (2nd ed., pp. 115–132). New York: Cambridge University Press.

Werner, E., & Smith, R. (1982). *Vulnerable but invincible: A longitudinal study of resilient children and youth.* New York: Adams, Bannister, & Cox.

Winfield, L.F. (1995). The knowledge base on resilience in African-American adolescents. In L.J. Crockett & A.C. Crouter (Eds.), *Pathways through adolescence* (pp. 87–118). State College, PA: Penn State University Press.

Zimmerman, M.A., Ramirez-Valles, J., & Maton, K.I. (1999). Resilience among urban African American male adolescents: A study of the protective effects of sociopolitical control on their mental health. *American Journal of Community Psychology, 37(6),* 733–751.

Chapter 7

Resilience in the Asian Context

GRACE WONG

An old Chinese folk tale tells of a father who gathered his sons around him as he was dying. Drawing an arrow from its sheath, he snapped it in two, and said to his sons, "If you stand alone, you are vulnerable and easily broken." Taking all the arrows from his sheath, he handed the bundle to his eldest and asked him to break it. His son could not. He asked the next and the next. None of the brothers could break the arrows. Then, he said, "If the arrows band together, it is not easily broken. My sons, if you stand united, you will live strong and protected." (Source unknown)

The story above sets the tone for this chapter that examines the concept of resilience as it relates to Asian Americans, specifically, from countries in Asia that were greatly influenced by Confucianism and include China, Japan, Korea, Vietnam, and other surrounding countries.

IMMIGRATION STRESS AND ITS CHALLENGE TO RESILIENCE

The discussion of resilience in the Asian context includes a focus on immigrant families. Recently, immigration stress and adjustment have become an area of study, especially among clinicians that work in communities where new arrivals settle. Existing research on Asian Americans has examined conditions prior to immigration and current psychopathology (Leong, 1986; Westermeyer, 1987). Other studies focused on immigration adjustment in the United States (Gaw, 1983). The literature, though growing, continues to be limited as further research on Asian immigration adjustment is still needed. At times, observations are anecdotal as systematic research is in its early development.

A commonly acknowledged phenomenon about immigration is the varying rates of acculturation between generations within the family (Cooper, Baker, Polichar, & Welsh, 1993). The youngest generation has the greatest facility to acquire the language, adopt new values, and has greater opportunity to interact with English speaking peers. The middle-age generation has more established values from their homeland and, depending on the level of English skills, may have varying degrees of exposure to American culture. The oldest generation generally retains the most from the original culture and adapts the slowest. Often, the older generation has less education and a higher incidence of illiteracy, especially among women (Yu, 1986). Issues such as ambulation and English proficiency also contribute to limit older adults from interacting with the English-speaking world.

Over time, the culture gap between the generations grows wider to where some grandchildren cannot communicate with their grandparents except in rudimentary Asian language. Conversations are reduced to "Have you eaten?" and "It's cold outside." Deeper discussions are restricted by the limits of the common language. Value differences between the Asian and American cultures, educational differences, and mastery over the environment contribute to a growing discrepancy between the younger and the older. Grandparents and parents are proud of their off springs' accomplishments, but sometimes have little idea what their children do or what their world is like.

The generations sometimes do not see eye-to-eye about values and clash in areas such as degrees of independence, dating, marriage, and methods of raising children. However, Asian parents also modify their views and practices as they themselves acculturate (Uba, 1992). Chinese parents sometimes evoke the imagery of a bending willow to deal with changes. A willow that bends has more resilience than a stiff tree branch which breaks when bent beyond limit.

As the power differential within the family shifts in favor of the younger generations (and sometimes women), the older generation commonly complains that the young are not "obedient," and lack "respect," traits that are highly valued in Confucian society. Behind the stereotype of "Model Minority" ascribed to Asian people, life is far from stress-free. Aside from daily survival requirements, the conscious or unconscious drives to recapture family "legacies" lost while fleeing the war in their homeland or succeed for the sake of parents who have sacrificed so much to make a better future for their children, lead to added pressure to excel. While statistics appear to suggest a rosy picture of Asian Americans as a group that has the highest percentage attending college, a higher rate of depression was consistently found in Asian American college students with the most frequent stresses being test pressures, financial problems, and relationships (Chang, 1996; Okazaki, 1997). Within the family, conflicts and power shifts bring disharmony.

Aldwin and Greenberger (1987)'s study on Korean American college students found that females were more likely to be in the severely depressed category. Factors contributing to depression for these Asian females included conflict with parent's traditional values, unhappy family relationships, and being away from home.

CONFUCIANISM AND ITS ROLE IN THE ASIAN CULTURE

Important major contributors to the way of life for Asian cultures include Buddhism, Taoism, Hinduism, and Confucianism, among others, but, Confucianism by far defines the practical rules of do's and don'ts of daily life. Even though Confucianism eventually became a religion of sorts, the teachings of Confucius were a set of philosophical ideas that successfully brought about some semblance of individual and social order. So significant were his teachings that although he taught 26 centuries ago, they continue to play a significant role in the worldview of many Asian countries through various political and dynastic changes (Hsu, 1976). Within these rules of social behavior, society benefited from the uniformity of expectations between ruler and subject, individuals' interpersonal duties toward others and to oneself, and between parents and children. Any discussion on resilience in Asian countries such as China, Japan, Korea, Vietnam, and other surrounding countries must take place in the context of Confucianism as his philosophy permeates through the cultures of these countries.

Basic Confucian Ideas

Confucius, known as Kung tzu in Chinese, was a scholar and a magistrate. He lived around 551–479 BC when feudalism degenerated in China and "intrigue," vice, and chaos were rampant (Lin, 1966). Confucius believed the only remedy was to convert people to the principles and precepts of the sages of antiquity. Therefore, he taught the importance of moral principles as a way toward prosperity and happiness. His students later promulgated his teachings to the masses. So powerful was the presence of Confucianism that when Communism tried to eradicate some of the "reactionary attitudes" of the past in China, Confucianism was targeted because of its significant hold on the *Weltanshauung*—the world-view of the people.

The significance of Confucius' teachings over the centuries is that they provide the individual and society with the kind of stability that contributes to resilience. However, he was a man of his times and can be currently criticized for being authoritarian, sexist, and somewhat rigid. Shortcomings aside, his teachings provided the kind of backbone needed in times of social chaos and dynastic changes.

Confucius taught that the moral person conducts himself in ways that would be beneficial to others by identifying characteristics that would be important to instill in one's own character. As one becomes a self-disciplined person who is able to benefit others, the whole of society benefits. Order occurs in society as well as families when individuals exercise their self-discipline and benevolence towards others. Self-discipline includes exercising self-control over one's words, actions, and moods when interacting with others. In a society where families live in close quarters, this teaching takes on a practical aspect. When there is order, everyone benefits. In Confucius' teachings, the moral human being must have "*ren*" which can also be translated as kindness, love, goodness, humanity, and human-heartedness. He believed that having a concern for others is something that can be fostered and allowed to bloom, regardless of class and family background. To a certain extent, he believed in the malleability of human beings. A child can be shaped at a young age to become a moral being.

The "ren" above differs from the other character "ren" (different tone), which encompasses the meaning of holding in, tolerating, enduring, and delaying gratification. The second character of ren is about learning to build endurance through difficult times and tolerating pain and suffering. A truly learned person develops this ability to exercise self-control. Secondly, "*decorum*" or self-regulation is a result of practicing "*ren.*" One uses ones self as a standard to regulate conduct and interactions with others. The two self-regulating principles are further divided into *altruism* and *conscientiousness*. *Altruism* is "Do unto others..." *Conscientiousness* is "Do not do unto others." The latter is a check on ones destructive impulses, which are believed to come from unrestricted expression. To some degree, this is in contrast to the encouragement in our western society toward individualism and self-expression.

Ren is manifested in *Chung* (faithfulness/loyalty) to self and others. Sometimes *Chung* is also translated as loyalty. When an individual is described as being *Chung*, it usually suggests that the person has integrity and can be counted upon during unfavorable times. While *Chung* is an internal quality, it is not self-focused. What it asks from the self is sacrifice for the sake of others. *Righteousness* or *oughtness* is the formal essence of the duties of men and women in society, which lies in the doing itself, not in any external result. Righteousness is the value that impels a person to comply with the *oughtness* of a situation. Therefore, the execution of one's obligation is defined as justice; the compliance to one's role is deemed fairness. When one intends to behave against justice, or acts against what one should do, the consequential experience is guilt. When one does not perform as he or she should, or violates fairness, he or she experiences shame. Whereas *altruism* and *conscientiousness* provide the directions for *righteousness*, guilt and shame inhibit behavior that strays from *oughtness* (Huang and Charter, 1996).

Wisdom is what every human being should strive for. Confucius himself loved education and often became so engrossed in his studies that he forgot to eat and sleep. He believed that if you apply all the ancient principles, one would acquire wisdom. Hence, education is highly valued to acquire wisdom. Confucius believed that education was for both the rich and poor. This was not applied equally to men and women, but over the centuries some political climates were more supportive of women and education (e.g., in the Tang dynasty). Over the centuries, education was the only means out of poverty in China. A formal three tier examination system was in place that allowed even the very poor the potential to become scholar-magistrates. The higher the tier, the closer one could access the inner core of government. This valuing of education can be seen in other Asian countries that were influenced by China, which for centuries, was the primary influence in Asia other than India (Miyazaki & Schirokauer, 1976).

In the Confucian society, a hierarchy is necessary. The Emperor is to rule over the people with benevolence. In turn, his subjects would be loyal to him. In the family, the head of the clan (usually the oldest male) has responsibility to the whole clan. Family members would act in ways that would not cause the family to lose face. Among members of the family, the older watches over the younger. The younger defer to the older. Men are given priority over women, but have responsibility to provide for them. Children are to learn deference to adults as they have lived longer and have acquired more life experience. Even in simple rituals such as passing out food at a table, the elderly are first served. The youngest is to say the appropriate words ("Li" or ritual) to honor them and request that they begin first. A primary reason for honoring the elders is the assumption that with greater life experience comes wisdom.

Within the family, the parents take care of the children when they are young. The children repay in kind when their parents become old. Honoring ones parents and grandparents (*filial piety*) extends beyond this life. Ancestors who have gone to the other world watch over the living, but the living must remember to prepare offerings at the family altar so that the ancestors would not be deprived and neglected. Children learn at a young age that they have a familial duty to their ancestors, parents, and their younger siblings. They also learn that their parents will take care of them and sacrifice their own wants and desires for the children's sake. Family responsibility is a deeply engrained teaching that family members carry within their psyche. Hence, despite unhappy marriages, many Asian men work long hours to pay for the family expenses even if they remove themselves emotionally from the family. Despite the hollowness of such a marriage, couples remain together for the sake of the children who are thought to benefit from a stable (albeit emotionally barren) family life. For some, marriage is not seen as a relationship of love and passion but a practical necessity and commitment.

Interestingly, the codes of behavior taught by Confucius also promote some of the necessary skills that contribute to resilience. Self and cognitive regulation, self-discipline and interpersonal harmony are basic skills of life that are foundational to orderly existence and acceptance by others. They contribute to academic and work success which are highly valued in society both east and west. Johnson's well-known study (1977) on Japanese-Americans in Hawaii examined the "obligatory" system that helped maintained family solidarity. She examined interdependence, reciprocity, and indebtedness and the fact that these qualities were still intact three generations after arriving in Hawaii. Johnson described Confucian values for families, but failed to emphasize that these values, Confucian or not, are passed on through generations because they have such an emotional life within them. Interdependence is about day to day ways of relating to each other. Reciprocity and indebtedness are also strongly emotional experiences. It is not surprising that these values remain intact over three generations because grandparent-parent-child relationships are passed on through emotional bonds.

Positive views of self and effectiveness over the environment, the other necessarily skills identified as present in resilient children (Masten, 2001), appear to find expression differently within the rules and demands of Asian cultures. Since Confucian teaching emphasizes humility and self-discipline, positive views of self and effectiveness would be identified primarily by confidence in that individual's action rather than verbal report, as the latter would appear vain and conceited in a Confucian society. An individual who "crows" about his/her achievement commits a social faux pas in Asian society.

CHALLENGES TO RESILIENCE AND THE CONFUCIAN MODEL

Historically, Confucianism provided organization to society and defined roles and rules of power within the family. Resilience is found in the strength of family members banding together and helping each other. "Family" is identified as the extended family rather than the nuclear family. Family members are responsible for each other and try to help each other, thereby insuring the survival of the clan.

The foremost virtue is filial piety and the responsibility of the family generations for each other (even beyond the grave). The concept of filial piety is really about sacrifice. Everyone in the family is called to sacrifice at one time or another. Parents care for young children and adult children care for aging parents. In some families, older siblings sacrifice their own education to work so that a younger or a brighter sibling may study. Ideally, the siblings who succeed may return the favor. Many immigrants "sacrifice" themselves for the sake of their children's (and thereby, family's) future by coming to the United States, giving up their own profession in the homeland. In turn, their children are expected to study hard, become successful, and care for the parents as they become old.

Many Asian parents try to bring up children by offering what they personally valued and are familiar with. These include the Confucian values of respect, obedience (which contributes to self-discipline and filial piety), and valuing of education. Research has found that Asian-American parents place a greater emphasis on parental control (Lin & Fu, 1990), since children are believed to be malleable.

Further, parental control is exercised because of the emphasis on "family teaching," (jia jao) the responsibility of the family to mold children into moral and disciplined adults. The role of Asian parents is to raise children who have self-discipline rather than children who are assertive and seek mastery over the environment. Generally, Asian parents also expect to have a greater say (compared to White parents) about teenagers' decision-making (Dornbusch, Ritter, Mont-Reynaud, & Chen, 1990.) For instance, O'Reilly, Tokuno, and Ebata (1986) found that Japanese American parents rank "behaves well" high on what was considered as social competence whereas White parents ranked "self-directed." If children do not behave well, their behavior is a reflection on the family. Poor behavior causes the family to "lose face" and bring shame upon the family. The flip side of this is family pride. Children are expected to present their family well and display an identity that is rooted in their family and the generations that came before it. This training of Asian children to "behave well" has traditionally eased the acceptance of children socially into classrooms and social settings, but occasionally draws the criticism that Asian children are quiet and not assertive enough.

As Asian children learn the need to become more assertive in American society to fit in, get one's needs met, and get ahead, the children adapt to this trait in order to navigate at school. At home, however, assertiveness may be experienced as disrespect and pushiness, leading to the criticism and lament by the older generation that children lose their sense of respect, propriety, politeness (li mao) and family teaching (jia jao) in America. As children encounter the reality outside of the house that things need to be handled differently than as their parents may suggest, children may also speak out directly to their parents in disagreement, (as other American children do) further confirming to parents that the children are "rebellious" against the old ways.

Some immigrant children experience a loss of efficacious adults. Children of immigrant parents who do not speak sufficient English feel as if their parents cannot protect them in the world outside of home. In fact, children find themselves believing they must protect their parents who they now see as powerless within the outside world. In addition to not being able to rely on their parents in the outside world, children also become "parentified" at an early age. A poignant example is a 6-year-old Chinese girl whose uncle had began to present serious mental health problems. Her parents brought her, her grandparents, and her uncle to the mental health clinic appointment. When the psychiatrist sent the family down to the hospital pharmacy to fill a prescription, the adults found themselves unable to understand the announced numbers in English to signal that the medication was ready. The whole family of adults turned to the 6-year-old and asked her to listen for the number as she alone was the who could understand. Many other immigrant children (not only Asian) have reported similar situations of helping parents prepare taxes, fill applications to buy homes, and answer phones. This dependence on children inevitably shifts the power structure of the traditional

Confucian family. Parents feel less power and control over their own lives, let alone their children's. The children may feel less inclined to listen to parents as traditionally expected. For children, response to additional responsibility is varied. Some children express resentment about having to take over adult roles while others take on the role without complaint.

The middle generation loses their status in multiple ways. Aside from loss of power within the family structure, many heads of households come to the United States expecting a "land of opportunity" only to find a downward mobility. Many have to take jobs at a lower employment level due to differences in credentials, language, or having to enter a competitive workforce later in life. Conversations with waiters at different Asian restaurants inevitably uncover that many of them previously worked in a different profession in Asia such as teaching, accounting, law, or business. Many are surprisingly stoic about the loss of status as this is a choice made for a better future. Nevertheless, from day to day, the frustration of lower personal prestige can wear on self-esteem. The middle generation also loses the possibility of their children caring for them as their children might have in Asia. In the Confucian cycle, parents take care of children with the expectation that children would naturally do in kind. In America, their children are no longer locked into this responsibility. As nursing home care and independent living have become options for the geriatric population, children may select those options, especially when their careers become demanding or if their spouse is not in agreement for parents to move in. While choosing a nursing home may not be poorer care, the parents may feel abandoned; for the child, questions about whether one is sufficiently handling filial responsibilities is frequently asked.

Sometimes, unhappiness is expressed inside the family, avoiding dirty laundry to be aired outward. Domestic violence in the Asian community needs to be understood in the context of immigration stress and in the context of a collectivistic culture. Triandis (1995) defines collectivistic cultures (as opposed to individualistic cultures) as cultures where the detachment from family or group of origin is minimal and that personal goals are subordinated to that of the collective. Lum (1998) noted that because of this collectivistic orientation, family unity may be considered a higher priority to sacrifice oneself for. Filial piety may also lead some to take abuse from parents without questioning the appropriateness of such behavior.

In the world outside of home, children deal with physical self-esteem issues. In her study of ethnic minority children, Phinney (1989) suggested that physical self-esteem has an impact on the ethnic identity development. Grove (1991) found that Asian American students identified that skin color was a salient characteristic of attractiveness. Given the general cultural tendency to regard certain features (i.e., blond hair, blue eyes, long legs, etc.) as attractive, Asian American children must contend with being outside of the standard of attractiveness. Some Asian children choose to sublimate energy toward academics while others try to move toward the physical ideal. In either direction, one is dealing with the quiet pain of not being the ideal.

Sometimes in situations that mitigate against family loyalty, against great odds, family members remain loyal to each other. For example, children who may have rarely seen their parents during their childhood, as their parents worked long hours in low paying jobs, manage to succeed in school, become professionals, and take care of their parents. This is helped along by the heavy emphasis in Confucian cultures about filial piety and the value of education and belief that education is traditionally a way out of poverty.

As, mentioned earlier, tradition and culture are passed on not only in didactic teaching, but also emotionally. Hence, the adherence to traditional values may not be easily apparent. Sacrifice is an observable behavior and is experienced emotionally. Watching parents come home after a long day, cooking, and asking about homework is an emotional experience even though affection is not frequently verbalized in Asian cultures. In this sense, the Confucian emphasis in the culture to sacrifice for each other and remain loyal contribute significantly to the resilience of the family that, in turn, provides a stable environment for the children in the face of immigration and acculturation stressors. That is, Confucian values help to buffer these stressors and promote resilience in Asian youth and families. Even though depth and mutual understanding through conversation may be lost, loyalty and the memory of the sacrificing behavior of family members for each other appear to provide key ingredients in promoting resilience.

AN EMPHASIS ON EDUCATION

As mentioned earlier, education is valued by Confucius and highly valued as a way a person can be internally transformed to understand morals and propriety. Practically speaking, Confucianism has traditionally been a way out of poverty. Asian parents may tend to push their children in academics whole providing less psychological support (Campbell & Mandel, 1990). As expected, this can lead to conflict between parental wishes and a child's desire. Children who are artistic or do not fit in easily to their parent's idea of what is good and practical for them (such as becoming a doctor or lawyer) face the most disapproval, especially with parents who are rigidly traditional. Asian parent's high emphasis on education, at times, puts unusual pressure on children to succeed. Some teenagers try to fulfill parental wishes and fail, leading to referrals to mental health centers to address depression.

Chin (1998) outlined three factors that clinicians should be aware of when the Asian client is seeking mental health services. They include a more somatic conceptualization of illness, the unfamiliarity to what mental health providers do, and expectation of the therapist to be an authority figure. In addition to the above, the fear of losing face contributes to the reluctance of Asian families to get assistance for family members with serious mental illness. Other factors observed in clinical settings include the attempt to manage the patient at home, lack of knowledge about resources, and concern about expenses. For the less serious psychiatric problems, the collectivistic cultural tendency to "defer to the group" can lead some individuals to neglect their own needs. The Confucian concept "ren" (to endure, tolerate) can lead individuals to attempt to deal with their own sufferings somewhat similarly to the British "stiff upper lip." The positive aspect of this concept is that people try to solve their own problems, the negative being that some suffer needlessly when help is available. In their research, Lin and Fu (1990) found a healthy balance between traditional values (parental control and emphasis on achievement) that were maintained by Chinese parents while encouragement of independence in school and achievement domains were also adapted. These researchers found this combination of values appeared to facilitate a bicultural socialization that encouraged effective functioning in both cultures.

A CLINICAL CASE IN PRIVATE PRACTICE

The following is a clinical vignette of a 21-year-old Korean-American female who attends a prestigious private college. She was referred to a private practice clinician by the university counseling center as she was returning to her hometown after she decided to take a year off from school. Her case vignette illustrates some of the typical problems of resilience encountered by young Asian Americans:

Having been successful in high school, "Tiffany" was accepted by a small women's college. In college, she found herself aimless and lost, missing classes and sleeping in her dormitory room. She missed midterms and missed further classes until her roommate reported her behavior to the freshmen counselor, who, in turn, sought help.

In session, she was articulate, but tearful. Tiffany missed home, but also hated being there. She described her father as rigid and traditionally "Korean" with an explosive temper who worked all day at a grocery store. As the oldest daughter, she was left with all the responsibilities of caring for her two younger siblings who only listened to her occasionally as she was not "mom." Her mother, when not working at the store, was active in church and ignored problems at home. She was fearful of her father's temper but loved him for sacrificing for the family by working long hours at the grocery store he ran with his wife. In her spare time, Tiffany was expected to help out at the grocery store. She couldn't understand why she was so depressed and aimless even though she felt that way since junior high school. It never occurred to her to talk to someone as no adults were around. She was in danger of failing all her courses and getting kicked out of the school. In response to that possibility, she went out and spent $700 dollars on her credit card. Now, she doesn't know how to face her father.

Family sacrifice engenders much loyalty, but also brings out feelings of ambivalence. Parental absence, value difference, imagined expectations, insufficient fostering of the child's own goal-direction, and potential object relations issues can lead to feelings of loss, lack of direction, and ambivalence about completing goals that the individual feels no ownership of. In the case of the student above, potential domestic abuse issues are also present, adding to her sense of insecurity when she is home as much as she longs for home. Her parents were able to come through for her financially, but whether they were able to connect with her emotionally remained uncertain. In this case, the clinician played a vital role in providing support and encouragement as Tiffany worked through multiple issues. Tiffany wanted to be loyal to her family, a reflection of the Confucian value instilled in her. She felt disloyal when she became angry with her family as they have sacrificed for her. She could not bring herself to articulate how empty her relationship to her parents is, but with permission, she was able to do so once therapy helped her realize that caring about herself was not being disloyal to the family. Rather, feeling anger was a sign that she cared about herself (which is permissible in the "western" side of her) and for things to be better in the family.

With time, Tiffany was also able to see how angry she was with her parents for "abandoning" her at home alone during childhood to care for her younger sisters. To encourage greater ownership over her college experience during therapy, she looked into her choice of majors and decided that she did not like her current decision. She identified a different major, asked her parents permission to find a job outside the grocery store, and moved out. Her choice to live with a roommate from church also made it easier for them to put their minds at ease. Tiffany's parents met her halfway. She was surprised that her parents understood she felt lost in school and felt encouraged to take steps toward a major of her choice. She feared losing her parents should she act contrary to their wishes, but was pleasantly surprised they were not as inflexible as she assumed.

SUMMARY AND CONCLUSION

For Asian youth and families, immigration adjustment is a lifelong process. Adaptability and flexibility are important characteristics to have in adjustment, but how one's old and new cultures form an integrated future culture is up to the individual. Successful adaptation is helped along by family stability, self-discipline, social skills, and the ability of family members to extend to each other. Outside intervention such as therapy, psychoeducation, and emotional support by professionals (i.e., teachers, therapists, coaches, clergy) is helpful in offering bridges for those times when resilience is severely tried. In the discussion on resilience and children, Asian communities look to the family system and values from the past to take the individual into the future. Confucianism plays a great role in the family, how the family structure is organized, the responsibility between family members, and what is regarded as valuable. Confucianism is often invisibly imbedded and unrecognized by those who practice its principles, and yet these principles may contribute to resilience for Asian youth and adults. These same principles can create tensions, and need to be understood in when psychosocial interventions for Asian people are developed. For instance, within the Asian context, discussion about children is inevitable about family.

Once in America, immigration may be a source of stress, but the new culture has offerings that can help immigrants deal with the future. While old and new cultures clash, they can also strengthen and diversify the individual so that one is no longer limited to solutions from one culture. Challenges to the resilience of Asian children and adolescents include losing parents to long work hours, contending with home and outside values, dealing with challenges to self-esteem and ethnic identity, concerns about disappointing parents, and trying to make sense of and integrate one's dual cultures. The last does not appear stressful on the surface, but cultural integration is akin to running the marathon. The process is long and testing of ones endurance.

Much of the material in this chapter is of an anecdotal nature. This is necessary because the psychological research literature and, particularly, the literature on resilience and Asian youth are limited. Hopefully, this chapter begins to capture a glimpse of how much Confucianism is a part of the psyche of those who come from cultures where his teachings have become so deeply embedded. The author hopes that the chapter points to important research directions such as developing methods to quantify the operation of Confucian values in the lives of Asian people and to investigate how these values promote resilience and lead to tensions. Such research will allow for greater understanding of the presence of such a powerful force as Confucianism, inform the development of mental health promotion and intervention strategies for Asian people in the United States, and add to the growing literature on resilience in children.

REFERENCES

Aldwin, C. & Greenberger, E. (1987). Cultural differences in the predictors of depression. *American Journal of Community Psychology, 15*, 789–813.

Campbell, J., & Mandel, F. (1990). Connecting math achievement to parental Influences: Annual meeting of the association for Research in Science Teaching. *Contemporary Educational Psychology, 15*(1), 64–74.

Chang, E.C. (1996). Cultural differences in optimism, pessimism, and coping: Predictors of subsequent adjustment in Asian American and Caucasian American college students. *Journal of Counseling Psychology, 43*, 113–123.

Chin, J.L. (1998). Mental health services and treatment. In L.C. Lee & N.W.S. Zane (Eds.), *Handbook of Asian American Psychology* (pp. 485–504). Sage Publications, Thousand Oaks, California.

Cooper, C.R., Baker, H., Polichar, D., & Welsh, M. (1993). Values and Communication of Chinese, Filipino, European, Mexican, and Vietnamese American adolescents with their families and friends. *New Directions for Child Development, 62,* 73–89.

Dornbusch, S.M., Ritter, P.L., Mont-Reynaud, R., & Chen, Z.Y. (1990). Family Decision making and academic performance in a diverse high school Population. *Journal of Adolescent Research, 5,* 143–160.

Gaw, A. (1982). Chinese Americans. In A. Gaw (Ed.), *Cross-Cultural Psychiatry* (pp. 1–29). John Wright: Littleton, MA.

Grove, K.J. (1991). Identity development in interracial, Asian/White late adolescents: Must it be so problematic? *Journal of Youth and Adolescence, 20,* 617–628.

Hsu, I.C.Y. (1976). *The Rise of Modern China.* Oxford University Press.

Huang, D.D., & Charter, R.A. (1996). The origin and formulation of Chinese character: An introduction to Confucianism and its influence on Chinese behavior patterns. *Cultural diversity and mental health, 2*(1), 35–42.

Johnson, C.L. (1977). Interdependence, reciprocity and indebtedness: An analysis of Japanese American kinship relationships. *Journal of Marriage and the Family, 39,* 351–363.

Leong, F.T.L. (1986). Counseling and psychotherapy with Asian-American: Review of the Literature. *Journal of Counseling Psychology, 33,* 196–206.

Lin, C.Y.C. & Fu, V.R. (1990). A comparison of child-rearing practices among immigrant Chinese, and Caucasian-American parents. *Child Development, 61,* 429–433.

Lin, Y.T. (1966). *The Wisdom of Confucius.* The Modern Library. New York.

Lum, J.L. (1998). Family violence. In L.C. Lee & N.W.S. Zane (eds.) *Handbook of Asian American psychology.* (pp. 505–526) Sage Publishers: Thousand Oaks, California.

Masten, A.S. (2001). Ordinary Magic: resilience processes in development, American Psychologist, 56, 227–238.

Miyazaki, I., & Schirokauer, C. (translator) (1981). *China's Examination Hell: The Civil Service Exams of Imperial China.* Yale University Press, New Haven.

Okazaki, S. (1997). Sources of ethnic differences between Asian American and White American college students on measures of depression and social anxiety. *Journal of Abnormal Psychology, 106*(1), 52–60.

O'Reilly, J.P., Tokuno, K.A., & Ebata, A.T. (1986). Cultural differences between Americans of Japanese and European ancestry in parental valuing of social competence. *Journal of Comparative Family Studies, 17*(1), 87–97.

Phinney, J.S. (1989). Stages of ethnic identity development in minority group adolescents. *Journal of Early Adolescence, 9* (1/2), 34–49.

Triandis, H.C. (1995). *Individualism and Collectivism.* Boulder, Colorado: Westview Press.

Uba, L. (1992). Cultural barriers to American health care among Southeast Asian refugees. *Public Health Reports, 107,* 544–548.

Westermeyer, J. (1987). Clinical Considerations in cross-cultural diagnosis. *Hospital and community psychiatry, 38*(2), 160–165.

Yu, E.S. (1986). Health of the Chinese Elderly in America. *Research on Aging, 8,* 84–109.

Chapter 8

Risk and Resilience During the Teenage Years for Diverse Youth

EDITH G. ARRINGTON AND MELVIN N. WILSON

Developmental trajectories for youth in today's society occur in a myriad of contexts and range along a continuum (Crockett & Crouter, 1995). At one end of the continuum lie positive behaviors and situations that are indicative of stable adaptive functioning (Compas, Hinden, & Gerhardt, 1995) such as: nurturing parent relationships, academic achievement, involvement in community as well as school activities, and supportive peer relationships. At the other end of the continuum lie behaviors and situations that have the potential to compromise stable adaptive functioning. Compromising behaviors and situations include: strained parent-child relationships, academic underachievement, disengagement from community and school activities and maladaptive peer relationships. A substantial portion of today's youth are involved in various situations or engage in behaviors that have the potential to restrict their ability to lead productive and healthy lives. For example, 25% of people with sexually transmitted diseases are 15–19 year-old, while 25% of youth aged 12–17 use drugs (Lerner, 1995). In 2001, adolescent females between the age of 15 and 19 had the highest rate of gonorrhea than any other age group. Additionally, adolescents are more likely to contract sexually transmitted diseases than any other age group (Centers for Disease Control and Prevention, 2001). In terms of teens' alcohol consumption and drug use, 54% of students have tried an illicit drug and 80% have consumed alcohol during high school (Johnston, O'Malley, Bachman, 2002). The Substance Abuse and Mental Health Services Administration (SAMHSA, 2003) estimates that approximately 9% of youth between the ages of 12 and 17 are addicted to alcohol and drugs. Although the percentage of youth drug or alcohol addiction is lower than youth drug or alcohol ever-use, there are still other negative health consequences for youth substance use. Additionally, other people may also be affected by teens' actions when they have consumed alcohol or experimented with an illicit drug. The statistics on adolescent substance use clearly indicate the tenuous situation in which all youth have to cope with and develop within contemporary society.

The increasing racial and ethnic diversity in the United States has been most pronounced in the population of children and youth. The 2000 Census indicates that one-third of the youth population comprises of African-, Asian-, Latino-, and Native-American children and youth which is approximately 16 million people (U.S. Census Bureau, 2000). Teenagers encounter people from different races and ethnicities in their schools, neighborhoods, and peer groups (Paul, 2001). Parents, educators, psychologists, and youth-oriented service providers need to understand the role of culture in the lives of diverse youth. Several recent publications have called for an increased understanding and incorporation of diversity and culture in the study of all youth (e.g., American Psychological Association, 2002; McLoyd & Steinberg, 1998). In particular, race and ethnicity has become important in understanding and improving the developmental experiences of all of America's adolescents.

Developmental trajectories that result in unhealthy or maladaptive outcomes for youth do not always arise because of behaviors or situations that youth engage in. For instance, youth of color experience educational and health disparities. As compared to Whites, Blacks and Latinos have lower levels of academic achievement as measured by a variety of indicators and higher dropout rates (Sanders, 2000). There are also striking differences in health indicators for White youth and youth of color during every development period of childhood. According to the Federal Interagency Forum on Child and Family Statistics (2003), Black infants have higher infant mortality rates (13.6 infant deaths/1000 live births) than do White infants (5.7 deaths/1000 births). In addition, the proportion of Black and Latino youth who are overweight is higher than the proportion of White children who are overweight. Ninety-four percent of youth with type-2 diabetes are youth from racial and ethnic minority communities (Callahan & Mansfield, 2000). Additionally, a higher percentage of Black children and adolescents are likely to be afflicted with asthma than are White youth (Lee, 2000). Clearly, racial and ethnic community membership is of considerable importance, particularly when we are focusing on health and physical well-being in both the context and outcome of developmental pathways for today's teens.

In fact, Dryfoos (1990) calls attention to the fact that because of socioeconomic and cultural differences; youth are having experiences that directly effect their development. For instance, while 25% of all youth live in single-parent homes, 50% of African-American youth do not have both parents in their homes. Also, while 11% of White youth were poor, 44% of African-American, 17% of Asian-American, 38% of Latino-American, and 25% of Native-American children were poor (Lerner, 1995). Hence, socioeconomic status (SES) and culture appear to be of considerable importance in both the outcome and context of developmental trajectories for today's youth.

Even when considering many of the negative circumstances in which youth develop, (e.g., poverty), youth *do* exhibit competency in a wide variety of behavioral and mental health outcomes. This exhibition of competence in spite of adversity has been conceptualized as resiliency by a number of researchers (e.g., Masten, 1994; Taylor, 1994). There are different perspectives on the definition and validity of resilience (Franklin, 2000; Tolan, 1996). Not surprisingly, researchers are asserting that socioeconomic status and culture play critical roles in the expression of resiliency for youth (Cicchetti & Rogosch, 2002; Nettles & Pleck, 1994). We examine the concepts of risk and resilience in a manner that incorporates culture and diversity. We consider the context of youths' developmental trajectories and the adaptive or maladaptive outcomes of the trajectories. Our intent is to broaden the perspective of those who seek to understand how risk and resilience are displayed within the youth population.

DEFINITION AND ASSESSMENT OF RISK

All youth encounter stressful events during their development. Stressful events pose a threat to the development of competent behavioral and mental health outcomes. Examples of stressful events that are considered to be normative during adolescence include: a need to feel independent from one's family, an increase in intimate relationships with peers, and school-related pressures (Hauser & Bowlds, 1990). A normative stressor for African-, Asian-, Latino-, and Native-American youth is the experience of prejudice, racism and discrimination (Hauser & Bowlds, 1990; Spencer, 1995). Munsch and Wampler (1993) found that African-American and Mexican-American youth experience more stressors than did their European-American counterparts. However, Munsch and Wampler did not assess for stressful events that may be related to prejudice, discrimination and racism and may underestimate how much stress youth of African-, Asian-, Latino-, and Native-American descent are experiencing.

It is important to distinguish between risk and vulnerability when discussing stress. Risk is a more appropriate term for groups whereas, vulnerability is a term best suited for individuals (Gordon & Song, 1994; Masten, 1994). Risk has been conceptualized in broad terms (Gore & Eckenrode, 1994). For example, low SES is often used as a broad indicator of risk because of the simplicity of ascertaining whether someone is of low SES (Luthar, Doernberger, & Zigler, 1991). However the broad indicator of stress has the disadvantage of not specifying the rationale of an at-risk status. That is, we know that a low SES reflects a risk for a number of social issues, but we do not know the process by which SES places a person at-risk. Risk has also been determined by assessing the impact of a variety of life events (Gore & Eckenrode, 1994). It is thought that youths' likelihood of manifesting maladaptive behavioral and mental health outcomes increases due to the amount of stress they encounter via negative life events. Caution must be used with the enumerating approach for several reasons. First, negative life events may be differentially perceived as stressful according to the individual youth or a specific group (i.e., females or African-Americans). Second, negative life events may be differentially experienced across groups. To illustrate, young women are more likely be confronted with the trauma of date rape as opposed to African-, Asian-, Latino- and Native-American young men who may confront racist behavior in the work place.

Another definition of risk may be ascertained by focusing on a singular critical event (Gore & Eckenrode, 1994). Examples would include surviving or witnessing a violent episode such as a drive-by shooting in the low-income inner-city area or a shooting spree in a suburban school. Yet another definition of risk involves the one-time occurrence of problem behaviors by youth where they may exhibit behaviors or end up in situations that place them at-risk. As Franklin (2000) asserts, "... youth are disproportionately *placed* at risk (p. 6)" based on their demographic characteristics and others' perceptions of their demographic characteristics. Finally, risk is generally defined as a psychosocial adversity or event that would be considered a stressor to most people and that may hinder normal functioning (Masten, 1994). With the variety of ways in which risk can be defined, it is likely that when social and behavioral scientists are discussing the "at-risk" status of youth, they are discussing different constructs of risk (Luthar, Cicchetti, & Becker, 2000; Wang, Haertel & Walberg, 1998).

Resnick and Burt (1996) argue that the multiple definitions of risk result in an imprecise conceptualization of risk being used in research and in service delivery. Often risk is defined in a limited fashion, such as citing a one-time occurrence of problem behaviors. The behaviors can be those that youth are exhibiting presently or that youth previously displayed. If either the events that have occurred prior to youths' display of problem behaviors or the environment in which the behaviors have occurred are assessed, they are often used in a manner that is stigmatizing.

Hixson and Tinzmann (1990) cite two critical concerns with the term "at-risk" as it is used with youth. First, youth deemed "at-risk" often come from groups that differ from the majority White population. Second, deficits exist in the four commonly used definitions of risk: predictive, descriptive, unilateral, and school. The predictive approach assesses youth risk by examining those characteristics of youth that are often considered negative. The predictive approach does not explore the structure or process of risk and may lead to blaming the victim. The descriptive approach assesses risk by examining youth already exhibiting problem behaviors. The limitation to the descriptive approach is that it waits until youth are already having problems. The unilateral approach asserts that all youth are at-risk because of the problems that exist in society. The unilateral approach does not recognize the differential experiences of youth, particularly those youth that have been exposed to the most negative of society's problems. Finally, a school approach to assessing risk examines factors that exist in the school (e.g., tracking and teacher and administrator beliefs) and assigns risk based on the presence of those factors. The school approach does not address the role of students or parents in risk.

Some authors suggest an ecological perspective on risk (Hixson & Tinzmann, 1990; Resnick & Burt, 1996). Resnick and Burt (1996) assert that youth risk is increased when their environments make them vulnerable. Environments can make youth vulnerable when social resources are lacking, stress is high and institutions are not supportive. Specifically, Resnick and Burt suggest that risk is the presence of negative antecedent conditions (risk antecedents), which create vulnerabilities combined with the presence of specific early negative behavior or experiences (risk markers) that are likely to lead to problem behavior that will have more serious long-term health consequences (risk outcomes). Hixson and Tinzmann's (1990) ecological definition of risk uses a multidimensional approach that assesses the school, the student or family characteristics, the community context and the interrelation between the school, student and family, and community. They consider youth to be at-risk if one of the areas is not functioning optimally and is not offset by the other areas.

Although ecological definitions of risk are more inclusive than the other definitions reviewed, they are limited as well. First, Cowan, Cowan and Schulz (1996) point out that most definitions of risk are conceptualized in a static manner. They assert that risk and the outcomes that may arise from risk should be viewed in "processual" terms. Second, the definitions do not address the diversity that arises due to cultural context. In the Hixson and Tinzmann's (1990) definition of risk, for instance, cultural differences that may exist within and between assessable areas are not addressed. Similarly, the Resnick and Burt (1996) definition does not include any reference to how risk antecedents, risk markers or risk outcomes may be differentially experienced by diverse youth across contexts and cultures. The limitations of risk definitions influence our ability to accurately assess the risk status of youth. Without accurate knowledge of the risk status of youth, not only are interventions hampered, the discussion and understanding of the process of resilience is also limited.

DEFINITION AND ASSESSMENT OF RESILIENCE

As is the case with the conceptualization of risk, there is no consensus among researchers in regard to a singular definition of resilience. Chapter Two talks about a variety of definitions that exist that include: the lack of developmental impairment, or adaptation, despite exposure to risk (Masten, 1994; Masten & Coatsworth, 1995; Taylor, 1994), maintenance of adjustment despite the effects of negative life events (Cohler, Scott, & Musick, 1995), and achievement beyond expectations given the amount of stress experienced (Bartelt, 1994). More often than not, resilience is viewed simply as adaptation despite risk.

There are some caveats to be aware of when one speaks of resilience in terms of adaptation despite risk. First, resilience does not mean invulnerability. Luthar, Doernberger, and Zigler (1993) show that children who have high social competence despite high stress still have difficulty in some areas. Second, as highlighted in Chapter Three, Bartelt (1994) notes that resilience is often conceptualized in individual terms or as a trait of individuals. He cautions against viewing resilience as a trait and instead asserts that resilience is *relational*. That is, research should be examined in reference to: a subjective experience of stress, an inventory of resources, and what he terms a biography of success and failure. Resilience would then be inferred when a person exceeds the expectations that is warranted by an individual's (or community's) biographical field. Bartelt's perspective is one which heeds the importance of context in development because resilience is inferred only when an individual's or community's biography is taken into account.

Whereas Winfield (1994) agrees with Bartlet's statement that resilience is often conceptualized in reference to characteristics and attributes of an individual, she moves away from a static definition of resilience where the focus is still solely on the individual's display of resilience. She instead views resilience as a *process* that results when an individual reacts to risk factors, or vulnerabilities, that are present in their environment. As a result, resilience is an interactional process consisting of individual characteristics and the environment. The process of resilience can be fostered by correlates, or protective processes. Incorporating the interactions between the individual and their environment creates a more dynamic definition of resilience (Winfield, 1994).

Adding to a dynamic definition of resilience, Benard (1995) asserts that resilience is not only fostered by the individual, environment and protective processes but can itself foster positive attributes in individuals. She states that resilience can enable people to develop social competency, skills in problem-solving, a critical consciousness in relation to oppression, autonomy, and a sense of purpose. As such, resilience involves traits such as self-esteem, self-efficacy, autonomy and optimism. Richmond and Beardslee (1988) emphasize youth relationships with others, such as the family, as an important part of resilience.

The "processual" definitions of resilience attest to the importance of understanding interactions between the individual, their environment and the processes that either make youth vulnerable or foster resilience. Cowan, Cowan and Schulz (1996) suggest that risk processes predispose individuals and populations to specific negative or undesirable outcomes. They stress that children should not be considered to be "at-risk" unless there exists a specific negative outcome to which a risk is linked. Along that vein, Cowan and his colleagues (1996) make a distinction between risk and vulnerability processes. They state: "Vulnerability processes increase the probability of a specific negative or undesirable outcome in the presence of risk ... without the risk, vulnerability has no effect" (p. 10). In other words, risk must be assessed prior to discussing vulnerabilities of youth.

Processes that foster resilience in youth are defined as protective processes. A concise definition of protective processes comes from Cowan et al. (1996). They state that protective processes act to decrease the likelihood of a negative outcome. Benard (1995) elaborates on the Cowan et al. (1996) definition by stating that protective processes are those characteristics of the family, school and community that can change a negative outcome. Werner (1990) asserts that protective factors or processes help reduce negative outcomes by serving a compensating function, operating as a challenge to an individual or serving an immunization function. Winfield (1991) offers self-esteem and self-efficacy as examples of protective processes in the process of resilience.

Although many researchers have not attempted to address culture and context as important concepts in defining and displaying resilience, there has been some discussion of culture and diversity in the area of risk and resilience. Cohler, Scott, and Musick (1995) highlight the role that culture and ethnicity can play in the etiology and manifestation of psychological distress. Culture interacts with psychological development and adversity so that people experience risk differently. Bartlet (1994) suggests that the resources and adversities that are involved in the process of resilience are embedded in social contexts. Keogh and Weisner (1993) state that in order to understand risk and protective factors that the ecological and cultural context in which individuals reside must also be understood. They assert that the assessment of risk and protective processes should not be limited to an individual or family level, but should include levels such as the community, subculture and socioeconomic strata.

Although this chapter has clarified a definition of resilience and illustrated the modest amount of work on the interaction of resilience, culture, and context, the research on resilience is limited by its emphasis on European-Americans. There is a dearth of studies that have examined the concept of resilience in relation to the experiences of people who are of African-, Asian-, Latino- or Native-American descent (Winfield, 1995). A question not fully addressed within research, or theory relates to how to define resilience within the contextual biographies of ethnically diverse youth.

CULTURE AND DIVERSITY INCORPORATED INTO RISK AND RESILIENCE

Culture and diversity are gradually being acknowledged as relevant in the social and behavioral sciences (Basic Behavioral Science Task Force of the National

Advisory Mental Health Council, 1996). Culture reflects contexts of shared world-views, meanings, and adaptive behaviors derived from simultaneous membership and participation in multiple settings and situations (Falicov, 1995). Cultural contexts include race, ethnicity, gender, socioeconomic status, sexual orientation, and religion, among others. Diversity is defined as a variation in race, ethnicity, gender, physical handicap, nationality and culture (Lerner, 1995).

Trickett, Watts, and Birman (1994) address diversity in relation to psychology and assert that psychology must learn to address diversity as a psychological and sociopolitical construct that is relevant for all people regardless of the cultural or ethnic group of which they are a member. According to Trickett and his colleagues, a critical aspect of diversity is that individuals are located within cultural contexts within which opportunities and challenges that must be acknowledged. For example, Asian youth are often viewed using the stereotypical "model minority" lens where all Asian youth are perceived as high academic achievers with few psychological, social, or emotional challenges (Leong & Lau, 2001). However, there is a great deal of diversity within the Asian youth population such that youth from different ethnic groups within the Asian population will have unique experiences within their cultural context (Johnson-Powell, 1997).

Several theories have been posited that incorporate culture and diversity while addressing issues relevant to the study of risk and resilience. For example, The Phenomenological Variant of Ecological Systems Theory (PVEST) and the Integrative Model of Developmental Competencies (IMDC) are two theories that build on the notion that risk and resilience for youth exist within contexts and incorporate culture and diversity. Central to PVEST is "ecocultural character," which is defined as the embedded ecological niche and interactively linked cultural patterns, practices, traditions, values and beliefs that reciprocally influence individual developmental processes and social interactions among members (Spencer, 1995; Spencer, Harpalani, Fegley, Dell'Angelo, & Seaton, 2002). Aspects of culture and diversity such as race, gender, and socioeconomic status are conceived of as risk and protective factors in the PVEST model. A net stress engagement represents a youth engagement of culture in their immediate contexts. The net stress engagement influences, and is influenced by, teens' coping strategies. According to PVEST the outcomes of identity formation processes can be either adaptive or maladaptive. Resilience is conceptualized as the continuing ability of adolescents to achieve productive outcomes through the use of adaptive coping skills despite exposure to the stress. Resilience is continually achieved and negotiated as an ongoing process of adolescence.

As an illustration, Black youth attending private, elite schools find themselves in racially dissonant contexts where twenty percent or less of the student body is comprised of Black students (Gray-Little & Carels, 1997). Additionally, private schools are often economically privileged contexts with histories of exclusiveness based on race, ethnicity, or religion (Datnow & Cooper, 1999). Thus, racial status is conceived as a risk factor for stress for Black students. Any supportive relationships with peers and adults that are developed, served as potential protective factors. The net stress engagement for Black students in independent schools will be enhanced or reduced by the coping skills they develop within their school contexts. Arrington, Hall, and Stevenson (2003) reported that Black students attending exclusive private schools felt a psychological sense of school membership mediated any reported encountering racism-related stress in their schools. Resilience in the face of racism-related stress was expressed when students were able to engage meaningfully within their school communities.

DEVELOPMENTAL COMPETENCIES IN CHILDREN OF COLOR

Another cultural diversity perspective of risk and resilience is the integrative model of developmental competencies (Garcia Coll, Lamberty, Jenkins, McAdoo, Crnic, Wasik, & Vasquez Garcia, 1996). Garcia Coll and her associates (1996) suggest that background variables such as socioeconomic status, culture, ethnicity and race and stratification processes such as racism and discrimination are critical factors in the development of youth. Background variables are posited to be mediated by stratification processes. As a result, contexts in which youth develop are created that are often segregated along residential, economic, social and psychological dimensions. Garcia Coll et al. (1996) assert that it is necessary for the social and behavioral sciences to begin to address these ecological contexts, particularly for youth of color, in the development of theories and in research that is conducted.

The contexts that arise as a result of stratification processes are conceptualized by Garcia Coll et al. (1996) to be either inhibiting or promoting environments. Examples of promoting or inhibiting environments are the neighborhood or the school. The adaptive cultures of communities of color are the results of the ways in which youth and their families respond to the promoting or inhibiting environments that have existed in the past or that currently exist. Adaptive culture, along with family processes and individual child characteristics, have direct and interactional effects on the developmental competencies that youth of color display. Garcia Coll and her associates (1996) define developmental competencies as the functional competencies of a child at any one point in time and the developing skills that children bring to the multiple ecologies in which they exist.

Several concepts from the integrative model of developmental competencies augment the application and relevance of the traditional risk and resilience definitions to culturally diverse youth. For instance, Resnick and Burt (1996) define risk as the presence of negative antecedent conditions (risk antecedents), which create vulnerabilities combined with the presence of specific early negative behavior or experiences (risk markers) that are likely to lead, in time, to problem behavior that will have more serious long-term health consequences (risk outcomes). Although background variables are not considered to be inherently negative, they are thought to be risk antecedents. Background variables represent a potential mediating relationship between negative outcomes for youth and stratification processes. Stratification processes, such as racism and discrimination, are risk markers in that they lead to or create segregated contexts. Segregated contexts have the potential to make environments less promoting and more inhibiting and, as such, can be conceptualized as risk outcomes. The display of developmental competencies by youth of color despite the inhibiting environments that may exist constitutes successful adaptation despite adversity, or resilience.

CONCLUSION

The integrative model for studying developmental competencies in youth of color and the identity-focused cultural ecological perspective serve as model frameworks for those in the social and behavioral sciences that seek to understand how culture and diversity can contribute to a more comprehensive understanding of the processes of risk and resilience in the lives of youth in our society. Future work on risk and resilience with populations of youth of color would be more relevant and complete if theories that incorporate culture and diversity are used as a framework for research. Youth of color, as well as the social and behavioral sciences in general, will benefit from such endeavors.

It is clear that community and clinical interventions that are relevant and germane will take a perspective that considers and incorporates the context in which youth develop. More research is needed that accurately describes and utilizes the developmental contexts of youth of African-, Asian-, Latino-, and Native-American descent. A hallmark of community psychology is its sensitivity to cultural diversity, ecological perspectives, and individual-environment fit. This chapter addresses these points and recommends that the study of risk and resilience, as well as the interventions and research that arise from such study, include a perspective that includes the culture and diversity of youth of African-, Asian-, Latino-, and Native-American descent.

REFERENCES

American Psychological Association. (2002). *Developing adolescents: A reference for professionals.* Washington D.C.: American Psychological Association.
Arrington, E.G., Hall, D.M., & Stevenson, H.C. (2003). The Success of African American Students in Independent Schools Project. *Independent School Magazine, 62(4),* 11–21.

Bartelt, D. (1994). On resilience: Questions of validity. In M.C. Wang & E.W. Gordon (Eds.), *Educational resilience in inner-city America: Challenges and Prospects* (pp. 97–108). Hillsdale, NJ: Lawrence Erlbaum Associates.

Basic Behavioral Science Task Force of the National Advisory Mental Health Council. (1996). Basic Behavioral Science Research for mental health: Sociocultural and environmental processes. *American Psychologist, 51*, 722–731.

Benard, B. (1995). Fostering resilience in children, *Eric Digest*, EDO-PS-95-9, University of Illinois: Urbana, IL.

Callahan, S.T., & Mansfield, M.J. (2000). Type 2 diabetes mellitus in adolescents. Current Opinion in Pediatrics. *12*: 310–315.

Centers for Disease Control and Prevention. (2001). STD Surveillance 2001. http://www.cdc.gov/std/stats/TOC2001.htm. Retrieved February 5, 2003.

Cicchetti, D. & Rogosch, F.A. (2002). A developmental psychopathology perspective on adolescence, *Journal of Consulting and Clinical Psychology, 70(1),* 6–20.

Cohler, B.J., Scott, F.M., & Musick, J.S. (1995). Adversity, vulnerability, and resilience: Cultural and developmental perspectives. In D. Cicchetti & D.J. Cohen (Eds.), *Developmental psychopathology, Volume 2: Risk, disorder, and adaptation* (pp. 753–800). NY: John Wiley.

Compas, B.E., Connor-Smith, J.K., Saltzman, H., Thomsen, A.H., & Wadsowrth, M.E. (2001). Coping with stress during childhood and adolescence: Problems, progress, and potential in theory and research. *Psychological Bulletin, 127 (1),* 87–127.

Cowan, P.A., Cowan, C.P., & Schulz, M.S. (1996). Thinking about risk and resilience in families. In E.M Hetherington. & E.A. Blechman (Eds.), *Stress, coping, and resiliency in children and families* (pp. 1–34). Mahwah, NJ: Lawrence Erlbaum Associates.

Crockett, L.J. & Crouter, A.C. (1995). *Pathways through adolescence: Individual development in relation to social contexts.* Mahwah, NJ: Lawrence Erlbaum Associates.

Datnow, A., & Cooper, R. (2000). Creating a climate for diversity? Institutional responses of predominantly white independent schools to African-American students. In M. Sanders (Ed.), *Schooling Students Placed At Risk: Research and Practice in the Education of Poor and Minority Adolescents* (pp. 207–228). Mahwah, NJ: Lawrence Erlbaum.

Dryfoos, J.G. (1990). *Adolescents at risk: Prevalence and prevention.* New York: Oxford University Press.

Falicov, C.J. (1995). Training to think culturally: A multidimensional comparative framework, *Family Process, 34*, 373–387.

Franklin, W. (2000). Students at promise and resilient: A historical look at risk. In M.G. Sanders (Ed.). *Schooling students placed at risk: Research, policy, and practice in the education of poor and minority adolescents* (pp. 3–16). Mahwah, NJ: Lawrence Erlbaum Associates, Publishers.

Garcia Coll, C., Lamberty, G., Jenkins, R., McAdoo, H.P., Crnic, K., Wasik, B.H., & Vasquez Garcia, H. (1996). An integrative model for the study of developmental competencies in minority children, *Child Development, 67*, 1891–1914.

Gordon, E.W., & Song, L.D. (1994). Variations in the experience of resilience. In M.C. Wang & E.W. Gordon (Eds.), *Educational resilience in inner-city America: Challenges and prospects* (pp. 27–43). Hillsdale, NJ: Lawrence Erlbaum Associates.

Gore, S., & Eckenrode, J. (1994). Context and process in research on risk and resilience. In R. Haggerty, L. Sherrod, N. Garmezy, & M. Rutter (Eds.), *Stress, risk, and resilience in children and adolescents* (pp. 19–63). NY: Cambridge University Press.

Hixson, J., & Tinzmann, M.B. (1990). Who are the "at-risk" students of the 1990s?, *NCREL Monograph*: Oak Brook.

Johnston, L.D., O'Malley, P.M., & Bachman, J.G. (2002). *Monitoring the Future national results on adolescent drug use: Overview of key findings, 2001.* (NIH Publication No. 02-5105). Bethesda, MD: National Institute on Drug Abuse.

Keogh, B.K. & Weisner, T. (1993). An ecocultural perspective on risk and protective factors in children's development: Implications for learning disabilities, *Learning Disabilities Research and Practice, 8*, 3–10.

Lee, K. (2000). Asthma: HHS, Federal agencies focus on awareness. *Closing the Gap: A newsletter of the Office of Minority Health, Department of Health and Human Services, November/December 2000*, 11.

Leong, F.T.L., & Lau, A.S.L. (2001). Barriers to providing effective mental health services to Asian Americans. *Mental health services research, 3(4)*, 201–214.

Lerner, R.M. (1995). *Early adolescence: Perspectives on research, policy and intervention*. Hillsdale, NJ: Lawrence Erlbaum Associates.

Luthar, S.S, Cicchetti, D., & Becker, B. (2000). The construct of resilience: A critical evaluation and guidelines for future work. *Child Development, 71(3)*, 543–562.

Luthar, S.S., Doernberger, C.H., & Zigler, E. (1993). Resilience is not a unidimensional construct: Insights from a prospective study of inner-city adolescents, *Development and Psychopathology, 5*, 703–717.

Masten, A.S. (1994). Resilience in individual development: Successful adaptation despite risk and adversity. In M. Wang & E. Gordon (Eds.), *Risk and resilience in inner city America: Challenges and prospects* (pp. 3–25). Hillsdale, NJ: Erlbaum.

Masten, A.S., & Coatsworth, J.D. (1995). Competence, resilience, and psychopathology. In D. Cicchetti & D.J. Cohen (Eds.), *Developmental psychopathology- Volume 2: Risk, disorder, and adaptation* (pp. 715–752). NY: John Wiley.

McLoyd, V.C. & Steinberg, L. (1998). *Studying minority adolescents: Conceptual, methodological, and theoretical issues*. Mahwah, NJ: Lawrence Erlbaum Associates, Publishers.

Munsch, J., & Wampler, R. (1993). Ethnic differences in early adolescents = coping with stress, *American Journal of Orthopsychiatry, 63*, 633–646.

Nettles, S.M., & Pleck, J.H. (1994). Risk, resilience and development: The multiple ecologies of Black adolescents in the United States. In R. Haggerty, L. Sherrod, N. Garmezy, & M. Rutter (Eds.), *Stress, risk, and resilience in children and adolescents* (pp. 147–181). NY: Cambridge University Press.

Paul, P. (2001). Getting inside Gen Y. *American Demographics, 23(9)*, 42–29.

Resnick, G., & Burt, M.K. (1996). Youth at risk: Definitions and Implications for service delivery, *American Journal of Orthopsychiatry, 66*, 172–188.

Richmond, J.G., & Beardslee, W.R. (1988). Resiliency: Research and practical implications for pediatricians *Developmental and Behavioral Pediatrics, 9*, 157–163.

Sanders, M.G. (2000). Preface: Research, policy, and practice in the education of poor and minority adolescents. In M.G. Sanders (Ed.). *Schooling students placed at risk: Research, policy, and practice in the education of poor and minority adolescents* (pp. xv–xxi). Mahwah, NJ: Lawrence Erlbaum Associates, Publishers.

Spencer, M.B., Harpalani, V., Fegley, S., Dell'Angelo, T., & Seaton, G. (2002). Identity, self, and peers in context: A culturally sensitive, developmental framework for analysis. In R. Lerner, F. Jacobs, & D. Werlieb (Eds.) *Handbook of Applied Developmental Science*. (pp. 123–142). Thousand Oaks, CA: Sage Publications, Inc.

Spencer, M.B. (1999). Social and cultural influences on school adjustment: The application of an identity-focused cultural ecological perspective, *Educational Psychologist, 34 (1)*, 43–57.

Spencer, M.B. (1995). Old issues and new theorizing about African-American Youth: A phenomenological variant of ecological systems theory. In R. Taylor (Ed.), *African-American youth: Their social and economic status in the United States* (pp. 37–69). Westport, CT: Praeger Publishers.

Substance Abuse and Mental Health Services Administration. (2003). *Results from the 2002 National Survey on Drug Use and Health: National Findings* (Office of Applied Studies, NHSDA Series H-22, DHHS Publication No. SMA 03-3836). Rockville, MD.

Taylor, R.D. (1994). Risk and resilience: Contextual influences on the development of African-American adolescents. In M.C. Wang & E.W. Gordon (Eds.), *Educational resilience in inner-city America: Challenges and Prospects* (pp. 119–137). Hillsdale, NJ: Lawrence Erlbaum Associates.

Tolan, P.H. (1996). How resilient is the concept of resiliency. *The Community Psychologist, 29 (4),* 12–15.

Trickett, E.J., Watts, R.J., & Birman, D. (1994). *Human diversity: Perspectives on people in context.* San Francisco, CA.: Jossey-Bass.

U.S. Census Bureau. (2000). Census 2000 PHC-T-8. Race and Hispanic or Latino Origin by Age and Sex for the United States: 2000. *Census 2000 Summary File 1.* http:factfinder.census.gov. Retrieved February 5, 2003.

Wang, M.C., Haertel, G.D., & Walberg, H.J. (1998). *Educational Resilience. Publication Series No. 11.* Office of Educational Research and Improvement (ED), Washington, DC.

Winfield, L. (1991). Resilience, schooling, and development in African-American youth: A conceptual framework. *Education and Urban Society, 24,* 5–14.

Winfield, L.F. (1994). Developing resilience in urban youth, *NCREL Monograph.*

Winfield, L.F. (1995). The knowledge base on resilience in African-American adolescents. In L.J. Crockett & A.C. Crouter (Eds.), *Pathways through adolescence: Individual development in relation to social contexts* (pp. 87–118). Mahwah, NJ: Lawrence Erlbaum Associates.

Chapter 9

A Global Perspective on Youth Outreach

HAWTHORNE E. SMITH AND ADEYINKA M. AKINSULURE-SMITH

It is very challenging to be a young person in today's global climate. The harsh reality is that the competition for limited resources whether economic, political, cultural, or territorial have created a world where war and armed conflict can be found in virtually every corner. Children in conflict areas are exposed to many overwhelming experiences, including violence, death, torture, separation from family members, and multiple personal losses (Women's Commission for Refugee Women and Children, 2002).

These experiences may cause extensive physical and psychological trauma (Abdalla & Elklit, 2001; Amowitz, et al., 2002; Berman, 2001; Dyregrov, Gjestad, & Raundalen, 2002; Mollica, Poole, Son, Murray, & Tor, 1997; Lachman, et al., 2002; Smith, 2003; Smith, Perrin, Yule, Hacam, & Stuvland, 2002; Totozani, Kallaba & Sheremeti, 2001; Vizek-Vidović, Kuterovac-Jagodić & Arambašić, 2000). These stressors are in addition to the challenges that youth generally face, even during peaceful times, such as identity formation, socialization, and educational and professional development.

As a result of the conditions created by war and armed conflicts there are almost 20 million refugees and displaced persons worldwide (United Nations High Commissioner for Refugees [UNHCR], 2002). It is estimated that children made up more than half of the people fleeing their homes in search of safety. Not only do refugee children endure war or other forms of persecution in their countries of origin, many continue to suffer human rights abuses in countries of asylum and their rights and special protection needs are frequently ignored (Lachman, et al., 2002; Berman, 2001). Amnesty International reports that "since 1997 children have reportedly been tortured or ill-treated by state officials in more than 50 countries around the world" (Amnesty International, 2000, p. 62). Additionally, more than 300,000 children have been forced to serve as child soldiers in armed conflicts in over 30 countries (Amnesty International 2000, Human Rights Watch, 2002).

Unfortunately, wars and armed conflict create, maintain, and exacerbate many of the circumstances and pretexts for human rights abuses, such as poverty and social chaos, including those that allow the HIV/AIDS pandemic to thrive. The disintegration of social norms, laws, extensive physical and sexual violence all serve to put individuals at greater risk for HIV infection (Women's Commission, 2002). Here again, the youth suffer enormous consequences. At the end of 2002, an estimated 3.2 million children younger than 15 years are living with HIV/AIDS worldwide and 6,000 young people aged 15–24 years become infected with HIV every day (UNAIDS, 2002). It is important to note that these figures do not include children who have lost one or both parents to HIV/AIDS (Lachman, Poblete, Ebigbo, Nyandiya-Bundy, Bundy, Killian & Doek, 2002).

Sadly enough, the assault continues as throughout the world. Children such as Dalit children in India, Haratin children in Mauritania, Palestinian Arab children in Israel, Bidun children in Kuwait, non-citizen children in Greece, children of Haitian descent in the Dominican Republic (and many others—too numerous to list) were denied access to education or segregated in inferior educational programs. These denials limited their potential for growth and thereby limited their futures (Human Rights Watch, 2002; Punamaki, 1989). In essence, young people around the world are faced with many daunting challenges that assault them at every turn, leaving them deprived of physical, emotional, spiritual and cultural needs (Berman, 2001; Women's Commission, 2002). Furthermore, the lack of adult leaders created by such traumatic situations leave vast gaps with children and youth obliged to step in and confront realities, roles and tasks for which they are not always developmentally, emotionally or physically prepared. Youth are often obliged to make complex familial decisions, care for sick or dying parents, become the head of household and act as the main economic provider for other siblings (Lachman, et al., 2002).

Given the numerous crises faced by youth around the world—war, armed conflict, HIV/AIDS, terrorism, limited access to education and health care, sexual violence, poverty and lack of other basic necessities; how does one go about fostering resilience in such a population? Caregivers are encouraged to remember that just as the needs for this challenged population are vast, so are the areas and ways in which communities and individuals can intervene.

Human development has been described as taking place in an ecological context in which a young person is simultaneously involved in several intertwined levels of interaction, including the biological, individual-psychological, social-interpersonal, institutional, cultural, and historical (Brofenbrenner, 1979; Lerner & Galambos, 1998). Just as these multiple interactions pose a complex picture, so too do they afford multiple levels at which one can engage with youth around the daunting challenges they face.

Perhaps the primary area of challenge and opportunity is on the biological/health level, where issues of poverty, endemic diseases, nutrition, sexually transmitted infections (STI's), violence, and basic physical survival are played out. While it has been argued that "effective remedies for these children must include a reaffirmation of their civil and political rights . . . real protection from such abuses requires measures to ensure that children enjoy access to education and health services and protection for their other economic and social rights" (Human Rights Watch, 2002).

The focus on basic survival is not a misguided one considering the public health, security, and economic stressors facing today's youth. "Modern" warfare is now waged in such a way that civilian populations suffer an ever increasing percentage of the casualties. Children make up a large percentage of those casualties. The stressors of warfare are often exacerbated by the stressors of forced migration, living as a refugee, and struggling to integrate into a new society (Akinsulure-Smith & Porterfield, in press; Berman, 2001; Lachman, et al., 2002). Frequently, children are orphaned and struggling to make these adaptations without parental guidance.

The massive struggles for survival for youth are not limited to war-torn areas. Crushing poverty has significantly damaged family and social structures in many areas of the world. Tales of destitute "street children" and violent street gangs can be heard in cities from Jakarta to Johannesburg. "These phenomena are created by a necessity for survival which occurs when the family transfers the institutional role of the house to the street" (Eisenstein, 1993, p. S46). Often, gangs, rebel groups, and other violent organizations that are able to successfully recruit youth into their ranks do so by appealing to basic ideas of self-preservation and one's need for protection.

Children frequently have no choice but to turn to the streets for survival. For example, as AIDS takes a higher toll on the adult populations in sub-Saharan Africa, more and more children are orphaned. In the past, the extended family would have stepped in to care for these orphans. Now, the extended family is usually overburdened financially, and the stigma attached to AIDS may inhibit some family members from caring for the children of their deceased kin (Lachman et al., 2002). Many children, whether infected or just affected by the disease, find themselves on the street.

Street children are often placed in a context in which stealing for survival, engaging in exploitative and illicit sexual activity, and involvement in other criminal endeavors are the sole means for survival, but are also major threats to their health status. Often, these youth are forced to adopt nomadic life styles in order to avoid predatory gangs, vigilantes, or officers of the law, who are determined to exterminate them (Eisenstein, 1993).

Intervening on the biological/health level with meaningful public health initiatives is a complicated but crucial area of inquiry. Over 10 million children die every year from readily preventable diseases and roughly 150 million children are malnourished. Over a million children were sero-positive or had lost at least one parent to AIDS related illnesses in the year 2000 (Lachman et al., 2002). More than 20% of youth remain poor, and rates of substance abuse and delinquency appear to be rising around the world (Lerner & Galambos, 1998).

It is evident that systemic, international, government-based, change must be contemplated in order to provide access to safe environs, proper medical care, adequate food supplies, and educational opportunities for all children (Eisenstein, 1993; Lachman et al., 2002). While such change is complicated by political realities such as corruption, special interests, and differing priorities, there are a number of ways that community and programmatic interventions are making headway.

One of the hallmarks of successful health interventions with youth populations is the development of health education materials that evolve within the youth's cultural levels of comprehension (Eisenstein, 1993). Programs that promote youth autonomy and peer relatedness have also been shown to reduce problematic behaviors among young adolescents (Allen, Kuperminc, Philliber, & Herre, 1994). A study of effective interventions for HIV/AIDS services also found that youth involvement in the creation and dissemination of educational materials was important. Programs in which youth were involved at all levels of design, planning and implementation in an equal, dynamic partnership with adult professionals seemed to be much more effective at outreach and involving youth in the HIV/AIDS services offered (Huba & Melchior, 1998).

Researchers working with street children in Rio De Janeiro and war affected youth in Sierra Leone focused on creative and alternative ways for youth to be involved in public health initiatives, and that the information disseminated should go beyond general health issues and delve into areas of consciousness, personal values, self-esteem, and human rights (Eisenstein, 1993; Women's Commission, 2002). Researchers also stress that finding culturally syntonic ways to communicate accurate information to refute misinformation about sexually transmitted diseases may lead to decreased sexual risk taking behavior (Akinsulure-Smith, 1997).

Beyond youth involvement, the literature on effective health interventions focuses on a tightly integrated approach between different services and levels of contact. Social services, outreach, vocational training, medical services, counseling services, case management, and educational initiatives must be coordinated to be optimally effective (Eisenstein, 1993; Forman & Kalafat, 1998; Huba & Melchior, 1998, Lachman et al., 1998). This is especially important as the risk and protective factors for many of the challenges facing youth (e.g., suicidal behavior and substance abuse) overlap greatly (Forman & Kalafat, 1998). In order to create effective multi-modal, multidisciplinary interventions, on-going communication among and between various governmental, medical, educational, and community agencies must be facilitated and viewed as a priority of paramount importance.

What are the factors that allow youth to access and utilize public health services and otherwise survive in such harsh conditions? The literature speaks frequently of the notion of resilience in youth, and explores the nature of resilience and the factors that can promote positive proactive behavior in youth. Resilience is seen as a quality that stems from both genetic and ecological factors, including physical health (Bell, 2001; Mrazek & Mrazek, 1987). This section explores individual psychological aspects of resilience.

Some of the intra-psychic indicators of resilience described in the literature are: high self-esteem; having a sense of purpose in life; having the ability to attract and use support; precocious maturity; having the conviction of being loved; positive projective anticipation; having curiosity and intellectual mastery; obtaining the conviction of one's right to survive; possessing the ability to remember and invoke images of good and sustaining figures; having the need and ability to help others; and being resourceful; (e.g. Bell, 2001; Lachman et al., 2002; Lerner & Galambos, 1998; Mrazek & Mrazek, 1987). Mrazek & Mrazek (1987) go on to mention that some of the traits that facilitate resilience in the face of acute traumatic stressors may become maladaptive if overused, or used when the stressors no longer exist.

What are effective strategies for promoting resilience at this most basic, individual level? Research shows that war, refugee trauma, being orphaned, engaging in substance abuse, and many of the stressors facing today's youth can cause psychological distress that works to reduce one's resilience (Berman, 2001; Forman & Kalafat, 1998; Mrazek & Mrazek, 1998; Mollica, et al., 1997). Maladaptive responses to the stressors of war and poverty may include: compromised scholastic and cognitive functioning, hypervigilance, suicidal or homicidal behavior, distorted family relationships, complicated bereavement, a general lack of trust, substance abuse, distorted moral development, and revenge fantasies (Berman, 2001; Lachman et al., 2002).

As such, psychological interventions may be warranted. As noted in the psychological literature (e.g., Bell, 2001; Lachman et al., 2002), exploratory individual talk therapy may not be the optimal mode of intervention for traumatized youth. Supportive interventions, including directed play therapy, art therapy, and structured therapeutic activities with peers that help to build community ties, feelings of connectedness, feelings of efficacy, self-worth, and belonging, may be more effective. Through such activities youth may internalize the ability to cognitively and emotionally restructure some of their past experiences such that they transcend feelings of traumatic helplessness, and transform them to "learned helpfulness" (Bell, 2001, p. 376).

In addition to psychological interventions, it is clear that other community resources can be brought to bear to facilitate positive coping and resilience among youth in challenging situations. Within the educational context, guidance and occupational counselors are encouraged to pay close attention to poor academic performance, difficulty interacting with peers, or gross motor problems that may signal that a student is having difficulties (Driver & Beltran, 1998).

There are several other ways to have impact on the individual psychological world of a young person. Community supports such as the extended family, religious groups, mentoring relationships, and other community groups are important means of intervention. The next section of this chapter will look at the social-interpersonal level of engagement. The social-interpersonal level may be the area in which caregivers in the community may find the greatest opportunities to intervene effectively with youth who are struggling to make sense of environments they may perceive as being hostile.

The community begins with the family, and a strong relationship with one's parents is one of the predominant factors in a child developing a resilient personality. When both parents are not available to the child, a strong, single parent or other members of the extended family may fill the parental void in an emotional sense. The notion of an effective and caring extended family is especially powerful in non-Western societies (Lerner & Galambos, 1998; McAdoo, 1993).

Unfortunately, many of today's youth may have lost their parents during war, forced migration, or to the HIV/AIDS epidemic. The literature shows that many youth report losing or being separated from their parents as being more distressing than air raids or bombings (Berman, 2001). Children may have seen their parents humiliated or killed, they may have been forced to care for dying parents, and as their family fabric has been torn, new collateral ties must be forged before the "streets" or other criminal elements fill the void. The importance of familial and community ties in the face of adversity is stressed in the psychological literature (Berman, 2001; Eisenstein, 1993; Lachman et al., 2002).

One potential intervention in this domain is the effective use of mentoring relationships. Mentoring is a relationship-based intervention that is often naturally occurring outside of any formal intervention by a community group (Darling, Hamilton, Toyokawa, & Matsuda, 2002; Rhodes, Grossman, & Roffman, 2002; Zimmerman, Bingenheimer, & Notaro, 2002). So called "natural mentors" may exist within the extended family, or may be adults with whom the child has contact in the school setting or elsewhere in the community. Natural mentors may be found in religious institutions, cultural institutions, sporting clubs, or may be found in the vocational realm, as when youth engage in informal apprenticeships (Rhodes, et al., 2002).

Natural mentors have been shown to be effective at helping to reduce levels of substance abuse and non-violent delinquency in adolescents, increasing youth's levels of self-esteem, and fostering more positive attitudes toward school (Rhodes et al., 2002; Zimmerman et al., 2002). The positive impact of mentoring seems to increase with time, frequency of contact, and the closeness of the relationship (Dubois, Holloway, Valentine, & Cooper, 2002; Grossman & Rhodes, 2002). The availability of caring adults to perform this critical role has unfortunately not kept pace with the need for such interventions. As such, mentoring practices have evolved to meet the new realities. Site based approaches, which are usually based in the schools, seem to draw on older, less educated members of the community who are more likely to be part of the youth's cultural or ethnic group. This helps to expand the pool of mentors, gives the children access to people who have valuable experience in navigating similar social circumstances, and these school-based initiatives tend to be cost effective. One drawback with school based mentoring is that they are often not year-round services, and the youth may go several months without support (Rhodes et al., 2002). Group mentoring has also become more widely used. Although each child may not have as much one on one time with their mentor in a group setting, there are more opportunities to observe the youth interacting with their peers and intervene and provide feedback in "real time" to any problematic or positive behaviors (Rhodes et al., 2002).

Statistical analyses show that mentoring relationships seem to have increased positive impact when they last for 12 months or more (Grossman & Rhodes, 2002). These researchers also found that traumatized youth may have a more difficult time engaging in meaningful relationships, so special support to help ensure that their mentoring relationships survive the first few difficult months, is indicated. Such support may take the form of visits to the home or school, or follow-up phone calls, if the young person misses sessions. Increasing the frequency of activities early in the relationship may also help to ensure that an effective connection takes root.

Successful mentoring initiatives share certain characteristics beyond the duration of the relationship. In a large meta-analytic review of formal mentoring programs in the US, DuBois, Holloway, Valentine, & Cooper et al. (2002) evaluated 55 diverse programs. There were no significant findings in terms of the age, gender, ethnicity, race, or family structure of the youth, which may speak to some generalizability of their findings to programs for use with different populations.

DuBois et al. (2002) found that certain of the "best practices" identified in the mentoring literature were linked to more positive outcomes. Such practices included: utilizing mentors who have a background in a helping profession (e.g.; teachers, coaches, counselors, etc.); providing on-going training and support for mentors beyond an initial orientation or screening process; and having expectations regarding the frequency of mentor-mentee contacts. Clearly communicating that a specific number of contacts are required for the mentoring relationship helps to clarify expectations, and helps to facilitate increased mentor involvement.

Other important factors in successful mentoring relationships were having structured activities for the mentors and youth; having parent/familial involvement in the program; and holding the mentoring sessions outside of the school environment. The programs that engaged in a majority of these practices

demonstrated positive effects of mentoring in five different domains of youth functioning: problem/high risk behavior; social competence; academic/educational;
career/employment; and emotional/psychological. Beyond counseling, mentoring
and other child-adult relationships, youth to youth interventions have shown
increasing promise as effective interventions. Research has shown that peer
emotional support is linked with school competence and social competence
(Lerner & Galambos, 1998).

Youth organizations have multiple opportunities to intervene in many of the
areas identified as fostering resilience in youth. Utilizing some of the aspects of
youth resilience identified by Mrazek & Mrazek (1998), we can explore how youth
programs may intercede as indicated by the following:

- *Rapid responsivity to danger*—Youth groups may serve as reservoirs of
  pertinent information, to keep youth well informed of the dynamic challenges they and their communities face. Youth organizations may also
  serve as a base of action, by which youth may utilize their collective
  energy to make a tangible positive difference.
- *Information seeking*—Again, youth groups may serve not only as a reservoir of information, but young people may be instructed in more effective
  ways of finding, collecting, and utilizing information. Adult mentors and
  advocates may be useful in helping youth groups in this endeavor.
- *Formation and utilization of relationships for survival*—The ability to
  create and sustain relationships, particularly during times of crisis is a
  critical skill for survival. The increased confidence of not being alone in
  the world also fosters resilience. It has been said that "Two watchdogs are
  ten times better than one."
- *Positive projective anticipation*—Youth groups that engage in skill building and training that will help its members not only survive, but potentially
  thrive, in the world offer hope for a better future. It has been shown in the
  psychological and educational literature that youth are likely to put forth
  more effort, and will learn skills better, if they have been demonstrated to
  have significant "real-world" applicability (Smith, 1999). The skills may
  be in the social realm, the academic realm, or in the vocational realm.
- *Decisive risk taking*—Youth groups can help facilitate improved critical
  thinking and problem solving skills. These skills, and the confidence they
  bring, will hopefully encourage youth to make well-founded decisions,
  and then follow-up on these decisions with purposeful action.
- *The conviction of being loved*—Belonging to something larger than one's
  self is of crucial importance, particularly for youth who have had much
  of their familial and community roots disrupted if not entirely destroyed.
  Collateral ties may be especially important for youth coming from non-
  Western societies.

Theorists (e.g. Allen et al., 1994; Bell, 2001; Lachman et al., 2002), focus on the adaptive ways in which bonding, attachment, community interaction, networking, and connection with other peers help to facilitate self-esteem, resilience, community development, and fewer problematic behaviors. Bell (2001) speaks of "rebuilding the village" in an emotional sense, such that a feeling of connectedness can foster increased emotional strength (p. 375). Others conceive of a youth empowerment process by which youth groups provide opportunities to learn skills, assume responsibilities, and participate in social/public affairs. As such, these initiatives provide opportunities to demonstrate success, reinforce notions of achievement, and provide social support (Kim, Crutchfield, Williams, & Hepler, 1998).

Increasingly, theorists are moving away from notions of deficits and inadequacies, and are looking more at the notion of youth empowerment and development that focuses on strengths and assets (Kim et. al., 1998; Rhodes et al., 2002). The next section of this chapter will focus on the tenets of youth empowerment, and give an example of a youth program that is utilizing these ideas effectively in a crisis situation.

Much of the theory behind the youth development and empowerment approach comes from the substance abuse field. As Kim et al. (1998) describe, the struggle against substance abuse in Western countries has gone thorough several phases. At first, prevention efforts in the 1960's were predominantly based on information deficit models. The subsequent interventions had essentially no impact on drug abuse levels. During the seventies and eighties, a movement toward more affective-humanistic approaches that emphasized self-esteem and values were used. The results were mixed in terms of effective prevention strategies.

In essence, three decades of strategy were based on the notion of protecting youth from risks that exist in the environment. Slowly a shift has taken place in which emphasis is being placed on promoting youth development and providing them with positive skills and opportunities, as opposed to simply focusing on a risk-factor paradigm. As such, the field is shifting from the traditional prevention strategy of "problem-free youth" to the new approach of "fully prepared youth" (Kim et al., 1998, p. 5).

As the field shifts, there are several suggestions for creating effective youth programs that help facilitate the notion of empowered youth. Incorporating some sort of *individualized attention* from a caring adult, whether it be mentoring, coaching, training, or counseling is recommended (Lerner & Galambos, 1998). *Community wide, multi-agency collaboration* has already been identified as a necessary for the effective coordination of services (Eisenstein, 1993; Forman & Kalafat, 1998; Huba & Melchior, 1998, Lachman et al., 1998).

Early involvement with the youth is important. The mentoring literature shows that the earlier the relationship begins, the more likely it is to last and have positive effects (Grossman & Rhodes, 2002). *Continued training* for adults working with individual youths or youth groups leads to more positive outcomes (DuBois et al., 2002). *Involvement of peers* in designing and implementing interventions targeted at youth and *parental support and involvement* have also been identified as factors that positively contribute to successful youth outreach programs (DuBois et al., 2002; Eisenstein, 1993; Lachman et al., 2002).

One other factor identified as being important in developing youth interventions is that there should be some tangible connection to the world of work (Lerner & Galambos, 1998). Studies have shown that adolescents will put forth more academic effort and improve their academic performance when they feel that their behavior will result in some tangible life benefit, such as a higher paying job or better career choices (Smith, 1999). Subsequently, youth programs should offer some sort of potential "real world" benefit to help engage youth in the activities.

An example of a youth program that has arisen in a situation of social catastrophe and has successfully implemented many of the "best-practices" of a successful youth program is the Texas Community Center in Sierra Leone. The community got its unique name from the fact that it was formed in a notorious ghetto of Freetown that was known for its "Wild West" level of violence. In this context of violence, that predated Sierra Leone's recent war, the youth responded by starting their own community reclamation group.

Several young members of the community began the Texas group by forming a single football club. Soon, they had formed two leagues with 20 teams for adolescents and younger children from throughout the community. They used an intervention that the youth saw as attractive and fun (and therefore worth their time), and they targeted youth of a young age as well as those adolescents at most risk for delinquent behavior.

As their numbers grew, Texas began providing social services with volunteer labor from its members. They expanded beyond youth and reached out to the entire community. They began providing training and support for young mothers and cleaning up the neighborhood. They began to garner more community support as they demonstrated their value to the community at large. Consequently, more adults and community leaders were inclined to offer time, advice, and support to the Texas program.

As the situation in Sierra Leone deteriorated and descended into war and chaos, and as the country now attempts to rebuild itself, the Texas Community Center has taken on even more challenges. They provide basic education for school age children; training in micro business creation; supportive therapeutic services; social advocacy, training in weaving, plumbing, and tailoring; and engage in conflict resolution. In order to achieve these diverse yet intertwined objectives they have collaborated with international NGO's (non-governmental organizations that provide aid during crises and other developmental assistance) in terms of the cutting edge interventions in the psychosocial realm, but they have tailored their interventions to meet the cultural sensitivities of their community. Youth have been included in all phases of the organization's development, and they feel invested in its continued growth and effectiveness.

Practical issues, such as vocational training, are treated in addition to the psychosocial challenges facing a war-affected population. Real-world considerations like employment and economic concerns are seen as crucial factors in the overall context of social reintegration. Advocacy work is another vehicle by which youth feel involved in the struggle for justice and human rights (Women's Commission, 2002). By utilizing theater, music, story telling and other cultural appropriate vehicles to communicate their pro-social messages, program participants increase their ability to affect change and foster understanding among community members from different generations.

Perhaps some of the most important work done at the Texas Community Center is the provision of a venue where issues of social reconstruction and reconciliation can be addressed. Supportive group meetings in which people can communicate regarding their current challenges they are in the aftermath of the war; where feelings of loss and pain mix with the necessity for the rebuilding a decimated society. Meetings may be attended by former rebels (who waged a brutal guerilla campaign against the general population), former pro-government vigilantes (who fought against the rebels and may have committed human rights abuses themselves), sexually abused women who were forced to serve as sex slaves or "rebel wives" during the conflict, war-wounded people, and people who lost loved ones and/or homes in the conflict. Complicated notions of acceptance, healing, and forgiveness are discussed in an open forum (Akinsulure-Smith, 2002).

Such sensitive and important therapeutic could not occur unless the organization possesses credibility on cultural, social, and interpersonal levels. Many of the tools for gaining such credibility, like encouraging youth to have a proactive impact on the institutional and political barriers they face (Bell, 2001; Punamaki, 1989); utilizing culturally syntonic interventions (Akinsulure-Smith, 1997; Eisenstein, 1993); and fostering a sense of belonging to something larger than one's self (Punamaki, 1996; Smith, 2003); have been used successfully by the Texas Community Center.

The notion of belonging to a family, a community, an organization, or some valued entity larger than one's self is of crucial importance considering the pressures facing today's youth. Creating a proactive sense of social attachment and connection in a child is akin to the proverbial "ounce of prevention" espoused by the youth empowerment literature (Bell, 2001; Rhodes et al., 2002). Whereas responding reactively to "troubled" or "isolated" youth similar to the "pound of cure" associated with the risk-factor paradigm of previous years (Kim et al., 1998).

In conclusion, the challenges facing youth around the world are daunting. Public health issues such as warfare, human rights abuses, refugee trauma, poverty, endemic diseases, STI's, and social dislocation complicate the lives of youth at the basic level of survival. These youth are also challenged at the individual psychosocial level, as well as interpersonal, societal and institutional levels (Eisenstein, 1993; Lachman et al., 2002).

As the challenges facing youth are multifaceted, so too are the ways in which caring members of the community can be involved and intervene. Initiatives that empower youth to proactively engage in activities that help them to foster resilience on multiple levels have been discussed, and ways in which community members can help facilitate and promote these activities have also been detailed.

It is hoped that professional care providers and other concerned members of the global community will commit themselves to helping youth navigate the challenging environments they face by developing and expanding community initiatives and partnerships. Additionally, we would like to emphasize the need to consider reaching out to youth in more creative, culturally syntonic, non-traditional ways in order to promote bio-psycho-social well-being.

REFERENCES

Abdalla, K., & Elklit, A. (2001). A nation-wide screening survey of refugee children from Kosovo. *Torture, 11*(2), 45–49.

Akinsulure-Smith, A. (1997). *The effects of HIV/AIDS knowledge, sexual self-efficacy, and susceptibility on sexual risk-taking behavior in Sierra Leonean students of higher education.* Unpublished doctoral dissertation, Columbia University, New York.

Allen, J.P., Kuperminc, G., Philliber, S., & Herre, K. (1994). Programmatic prevention of adolescent problem behaviors: The role of autonomy, relatedness, and volunteer service in the teen outreach program. *American Journal of Community Psychology, 22*(5), 617–638.

Amowitz, L.L., Reis, C., Lyons, K.H., Vann, B., Mansaray, B., Akinsulure-Smith, A.M., Taylor, L., & Iacopino, V. (2002). Prevalence of war-related sexual violence and other human rights abuses among internally displaced persons in Sierra Leone. *Journal of the American Medical Association, 287*(4), 513–521.

Amnesty International. (2000). *Torture Worldwide: An Affront to Human Dignity.* Amnesty International Publications.

Bell, C.C. (2001). Cultivating resiliency in youth. *Journal of Adolescent Health, 29,* 375–381.

Berman, H. (2001). Children and war: Current understandings and future directions. *Public Health Nursing, 18*(4), 243–252.

Brofenbrenner, U. (1979). *The ecology of human development: Experiments by nature and design.* Cambridge, MA: Harvard University Press.

Darling, N., Hamilton, S., Toyokawa, T., & Matsuda, S. (2002). Naturally occurring mentoring in Japan and the United States: Social roles and correlates. *American Journal of Community Psychology, 30*(2), 245–253.

DuBois, D.L., Holloway, B.E., Valentine, J.C., & Cooper, H. (2002). Effectiveness of mentoring programs for youth: A meta-analytic review. *American Journal of Community Psychology, 30*(2), 157–197.

Driver, C., & Beltran, R.O. (1998). Impact of refugee trauma on children's occupational role as school students. *Australian Occupational Therapy Journal, 45,* 23–38.

Dyregrov, A., Gjestad, R., & Raundalen, M. (2002). Children exposed to warfare: A longitudinal study. *Journal of Traumatic Stress Studies, 15*(1), 59–68.

Eisenstein, E. (1993). Street youth: Social imbalance and health risks. *Journal of Pediatric Child Health, 29*, Suppl. 1, S46–S49.

Foreman, S.G., & Kalafat, J. (1998). Substance abuse and suicide: Promoting resilience against self-destructive behavior in youth. *School Psychology Review, 27*(3), 398–406.

Grossman, J.B., & Rhodes, J.E. (2002). The test of time: Predictors of the effects of duration in youth mentoring relationships. *American Journal of Community Psychology, 30*(2), 199–219.

Huba, G.J., & Melchior, L.A. (1998). A model for targeted HIV/AIDS services: Conclusions from 10 adolescent targeted projects funded by the Special Projects of National Significance Program of the Health Resources and Services Administration. *Journal of Adolescent Health, 23S*, 11–27.

Human Rights Watch (2002). World report, 2002, from (www.hrw.org/wr2k2/children.html)

Kim, S., Crutchfield, C., Williams, C., & Helper, N. (1998). Toward a new paradigm in substance abuse and other problem behavior prevention for youth: Youth development and empowerment approach. *Journal of Drug Education, 28*(1), 1–17.

Lachman, P., Poblete, X., Ebigbo, P.O., Nyandiya-Bundy, S., Bundy, R.P., Killian B., & Doek, J. (2002). Challenges facing child protection. *Child Abuse & Neglect, 26*, 587–617.

Lerner, R.M., & Galambos, N.L. (1998). Adolescent development: Challenges and opportunities for research, programs, and policies. *Annual Review of Psychology, 49*, 413–446.

Mollica, R.F., Poole, C., Son, L., Murray, C.C., & Tor, S. (1997). Effects of war trauma on Cambodian refugee adolescents' functional health and mental health status. *Journal of the Academy of Child and Adolescent Psychiatry, 36*(8): 1098–1106.

McAdoo, H.P. (1993). *Family ethnicity: Strength in diversity.* Newbury Park, CA: Sage Publications.

Mrazek, P.J., & Mrazek, D.A. (1987). Resilience in child maltreatment victims: A conceptual exploration. *Child Abuse & Neglect, 11*, 357–366.

Mollica, R.F., Poole, C., Son, L., Murray, C.C., & Tor, S. (1997). Effects of war trauma on Cambodian refugee adolescents' functional health and mental health status. *Journal of the American Academy of Child & Adolescent Psychiatry, 36*(8), 1098–1106.

Punamaki, R. (1996). Can ideological commitment protect children's psychosocial well being in situations of political violence? *Child Development, 67*, 55–69.

Punamaki, R. (1989). Factors affecting the mental health of Palestinian children exposed to political violence. *International Journal of Mental Health, 18*, 63–79.

Rhodes, J.E., Grossman, J.B., & Roffman, J. (2002). The rhetoric and reality of youth mentoring. *New Directions for Youth Development, 93*, 9–20.

Smith, H. (1999). Psychological detachment from school: Its effects on the academic performance of Black adolescent students in inner-city schools. Doctoral Dissertation. Teachers College, Columbia University.

Smith, H. (2003). Despair, Resilience, and the Meaning of Family: Group Therapy with French-Speaking Survivors of Torture from Africa. In R. Carter & B. Wallace (Eds.) *Understanding and Dealing with Violence. Multicultural Perspectives* (pp. 291–319). Thousand Oaks, CA: Sage Press, Inc.

Smith, H. & Akinsulure-Smith, A. (2002). Mission to Freetown. *Mano Vision (26), 12–13.* London, UK.

Smith, P., Perrin, S., Yule, W., Hacam, B. & Stuvland, R. (2002) War exposure among children from Bosnia-Hercegovina: Psychological adjustment in a community sample. *Journal of Traumatic Stress Studies, 15*(2), pp. 147–156.

Totozani, D., Kallaba, M., & Sheremeti, A. A study of the psychological state of Kosovo refugee children settled in Shkallnur village in the Durrës District. *Torture, 11*(2), 42–44.

United Nations High Commissioner for Refugees (2002). *World Refugee Survey,* 2002. United Nations: New York.

UNAIDS, (2002). *AIDS Epidemic Update.* United Nations: New York.

Williams, R.M. (1994). The sociology of ethnic conflicts: Comparative and International perspectives. *Annual Review of Sociology, 20,* 49–79.

Vizek-Vidović, V., Kuterovac-Jagodić, G., & Arambašić, L. (2000). Posttraumatic symptomatology in children exposed to war. *Scandinavian Journal of Psychology, 41,* 297–306.

Women's Commission for Refugees, Women, and Children (2002). *Precious resources: Adolescents in the reconstruction of Sierra Leone. Paricipatory research study with adolescents and youth in Sierra Leone.* Women's Commission for Refugees, Women, and Children: New York.

Zimmerman, M.A., Bingenheimer, J.B., & Notaro, P.C. (2002). Natural mentors and adolescent resiliency: a study with urban youth. *American Journal of Community Psychology, 30*(2), 221, 221–243.

Part 3

Areas of Special Need

Chapter 10

Responses to Terrorism
The Voices of Two
Communities Speak Out

Caroline S. Clauss-Ehlers, Olga Acosta
and Mark D. Weist

Perhaps no other event in the history of our nation was as broadly traumatizing as the events of the September 11, 2001 disaster. Much of the population in the United States (U.S.) and in other nations were traumatized by the events related to their magnitude; tremendous loss of human life; constant media coverage and repeated exposure to horrific images; the heroic activities and injuries and deaths of police, fire-fighting and rescue staff; and the uncertainty of imminent or future terrorist attacks, among many factors (see Weist, et al., 2002). These traumatic events were followed relatively closely in time by Anthrax attacks, sniper shootings, continued escalation in terrorism in places around the world, especially the Middle East, war in Afghanistan, and now war in Iraq. In this new century and millennium, it indeed is a new world, characterized by stresses, concerns and traumas at levels unexperienced by many Americans and citizens of other nations. Terrorism and disaster have particularly strong effects on children and adolescents (Waddel & Thomas, 1999). However, even youth most affected by the September 11 disaster are resuming their lives, and showing resilience in their school, social and emotional functioning.

Importantly, the events of and subsequent to September 11, 2001 have both underscored that mental health issues are universal, and helped to destigmatize the receipt of mental health care, as people who normally would not seek such care have done so since the disaster (Weist et al., 2002). Relatedly, there is growing realization that we must do a better job of attending to the emotional and behavioral needs of children and adolescents, ideally in proactive ways in settings where "they are" (U.S. Public Health Service, 2000; Weist & Ghuman, 2002). In New York City and Washington, DC, schools supporting a more comprehensive mental health approach were better able to respond to the events of September 11 and after, and this response has helped to propel advocacy and coalition building that is contributing to the further growth and improvement of the programs (Center for School Mental Health Assistance [CSMHA], 2001).

A central feature in the efforts of school mental health programs in Washington, DC and New York and many other places in the nation is moving from a focus on finding and treating pathology to implementing a full continuum of mental health promotion, early intervention, and treatment that prioritizes the enhancement of existing strengths and the development of resilience. This chapter seeks to reach a contemporary understanding of youth affected by terrorism, disaster, and trauma. The cultural context of trauma will also be considered as we examine cultural manifestations of trauma in New York City and Washington DC in relation to the September 11th disaster.

CONTEMPORARY UNDERSTANDING OF YOUTH AFFECTED BY TERRORISM, DISASTER AND TRAUMA

Child and adolescent reactions to terrorism are variable, with reactions including anger, depression, loss of control, and isolation (Waddel & Thomas, 1999). In addition, when disaster leads to the loss of basic security needs such as food, supplies and shelter for children, such losses can lead to or compound feelings of vulnerability, anxiety and concern about their own safety and the safety of family members (Duffy, 1988). Schuster, et al. (2001) conducted a phone survey five days after September 11, asking parents to rate the emotional reactions of their children and found that 47% reported that their children had significant anxiety about their own personal safety.

Reactions to terrorism are associated with reactions similar to those experienced from other forms of trauma. When trauma is more intense it may lead to Post-traumatic Stress Disorder (PTSD). Youth with PTSD may present symptoms such as avoidance of stimuli and situations associated with the traumatic event, intrusive thoughts and nightmares, hyper-vigilance, increased startle response, and detachment and withdrawal from friends and family and normal activities (American Academy of Child and Adolescent Psychiatry [AACAP], 1998). When youth are exposed to repetitive and/or chronic traumas dissociative symptoms may be present, including feeling out of touch with reality, losing one's sense of self, engaging in risky and self-harmful behaviors, and presenting emotions that appear disconnected from events (e.g., laughing when talking about violence) (AACAP, 1998; Terr, 1991).

Traumatic events often have long lasting impacts on children and adolescents. For example, following Hurricane Andrew, 70% of youth from the area of primary impact continued to present noteworthy symptoms of PTSD over two years after the event (Shaw, Applegate, & Schorr, 1996). Similarly, youth affected by the Oklahoma City bombing showed signs of severe stress and trauma ten months after the event (Pfefferbaum, et al., 2000). Importantly, PTSD in youth is often associated with other problems such as depression and other mood disorders, adjustment disorders, and substance abuse (Shaw, 2000).

The events of September 11, 2001 had a strong influence on children and parents, with reactions by parents affecting reactions of children and vice versa (NIMH, 2001). For example, in the Schuster et al. (2001) phone survey five days after September 11, almost half of the parents reported experiencing substantial stress, with over 90% reporting at least one serious stress symptom. Another study found that the level of PTSD in parents was related to whether their children received counseling after the traumatic events of September 11th (Stuber, et al., 2002). In this study, parents with current PTSD were more likely to have their children seen for professional counseling. In another study, adolescents surveyed after the September 11th terrorist attacks were more likely to perceive the risk of dying from general causes (i.e., a tornado) as much higher than adolescents who were surveyed prior to the attacks (Halpern-Felsher & Milstein, 2002).

Alternatively, Fredrickson, Tugade, Waugh, and Larkin (2003) found that resilient individuals were buffered from becoming depressed after September 11th by positive emotions such as gratitude, love, and interest that were experienced in the face of the trauma. A study that looked at caregivers (i.e., psychologists) found more positive than negative responses regarding their interventions post September 11th, stating they felt they were truly helping individuals and the nation heal during a time of crisis (Eidelson, D'Alessio, & Eidelson, 2003). At the same time, the most negatively cited response on the survey was that practitioners felt inadequate or helpless in the face of such need.

Reactions to stress and trauma are partly determined by a child's age and developmental level (The American Academy of Experts in Traumatic Stress [AAETS], 1999). Research has shown that even the youngest members of our society, infants and toddlers, who may not comprehend the nature of a traumatic event, will still react to changes in routine or changes observed in their caregivers as a result of a distressing experience (Munson, 2002). Table 1 outlines such age-related traumatic symptoms.

YOUTH RESPONSES TO TREATMENT

Youth in New York City

In the report entitled *Effects of the World Trade Center attack on NYC public schools: Initial report to the NYC Board of Education* (Applied Research & Consulting [ARC], Columbia University Mailman School of Public Health, &

Table 1. Age-Related Traumatic Stress Reactions

Age Range	Relevant Traumatic Symptoms
1–5	• Feelings of helplessness and fear due to their dependence on others for protection and lack of understanding about the stressful situation (New York State Office of Mental Health [NYSOMH], 2000). • Often strongly affected by the emotional or behavioral reactions exhibited by their caregivers. • Fear of abandonment resulting in clingy behavior towards parents or caregivers or separation anxiety when being left alone or with strangers (NYSOMH, 2000). • Regressive behaviors (i.e., bed-wetting, a new fear of the dark, loss of bladder control if successfully potty-trained (AAETS, 1999).
5–11	• High levels of fear and anxiety related to a traumatic event as beginning to understand permanent change, loss, and death. • Preoccupied with the details of a disaster as a way to mitigate anxiety about the stressful situation (NYSOMH, 2000). • Irritability, school avoidance, poor concentration, physical complaints (AAETS, 1999). • Recurring nightmares, night terrors, and other sleep disturbances (Munson, 2002). • Need to discharge and gain mastery over stress that may result in aggressive behavior.
11–14	• Anxiety and depression may be expressed by an increase in oppositional behaviors. • School problems, unusual rebellion at home, and physical complaints (AAETS, 1999). • Engage in various activities, such as watching television or playing video games as a distraction (Munson, 2002).
14–18	• Stress and trauma may challenge developmental task of separation because families may feel a need to rely on each other more to cope with a traumatic event. • Adolescent responses may be mixed with childlike reactions, causing the adolescent to appear unpredictable and emotionally labile during stressful situations (NYSOMH, 2000). • Appearing withdrawn and unwilling to discuss their feelings with adults, which may indicate feeling overwhelmed by their emotions or an effort to assert their independence (Munson, 2002). • An increase in risk-taking behaviors, apathy and depressive feelings (AAETS, 1999).

New York State Psychiatric Institute, 2002), it was found that New York City children in public schools at or near Ground Zero were the most physically exposed to the events of September 11th. Children in New York City schools outside Ground Zero were more likely to have family members present at the World Trade Center on September 11th. The rates and estimated number of New York City public school students with specific mental health problems after September 11th from fourth to twelfth grades were high. Table 2 presents the seven

Table 2. Estimated Rates of NYC 4th–12th Graders with
Mental Health Problems Post 9–11

Disorder	# of Students (estimated)	Rate (%)
Agoraphobia	107,395	15%
Separation Anxiety	88,064	12.3%
Conduct	78,040	10.9%
PTSD	75,176	10.5%
Generalized Anxiety	73,744	10.3%
Panic	66,585	9.3%
Major Depression	60,141	8.4%

Note: Table based on date from the following source: Applied Research & Consulting, Columbia University Mailman School of Public Health, & New York State Psychiatric Institute (2002). *Effects of the World Trade Center attack on New York City public schools: Initial report to the New York City Board of Education.* New York: Applied Research & Consulting, Columbia University Mailman School of Public Health, & New York State Psychiatric Institute, p. 2.

most common problems that students in this age group faced, going from the most to least prevalent that include: Agoraphobia, Separation Anxiety, Conduct, PTSD, Generalized Anxiety, Panic, and Major Depression. Clearly these findings speak to the enormous mental health difficulties New York City youth face post September 11.

The report to the Board of Education also found several factors increased children's chances of developing PTSD. Being younger accounted for a 400% increase in the chance of having PTSD, followed by having a family member exposed (200%), being female (88%), having any prior trauma (65%), having personal physical exposure (64%), and identifying as being Latino, Mixed, or Other for cultural/ethnic background (22–28%). Despite these prevalence rates, the study found that the proportion of New York City school children with probable PTSD who sought help was much less than the prevalence of the disorder. Only 22% of children with probable PTSD sought help through a school counselor, only 22% sought help through an outside professional, and only 34% of youth sought help from either the school counselor or an outside professional (ARC, Columbia University Mailman School of Public Health, & New York State Psychiatric Institute 2002). This means that of the 75,176 students with probable PTSD, only 25,560 students sought some kind of help. The other 49,616 students never sought out or received services.

Youth in Washington, DC

The *Terrorism-Related Mental Health Needs Assessment Project* served as a basis for assessing need and planning for a mental health response in Washington DC (DC Department of Mental Health [DCDMH], 2001). Youth focus groups

Table 3. Percent of Students Referred with Various Mental Health Problems to the DC School Mental Health Program Pre- and Post-September 11, 2001

Referring Problem	Percent endorsed for September 2000 ($N = 132$)	Percent endorsed for September 2001 ($N = 110$)	Percent endorsed for October 2001 ($N = 84$)	Percent endorsed for September 2002 ($N = 188$)
Disruptive Behavior	53%	44%	36%	49%
Hyperactive/Impulsive	22%	15%	2%	13%
Depressed/Withdrawn	19%	12%	26%	14%
Poor Academics	20%	9%	17%	11%
Poor Peer Relations	33%	15%	11%	33%
Family Problems	14%	20%	42%	37%

Note: Figures represent a percentage of the number of referring problems endorsed by the number of students referred and seen that month (September 2000 = 16 schools, September 2001 = 12 schools, October 2001 = 12 schools, September 2002 = 20 schools). Referral sources can identify up to three (3) predominant issues to include on the referral form. This data does not account for changes in numbers of referrals or in presenting problems that may be accounted for by maturity of the mental health program, increases in knowledge about mental health issues among school staff, or fluctuations due to external events occurring during the academic year.

were comprised of 66 children and adolescents divided into three age groups (8–10, 11–13, and 14 and older) from the four quadrants of the city. Youth participating in focus groups reported a general increase in feelings of fear and anxiety and a greater reluctance to venture outdoors or to travel by subway immediately following the September 11th attacks. Youth participants also endorsed a heightened sensitivity to previously normal events (i.e., planes flying overhead) and reported an increase in risk-taking behaviors following their rationale to "live for the moment."

Utilization data from the Department of Mental Health, School Mental Health Program, operating in 16 public schools in the fall of 2000 and expanded into 24 schools by the spring of 2003, revealed increases in some categories of referring problems immediately following the tragic events of September 11th. However, by the following year, referral patterns mirrored pre-September 11 (see Table 3). In October 2001, there was an increase in the number of referrals to the program for students who were exhibiting depressive symptoms and/or were suspected of using substances. Interestingly, the number of students referred because they were having "family problems" also increased significantly after September 11th (from 20% to 42% of the referring problems) and has remained an area of concern for children and youth to date. This suggests that family units and family communication were adversely affected by the culmination of stressors that plagued the area.

Throughout the aftermath of September 11th there was a pervasive sentiment that services for youth in DC's low income neighborhoods were limited and generally poorly distributed across the city. The School Mental Health Program, in collaboration with other district agencies, community providers, and a district-wide crisis response team, offered crisis support throughout the city. Over the course of 18 months, mental health providers conducted crisis debriefings (as intensive as possible), group, family, and individual counseling/therapy, and school staff consultation to address the varied responses from children and adolescents to September 11th, and later to the anniversary of September 11th, the Anthrax incident, and the sniper attacks. Yet it soon became clear that the supply of qualified, child-trained mental health professionals available to perform community outreach, offer mental health education, and commit to ongoing support services was far below the overwhelming clinical demand.

THE CULTURAL CONTEXT OF TRAUMA

Other considerations for effective treatment concerned the cultural context in which services were provided. The Surgeon General's report entitled *Mental Health: Culture, Race, and Ethnicity*, broadly defines culture as "a common heritage or set of beliefs, norms, and values. It refers to the shared, and largely learned attributes of a group of people" (U.S. Department of Health and Human Services, 2001, p. 9). Given this definition, it would make sense that culture shapes how individuals interpret traumatic events as well as how distress manifests itself (Clauss-Ehlers & Lopez-Levi, 2002a; 2002b). The following sections highlight some of the specific cultural issues related to the aftermath of traumatic experience.

Cultural Manifestations of Trauma in New York and Washington, DC

Self-Blame, Gender Roles, & Interpretation of the Event

Understanding how the individual interprets the traumatic event was a critical aspect of work with one Latina woman, who will be called Miranda.* Miranda's husband was working in Tower One on September 11th. That morning he left for work like any other, hugging his wife and 5-year-old son good-bye. Miranda was out doing errands when the plane hit Tower One, unaware of the events that had unfolded.

Miranda was never able to communicate with her husband that morning. In treatment she blamed herself for her husband's death. She truly believed she was at fault because she hadn't called him in time, to warn him to leave. Had she been at home, Miranda believed she could have called right away and her husband could have evacuated the building. Despite the reality that her husband was on the

---

* Names and identifying information have been changed to protect confidentiality.

top floor and the plane hit the building in the 80s, it was important to understand Miranda's interpretation of this event within a cultural context.

The cultural concept of *marianismo* was one way to make sense of Miranda's experience. The idea of marianismo is that the women's role is to liken herself to the Virgin Mary, to sacrifice and suffer for the good of her husband and children (Chin, 1994). For Miranda, the tragic loss of her husband and her inability to save him through her own suffering were too overwhelming to bear. It was almost as though Miranda needed to believe the ability to save her husband was in her control (i.e., she was not at home) than come to terms with the reality that she had no control over such a tragic situation. Here education about the crisis was helpful and involved explaining the logistics of where the plane hit the building. It was also important to be a consistent caring person, giving witness to Miranda's story while insisting she was not to blame for her loss.

Stigma

In working with trauma from a culturally-focused framework, it was also important to recognize that individuals and families might have different thoughts about the helping process itself. According to the Surgeon General's Report, stigma was portrayed as the "most formidable obstacle to future progress in the arena of mental illness and health" (as quoted in USDHHS, 2001, p. 29). Stigma can be viewed as negative beliefs and attitudes about mental health problems and/or people who present them (see Clauss-Ehlers & Weist, 2002). When working across cultures it was important to consider the stigma issues at play for the individual and his or her family. For instance, when asking one Latina mother about getting support from extended family, she quickly shared that members didn't even know she was in therapy. This mother decided not to tell extended family she had sought help because she feared they would think she was "una loca" (a crazy person) who couldn't handle the loss of her husband within the context of family support.

Religious Persecution

On numerous occasions following the events of September 11th, Muslim residents reported that they were repeatedly threatened, harassed, and singled-out due to misunderstandings about their religion and questions posed about their national loyalty. These real and persistent threats caused some women to temporarily stop observing Hijab, a covering of the head and body that addresses the requirement for modesty among Muslim women, due to fear of continued persecution and misguided blame for the attacks on the Pentagon and the World Trade Centers. Hijab not only describes a particular style of dress among Muslims, but it connotes behavior, manners, and appearance in public that ties one to a common set of beliefs about being a Muslim "believer." The lack of cultural awareness and sensitivity on the part of the mainstream population caused a group of devout individuals to feel great reluctance to express pride in their heritage, culture, and religious customs for fear of persecution.

Children and adolescents from Muslim families expressed confusion and anger about how they and their families were being treated. A school-based clinician recalled one student who continuously lashed out at her teacher (who dressed in Hijab) after September 11th due to the dissonance she experienced over public messages telling her she should fear Muslims and the reality that she was attached to and dependent upon Muslim adults in her school. The same school-based mental health provider noted that another Muslim student's emotional and behavioral problems exacerbated following September 11th due to defensive encounters with his peers who made him feel different and unwelcome.

A general reluctance to look outside of one's group for help or support can be expected among a group of people that are targeted for persecution, especially if the helpers are believed to be aligned in any way with those within the mainstream population (and therefore may be potential victimizers). Members of the Muslim community, both children and adults, demonstrated reluctance to share their experiences with unfamiliar and historically culturally insensitive mental health providers. It was only through relationship building within the second author's community and school-based programs that trust was gained and successful outreach was performed for those demonstrating the greatest need for mental health support during this volatile time.

Incorporating Culture into Trauma Relief Efforts: New York City and Washington DC

As we reach out to diverse communities, we are challenged to look at how service provision might incorporate, or leave out, cultural diversity. The following highlights new areas we might begin to consider in attempts to incorporate cultural sensitivity into trauma relief efforts.

Police Presence

Access to services is one area that is relevant to cultural inclusion. Faced with the aftermath of September 11th, many organizations set up booths to provide various services. Due to the lock down state of New York City at that time, a police presence was in view of many of these service outlets. Unfortunately, the police presence acted as a deterrent to seeking services for many individuals and families from culturally diverse communities. Having escaped torture, come to the US for political refuge, or been victimized in their countries of origin, the police presence acted as an unintentional re-traumatization for many. It is a difficult position to try to balance security versus services during a time of crisis. A possible alternative might be to provide access to some services separate and apart from law enforcement, or if this is not appropriate, for security personnel to be dressed less formally.

Mistrust of Government Authorities

The *Terrorism-Related Mental Health Needs Assessment Project* underscored that residents of Washington, DC from all age groups harbored a general mistrust of the local and federal government, believed that the authorities were keeping information from them, and worried that the government was generally unprepared to protect them from future harm (DCDMH, 2001). This was a significant finding given the heightened state of alert for both Washington DC and New York City and the public's dependence on the government for information, protection, and services. The report also pointed to "an absence of a coordinated system for community outreach and information dissemination, particularly for those who are more isolated from the mainstream, including... immigrants..." (DCDMH, 2001, p. 11). This was particularly noteworthy given that Washington, DC ranks as the fifth most common destination for legal immigrants nationwide (Giorgis & Roberts, 2001).

Number of Sessions

Another issue concerned parameters of treatment, particularly the number of sessions offered. When the first author started to work with families affected by the tragedy, a mere three sessions were allowed by a mental health service contract. As families bonded with the clinician, it became apparent that ending treatment after three sessions would perpetuate, and even re-create the loss and acute crisis. To make a connection in the face of crisis and then be forced to disconnect when the family was not prepared to do so was counter to cultural values such as *personalismo* where the relationship is highly valued (see Clauss-Ehlers & Lopz Levi, 2002a). While advocacy led to an eight month extension with some families, this was certainly not the reality for many others.

Benefit Maze

Access to benefits was another complication for many families and often related to language barriers between services and families. Without Spanish-speaking service providers, for instance, many families were at a loss about how to negotiate the maze of benefits before them. This left some families feeling powerless. One family, for instance, shared that they weren't going to pursue benefit options because it was so stressful. Other families had their children translate—acting as the communicator between service system and family system. This new "role" in the face of trauma placed an additional burden on children and their families. One adolescent girl, for instance, shared that she became deeply saddened as she translated information about procedures that would be used in attempts to identify her father's body. Being too close to the information and taking on the responsibility of being the transmitter of knowledge were factors that risked re-traumatizing this girl (Clauss-Ehlers, 2003).

Language Barriers

As mentioned, the inability for a growing number of New York City and Washington, DC residents to communicate to officials in English caused significant frustration (Clauss, 1998; Giorgis & Roberts, 2001). The diversity of backgrounds and lack of non-English speaking mental health providers (especially child mental health providers) for youth and families who speak Chinese, Vietnamese, Amharic, and Spanish, represents an alarming gap in our service delivery infrastructure. Washington DC focus group participants urged government officials to make information available in multiple languages, using standard linguistic adaptations, and to use multiple formats for disseminating information (both oral and written) to increase the likelihood of reaching marginalized members of this diverse community.

Religion

In work with trauma across cultures, it was also important to consider faith and religious background (Owens, et al., 2004). Clinicians should explore the ways a family's religious beliefs may provide comfort to family members and the ways they may be a source of stress so that coping mechanisms can be incorporated successfully into valued family belief systems. Should the family agree, clergy and mental health professionals can work together as a crisis team. It may also be that the family doesn't want clergy present during treatment, but does want to participate in religious ceremonies outside the treatment forum. Certainly this will expand the family's support system and outlets for grieving.

The importance of integrating mental health practice and religious practice was particularly important when a family must cope with religious questions that result from the trauma. The first author worked with one family who was very distressed that the father's body was never found. They had deep concerns about what not having the physical body meant for life after death. The family also had questions related to not knowing whether their loved one jumped off the World Trade Center. They wondered if God would view this as suicide or understand the reasons for jumping. Family members themselves grappled with trying to comprehend the amount of pain their loved one must have suffered if jumping became the only option. Incorporating religion and mental health helped the family process and cope with the situation from a perspective of both religious commitment and personal well-being.

Family-centered Interventions

Finally, immediate and extended family members play a vital role in coping with trauma or stress. Non-traditional members of a family can provide significant support to children and youth, such as Godparents or neighbors that are affectionately called "tia" (aunt) or "tio" (uncle). Respondents in the Washington DC focus groups were quoted as saying "I thanked God my mother and grandmother were still alive" and "we went back to school too soon . . . there was not enough time with our family." Given the importance of the family unit in helping to counteract feelings of anxiety that accompany unpredictable events, a goal within the School Mental Health Program was to help families and caregivers be better able to support their children through the various crises. Clinicians defined their roles as educators and consultants and assisted caregivers through one on one family consultations that addressed how to talk to children about coping with the many feelings and reactions they might have.

It is from these experiences that valuable lessons can be learned about how to integrate culture into trauma response. Table 4 organizes culturally relevant recommendations based on the National Association of School Psychologists (NASP) website (www.nasponline.org, downloaded 9/3/02; Young, 1998). These recommendations are meant to provide general guidelines when working with issues of trauma in a cross-cultural context. Approaching diverse clients in crisis from a cultural framework that addresses practical problems and provides specific cross-cultural intervention is a starting point for being responsive to all our families.

CONCLUSION: THE SCHOOL RESPONSE

Reaching people in need following large scale traumatic events is uniquely challenging. For youth, school-based approaches to outreach present many advantages in reaching them as well as many adults "where they are" (Jamieson, Curry, & Martinez, 2001). In addition to educational and support functions, schools usually have elaborate communication mechanisms in place and often serve as a gathering place in communities and for emergency response (e.g., they are often the site where people are evacuated to during severe weather related events). Optimally, a full range of activities should be conducted in schools to prepare for and respond to terrorism and disaster. These activities include the development of crisis response plans and teams, ensuring that these teams and plans become part of the fabric of the school (versus unused documents), school-wide mental health educational activities before disaster (e.g., on strategies for positive mental health,

Table 4. Culturally-Inclusive Responses to Trauma

Cultural Framework	Practical Problems	Specific Cross-Cultural Intervention
Search for the meaning of suffering and pain relevant to the culture	Deal with immediate problems that the individual is having difficulty handling	Ask survivors what you would like to do to be of assistance to them and then tell them truthfully what you can and can't do
Search for the meaning of death in the culture	Build trust	Reduce isolation
Search for the meaning of life in the culture	Assist with financial resources if possible	Relaxation techniques/Meditation
Traditions may help survivors feel re-oriented	Help survivors focus on something tangible that they can accomplish over the next few days	Education About Crisis in Culturally Relevant Terms
Ask survivors what they would like you to do to be of assistance to them, tell them truthfully what you can and can't do		• Help Individual Develop Control • Increase Self-Esteem • Be Aware of Specific Communication Techniques: -Eye contact -Integration of food and drink -Pace of conversation -Body language

Note: Select recommendations are included here. See NASP website for a full listing of their recommendations. Table created for this chapter, not a reproduction of any NASP table.

trauma symptoms, strategies for effective trauma response), school-wide plans for response after disaster; and more intensive therapeutic services for affected students, families and staff. It is beyond the scope of this chapter to review each of these areas in detail. The interested reader is referred to two resources: a book on crisis response in schools by Jonathan Sandoval (Sandoval, 2002); and a comprehensive review of school preparedness and response to terrorism and disaster by the third author and collaborators (Weist et al., 2002).

A critical action for all schools to both assist in preparedness for disaster, and to promote resilience is to initiate programs that broadly train students, families and staff on mental health. There is a particular need for training on the impacts of trauma, for example, on topics such as the psychosocial impacts of disaster, cultural factors, PTSD symptoms, grief and bereavement, and holiday and anniversary reactions (Arman, 2000; NASP, 2001; Call & Pfefferbaum, 1999). It is critically important that this mental health training be provided in advance of crises, since once crises occur learning and motivation for training are impaired (see Sandoval, 2002). Unfortunately, such broad training on mental health in schools occurs very rarely; in reality even basic crisis preparation and response functions are often extremely limited in schools (Weist et al., 2002). These realities point to a significant need for advocacy, training, and resource enhancement to ensure that schools are equipped to take on the critically important tasks of mental health education and preparation for effective response to crises, trauma, terrorism and disaster.

Assuming school staff have had some level of mental health training and preparation for response to significant traumas, their actions can play an important role in helping students in the recovery and healing process. In discussions about the crisis, school staff should be honest with students, help them to feel safe, and allow them to express their concerns, questions and feelings (Waddell & Thomas, 1999). Also, following a significant trauma such as student or staff deaths and/or terrorism, school staff should convey that it is OK for students to express a range of emotions, including anger, sadness, worry, and even some level of acting out. This can be challenging for schools to basically tread a line that on the one hand allows students to express real emotion, yet on the other hand manages student behavior and avoids widespread discipline problems (see Poland, 1994). Following severe crises such as a terrorist attack the most helpful response to affected individuals often involves "assistance with physical needs, re-location and shelter, and financial matters" (Pfefferbaum, Flynn, Brandt, & Lensgraf, 1999, p. 110). Since people may be unlikely to seek these services in specialized health or mental health centers, schools may be looked on to provide these services (Weist, Evans, & Lever, 2003).

Finally, schools represent one of the most, if not most powerful communication mechanisms in communities. Following terrorism or disaster, a critical activity is to get information out to the public. While print, radio and television media can and do perform this function, these media can also cause harm, as in the repeated coverage of the September 11th disaster, including horrific images of people jumping out of buildings in some media. It is also critical to get information out to people deemed important by mental health, health and education experts. The Office for Victims of Crime (OVC, 2001) at the U.S. Department of Justice, for instance, has developed a *Handbook for Coping After Terrorism*, which reviews reactions to a traumatic disaster, and presents practical strategies for coping such as: 1) "Whenever possible, delay making any major decisions. You may think a big change will make you feel better, but it will not necessarily ease the pain. Give yourself time to get through the most hectic times and to adjust before making decisions that will affect the rest of your life" and 2) "Take care of your mind and body. Eat healthy food. Exercise regularly, even if it is only a long walk every day. Exercise will help lift depression and help you sleep better, too . . . " The handbook presents 15 additional strategies to assist in coping, as well as information on additional resources and sources of assistance. There are many other written resources that would be helpful in schools' response to disaster. However, interviews with schools and school staff members following September 11th indicated that many of them did not identify the most useful written materials for dissemination, or logistical issues such as making hundreds of copies, prevented their broad dissemination throughout the school (CSMHA, 2001). This underscores key infrastructure needs for schools to be able to assume a more prominent role in assisting students, families, staff and community members in recovering from trauma (Weist et al., 2002).

REFERENCES

American Academy of Child and Adolescent Psychiatry (1998). Practice parameters for the assessment and treatment of children and adolescents with Posttraumatic Stress Disorder. *Journal of the American Academy of Child and Adolescent Psychiatry, 37*(supplement), 4S–26S.

American Academy of Experts in Traumatic Stress (1999). *A Practical Guide for Crisis Response in Our Schools*. http://www.aaets.org

Applied Research & Consulting, Columbia University Mailman School of Public Health, & New York State Psychiatric Institute (2002). *Effects of the World Trade Center attack on New York City public schools: Initial report to the New York City Board of Education*. New York: Applied Research & Consulting, Columbia University Mailman School of Public Health, & New York State Psychiatric Institute.

Arman, J. (2000). In the wake of tragedy at Columbine High School *Professional School Counseling, 3*(3), 218–221.

Call, J., & Pfefferbaum, B. (1999). Health response to the 1995 bombing. *Psychiatric Services, 50*(7), 953–955.

Center for School Mental Health Assistance (2001, November). Coping and moving forward. *On the Move with School-Based Mental Health, 6*, 1–2.

Clauss, C.S. (1998). Language: The unspoken variable in psychotherapy practice. *Journal of Psychotherapy, 35*, 188–196.

Clauss-Ehlers, C.S. (2003). Promoting ecological health resilience for minority youth: Enhancing health care access through the school health center. *Psychology in the Schools, 40*(3), 265–278.

Clauss-Ehlers, C.S., & Lopez Levi, L. (2002a). Violence and community, terms in conflict: An ecological approach to resilience. *Journal of Social Distress and the Homeless, 11*(4), 265–278.

Clauss-Ehlers, C.S., & Lopez Levi, L. (2002). Working to promote resilience with Latino youth in schools: Perspectives from the U.S. and Mexico. *International Journal of Mental Health Promotion: Special Issue on School Mental Health, 4*(4), 14–20.

Clauss-Ehlers, C.S., & Weist, M.D. (2002). Children are newsworthy: Working effectively with the media to improve systems of child and adolescent mental health. In Ghuman, H., Weist, M., & Sarles, R. (Eds.), *Providing mental health services to youth where they are: School and community-based approaches*. New York: Brunner-Routledge.

District of Columbia Department of Mental Health (December, 2001), *Terrorism-Related Mental Health Needs Assessment Project*.

Eidelson, R.J., D'Alessio, G.R., & Eidelson, J.I. (2003). The impact of September 11 on psychologists. *Professional psychology: Research and practice, 34*(2), 144–150.

Fredrickson, B.L., Tugade, M.M., Waugh, C.E., & Larkin, G.R. (2003). What good are positive emotions in crises? A prospective study of resilience and emotions following the terrorist attacks on the United States on September 11th, 2001. *Journal of Personality and Social Psychology, 84*(2), 365–376.

Giorgis, T.W., & Roberts, L. (2001). *Multicultural Competence: A case study in mental health service delivery*. District of Columbia Department of Mental Health.

Halpern-Felsher, B.L., & Millstein, S.G. (2002). The effects of terrorism on teens' perceptions of dying: The new world is riskier than ever. *Journal of Adolescent Health, 30*(5), 308–311.

Jamieson, A., Curry, A., & Martinez, G. (2001). School enrollment in the United States: Social and economic characteristics of students. *Current population reports*. Washington, DC: U.S. Census Bureau.

Munson, C.E. (2002). Child and adolescent needs in a time of national disaster: Perspectives for mental health professionals and parents. *Brief Treatment and Crisis Intervention 2*, 135–151.

National Association of School Psychologists. (2001). *Children and fear of war and terrorism: Tips for parents and teachers*. Bethesda, MD: Author.

New York State Office of Mental Health. (2000). *Crisis Counseling Guide to Children and Families in Disasters*. http://www.omh.state.ny.us/omhweb/crisis/crisiscounselingguide.

Office for Victims of Crime (2001). *OVC handbook for coping after terrorism: A guide to healing and recovery*. Washington, DC: U.S. Department of Justice, Office for Justice Programs.

Owens, C., Bryant, T., Sloane, T., Hatahway, A., Moore, E., Huntley, S., & Weist, M.D. (2004). Enhancing faith, education, and mental health partnerships to promote resilience in youth. In C.S. Clauss-Ehlers & M.D. Weist (Eds.), *Community planning to foster resilience in children* (pp. 283–296). New York: Kluwer Academic/Plenum Publishers.

Pfefferbaum, B., Flynn, B., Brandt, E., & Lensgraf, J. (1999). Organizing the mental health response to human-caused community disasters with reference to the Oklahoma City bombing. *Psychiatric Annals, 29*(2), 109–113.

Pfefferbaum, B., Gurwitch, R., McDonald, N., Lefwich, M., Micheal, J., Sconzo, G., Messenbaugh, A., & Schultz, R. (2000). Posttraumatic stress among young children after the death of a friend or acquaintance in a terrorist bombing. *Psychiatric Services, 51*(3), 386–388.

Poland, S. (1994). The role of school crisis intervention teams to prevent and reduce school violence and trauma. *School Psychology Review, 23*, 175–189.

Sandoval, J. (2002). *Handbook of crisis counseling, intervention, and prevention in the schools, 2nd edition*. Mahwah, NJ: Erlbaum.

Schuster, M., Stein, B., Jaycox, L., Collins, R., Marshall, G., Elliott, M., Zhou, A., Kanouse, D., Morrison, J., & Berry, S.H. (2001). A national survey of stress reactions after the September 11, 2001, terrorist attacks. *The New England Journal of Medicine, 345*(20), 1507–1512.

Shaw, J.A. (2000). Children, adolescents and trauma. *Psychiatric Quarterly, 71*(3), 227–243.

Shaw, J.A., Applegate, B., Schorr, C. (1996). Twenty-one month follow-up study of school-age children exposed to Hurricane Andrew. *Journal of the American Academy of Child and Adolescent Psychiatry, 35*, 359–364.

Sieckert, K., & National Association of School Psychologists, (n.d.). Cultural perspectives on trauma and critical response. Retrieved September 3, 2002, from http://www.nasponline.org

Singer, T.J. (1982). An introduction to disaster: Some considerations of a psychological nature. *Aviation, Space and Environmental Medicine, 53*, 245–250.

Starfield, B., Robertson, J., & Riley, A.W. (2002). Social class gradients and health in childhood. *Ambulatory Pediatrics, 2* (4), 238–246.

Stuber, J., Fairbrother, G., Galea, S., Pfefferbaum, B., Wilson-Genderson, M., & Vlahov, D. (2002). Determinants of counseling for children in Manhattan after the September 11 attacks. *Psychiatric Services, 53*(7), 815–822.

Tashman, N.A., Acosta, O.M., & Weist, M.D. (1998). *Fostering resilience among youth in schools: The school resiliency approach*. Unpublished manuscript.

Terr, L.C. (1991). Childhood traumas: An outline and overview. *American Journal of Psychiatry, 148*, 10–20.

U.S. Department of Health and Human Services (2001). *Mental health: Culture, race, and ethnicity—A supplement to mental health: A report of the Surgeon General*. Rockville, MD: U.S. Department of Health and Human Services, Public Health Service, Office of the Surgeon General.

U.S. Public Health Service (2000). *Report on the Surgeon General's Conference on Children's Mental Health: A national action agenda.* Washington, DC: Author.

Waddell, D., & Thomas, A. (1999, Spring). Disaster: Helping children cope. *National Association of School Psychologists' Communiqué,* 6–7.

Weist, M.D., Evans, S.W., & Lever, N.A. (2003). Advancing mental health practice and research in schools. In M.D. Weist, S.W. Evans, & N.A. Lever (Eds.), *Handbook of school mental health: Advancing practice and research* (pp. 1–8). New York, NY: Kluwer Academic/Plenum Publishers.

Weist, M.D., & Ghuman, H.S. (2002). Principles behind the proactive delivery of mental health services to youth where they are. In M. Weist, H. Ghuman, and R. Sarles (Eds.), *Providing mental health services to youth where they are: School- and community-based approaches (pp. 1–14).* New York, NY: Taylor Francis.

Weist, M.D., Sander, M.A., Lever, N.A., Rosner, L.E., Pruitt, D.B., Lowie, J.A., Hill, S., Lombardo, S., & Christodulu, K.V. (2002). School mental health's response to terrorism and disaster. *Journal of School Violence, 1 (4),* 5–31.

Young, M. (1998). *Community response team training manual (2nd Ed.).* Washington, DC: NOVA.

Chapter 11

Environmental Factors that Foster Resilience for Medically Handicapped Children

Jeannette M. Maluf

Children deemed to be medically or emotionally handicapped have been the focus of much of the research in the past 25 years, guiding the development of educational laws, child advocacy, and the implementation of prevention programs at the Federal and State levels (Albee, 1982; Canino & Spurlock, 1994; Luthar, Cicchetti, & Becker, 2000; Masten, 2001; Rutter, 1979).

The implementation of the landmark Education of the Handicapped Act of the Federal Education Public Law (PL94-142) in 1975, which advocated for the education of all handicapped children, heralded the onset of various models of intervention. These intervention models aimed at ameliorating the child's handicap, as well as fostering supportive environmental factors, thereby allowing the child to reach their maximum developmental and academic potential. In so doing, the Education of the Handicapped Act established specific guidelines for providing handicapped children with an adequate and meaningful education. More importantly, this Federal Education Public Law altered the manner in which children are evaluated, diagnosed, classified and placed within the educational system. It also required the development of individual educational programs (IEP); and accorded parents the authority to review records and participate in the educational objectives for their child (Sattler, 2001).

The 1975 Law PL94-142 set the precedent for defining a child's disability and provided the forum for developing environmental support, which included educational and parental intervention. In setting this precedent, this law inadvertently brought about the convergence of various systems to work in tandem and to intervene in providing a protective layer of support for a child considered handicapped.

In recognition of the need to provide support early in the life of the handicapped child, an amendment to the Education of the Handicapped Act (PL94-142) was made in 1986. This amendment, Federal Educational Public Law (PL99-457), authorized the creation of "early intervention programs for handicapped infants and toddlers ages 3 to 5 years." In 1992, PL99-457 was further amended to include "an infant or toddler from birth," who has a disability (Sattler, 2001).

The policy behind the Education of the Handicapped Act (PL94-142 and PL99-457) required the development and implementation of a "statewide, comprehensive, coordinated multidisciplinary, interagency program of early intervention services for handicapped infants, toddlers and their families" financed, in part by the Federal government. The Education of the Handicapped Act (PL94-142) was further updated and amended in 1997, and 1999 and is currently known as the Individuals with Disabilities Education Act (PL105-17), also know as IDEA'97 and IDEA'99 (Federal Register, 1997 & 1999).

The Individual with Disabilities Education Act (IDEA'97) defines 12 categories, which qualified as a disability under the mandate of the education law. The disabilities are "mental retardation, a hearing impairment, deafness, a speech or language impairment, a visual impairment, serious emotional disturbance, an orthopedic impairment, autism, traumatic brain injury, deaf-blindness, specific learning disability, and multiple disabilities (Federal Register, 1997).

Table 1. Evolution of the Federal Educational Public Laws

YEAR	LAW	
1975	PL94-142	EDUCATION OF THE HANDICAPPED ACT: defining the child's disability, development of individual educational programs (IEP), and environmental support with parental intervention.
1986	PL99-457	1st AMENDMENT: included early intervention for infants and toddlers, ages 3–5.
1992	PL99-457	2nd AMENDMENT: included early intervention for infants and toddlers from birth.
1997	IDEA'97	3rd AMENDMENT: defined 12 additional qualifying disabilities
1999	IDEA'99	4th AMENDMENT: included developmental delays and other health impairments, such as ADHD; does not include the category of non-verbal learning disability and sensory integration dysfunction.

Table 2. Disability Categories

Medical Impairments	Other Health Impairments
1. Mental Retardation	13. Attention Deficit/Hyperactivity
2. Serious Emotional Disturbance	14. Developmental Delay
3. Autism	15. Lead Poisoning
4. Traumatic Brain Injury	16. Epilepsy
5. Deafness	17. Asthma
6. Deaf-Blindness	18. Diabetes
7. Orthopedic impairment	19. Leukemia
8. Visual impairment	20. Nephritis
9. Hearing Impairment	21. Rheumatic Fever
10. Speech/language impairment	22. Sickle Cell Anemia
11. Specific Learning Disability	23. Heart Condition
12. Multiple Disabilities	

In 1999, further amendments were made which include the categories of "developmental delays, and other health impairments" (Federal Register, 1999). The disability category of "other health impairment" specifically includes attention deficit/hyperactivity disorder, as well as other chronic or acute health problems such as lead poisoning, epilepsy, asthma, diabetes, leukemia, nephritis, rheumatic fever, sickle cell anemia or a heart condition (Federal Register, 1999).

However, the syndrome of learning disabilities referred to, as "nonverbal learning disability" which consists of difficulty with tactile perception, psychomotor coordination, visual-spatial organization, and nonverbal problem solving is not considered a separate type of disability listed in the IDEA (Sattler, 2001). Similarly in younger children, the diagnosis of "sensory integration dysfunction," which refers to difficulty by the brain to process and make sense of stimuli derived from the senses, is a diagnostic entity not included in IDEA, nor in the Diagnostic and Statistical Manual of Mental Disorders (DSM-IV) (American Psychiatric Association, 1994; Stolberg, 2002).

If a child through the use of psychological, educational and medical assessment is diagnosed to have one of the eligible disabilities, and it is found that this disability negatively affects the child's educational performance, then the law mandates the child to receive all the necessary services under special education. Under this mandate a child who has a physical or emotional disability/delay that hinders the achievement of developmental markers, and who meet the psychological, educational and medical eligibility requirements, as stipulated by law IDEA'97 and IDEA'99, is considered to be "medically handicapped" or "a special needs child" or a "child with special health care needs." A working definition, used by some government agencies, defines "children with special health care needs" as children who "have or are suspected of having a serious or chronic physical, developmental, behavioral, or emotional condition and who also require health and related services of a type or amount beyond that required by children generally" (Office of Special Education Programs, 2003).

In addition to the Education law governing special education, the Federal government provided incentives at the state and city levels throughout the country to devise programs for children aimed at intervention and adaptation (Canino & Spurlock, 1994; Rutter, 1990; Munk & Maluf, 1991). Thus, intervention and adaptation became important variables defining much of the research on childhood development, psychopathology and resilience (Fonagy & Target, 2002; Luthar, Cicchetti & Becker, 2000). Additionally, many of the mental health initiative programs developed in the last twenty years have focused on prevention, intervention, and stress-reduction models (Canino & Spurlock, 1994; Ferran & Maluf, 1991; Munk, 1993).

Masten (2001) has noted in her seminal review of the research on resilience for the past twenty-five years, that the concept of resilience is "thought to be a systemic component of human adaptation." However, embedded in this systemic notion of an intrinsic human capacity of adaptation, is the notion that in order to assess the quality of the adaptation; one must do so along a developmental continuum. For example, the "early intervention" programs tend to quantify a child's adaptation to adversity by assessing how the child meets the expected developmental markers, or by the absence of clinical symptomatology (Canino & Spurlock, 1994; Munk, 1993). Thus, environmental variables are considered essential and intrinsic in assessing how a child adapts, as well as, actively contributing to the process of a child's adaptation (Calhoun & Tedeschi, 1999; Chatigny, 1994; Frederick, 1985; Hembree & Foa, 2000).

The environmental variables typically considered essential in fostering and developing a child's adaptation, are most notably parents, the school and the community (Masten, 2000). Although parents influence the development of behavior in children and thereby moderate the impact of any adversity on the child (Fonagy & Target, 2002; Dikengil, Morganstein, Smith, & Thut, 1994; Werner & Smith, 2001), nonetheless it is recognized that the environmental variables impinging on the parents begins as early as the prenatal phase of a child's development (Masten, 2001; Munk, 1993). Thus the medical and healthcare community contribute significantly at the earliest, and perhaps most critically sensitive part of a child's development.

The models for early intervention programs proposed in the late 1980's acknowledged the importance of prenatal care, and focused on assessing the strengths, risks, and protective factors of the environment as a way to modulate the adverse effect of a physical and/or emotional trauma and/or stress on a child (Fonagy & Target, 2002; Dikengil, Morganstein et al., 1994; Werner & Smith, 2001). Many prevention program models focused on strengthening the environmental variables, also known as "protective" factors to help facilitate the naturally occurring developmental markers of a child, as well as, to minimize the impact of a toxic or stress-related event on a child's adaptation (Canino & Spurlock, 1994).

Masten (2001) further notes that perhaps the most important aspect to creating effective adaptive systems for a child, in addition to parenting, is the notion that cognition and intellectual functioning be preserved, since research indicates that if these are "compromised prior to, or as a result of the adversity," then "major or long-lasting effects on adaptive behaviors in the environment may occur." Medically handicapped children whose cognitive and/or intellectual functioning has been compromised pose the most difficult challenge to educators and mental healthcare workers in providing them and their families with adequate care and in fostering resilience (Dikengil, Morganstein, et al., 1994; Sattler, 2002). The medically handicapped child is required to learn to cope with any limits of a medically handicapping condition, while simultaneously attempting to achieve all developmental milestones, even if these occur at a different rate than what is considered typical for the non-medically handicapped child (Blosser & DePompei, 1994; Frederick, 1985; Sattler, 2001, 2002).

To foster resilience for the medically handicapped child, it is important to understand the complex interplay of the child's medical condition with the pharmacological, behavioral, cognitive, educational and family interventions available for each child (Blosser, 1994; Dikengil, Morganstein et al., 1994; Lewis, 1994; Sattler, 2001). Furthermore, children deemed medically handicapped usually have multiple or comorbid disorders, which may greatly increase the family's ability to cope, as well as limiting the development of the child's cognitive, affective, and interpersonal coping skills (Hartshorne, 2002; Sattler, 2002). Any environmental support given the medically handicapped child needs to be mediated by the parent's involvement, and their perception of their child's handicap. These parental perceptions, as well as parental expectations, will influence the child's self-concept and their motivation to adapt to their handicap (Frederick, 1985; Hartshorne, 2002; Hembree & Foa, 2000; Sattler, 2002).

From the family's perspective, taking care of a medically handicapped child incurs great psychological and financial strain. A parent may have to stop working and care exclusively for their child. Other children in the family may feel neglected of attention, becoming angry and rebellious, or they may compensate by becoming a parentified child, helping the parent in taking care of the handicapped sibling (Safer, 2002). Parents may also feel guilt, and/or shame; and often may feel afraid, alone, and incompetent. The marital couple may not be able to withstand the financial, social and emotional stress of coping with the special needs of their handicapped child, and some marriages dissolve, creating further stressors for the family (Dewan, 2003; Hartshorne, 2002; Milliren & Barrett-Kruse, 2002).

Brooks and Goldstein (2001) have developed a ten-step strategy to teach parents to nurture resilience in their children. They recommend "being empathic,

Table 3. Early Developmental Variables Related to Fostering Resilience

1. **Early intervention programs:** aimed at the handicapped child to assess degree of disability, appropriate cognitive skills, self-esteem, and motivation in being able to adapt effectively to the environment. Particular emphasis is on preserving cognitive/intellectual functioning.
2. **Teaching parents to nurture resilience:** by being empathic, being accepting of limitations of handicap, increase child's positive view of self, fostering the development of realistic expectations and goals, reinforcing the child's areas of competence, and providing opportunities for child to contribute to society.
3. **Protective environmental factors:** interplay of parents, schools and community of professionals working together to ameliorate the adverse effects of the handicap by the implementation of pharmacological, cognitive-behavioral, educational and family interventions.

communicating effectively and listening actively, identifying and rewriting negative scripts" (p. 7). In addition, their model for building resilience includes, "accepting our children for who they are and helping them to set realistic expectation and goals, helping our children experience success by identifying and reinforcing their 'islands of competence,' helping children recognize that mistakes are experiences from which to learn, [foster the development of] responsibility, compassion, and a social conscience by providing [them] with opportunities to contribute, teaching our children to solve problems and make decisions, and disciplining in a way that promotes self-discipline and self-worth" (Brooks & Goldstein, 2002, pp. 8–9).

Parents with a medically handicapped child may need additional support and guidance to learn to implement some of these strategies (Blosser & DePompei, 1994; Sattler, 2002). Cognitive-behavioral therapeutic approaches have been successful in providing concrete goals and objectives for helping the parent develop the coping skills necessary to foster salient strategies for their child. For example, educators and healthcare workers teach parents to focus on the assets of their child, empower the parent to take an active role, teach the child the meaning and the parameters of their disability, accept the limitations imposed by the disability, reduce limitations of their medical, social and physical environment as realistically as possible while encouraging the use of environmental support, assistive devices, and enlisting the cooperation of the school and community (Safran & Segal, 1990; Sattler, 1992; Wright, 1983). It is important to encourage parents to accept and not deny their child's disability (Hartshorne, 2002), and to "live on satisfactory terms" with the disability while believing that despite these, their child may live "meaningful lives [as] indicated by their [child's] participation in valued activities and by their sharing in the satisfactions of living" (Sattler, 1992, p. 782; Wright, 1983, p. 195).

Following are two clinical case vignettes, that highlight different aspects of parental coping and fostering resilience with their medically handicapped child.

It is important to note that identifying information for all case material has been changed so that clients cannot be identified and confidentiality has been maintained.

CLINICAL VIGNETTE 1

Michael is an 11 year-old boy who suffered severe head injury as a result of a motor vehicle accident at the age of 1 year and 7 month-old. At the time of the accident, Michael suffered multiple injuries, including a fracture of the skull and he remained in a coma for over 72 hours. He underwent a number of medical procedures, among which, a laryngoscopy and tracheoscopy produced trauma to his vocal chords, requiring multiple reconstructive surgeries. He remained hospitalized for six months. Prior to the accident, Michael was considered a healthy child, pre and post-natal complications were reported absent and his developmental milestones had been achieved within normal limits.

The trauma Michael suffered occurred at a developmental age where he was just beginning to acquire language skills. The medical procedures he underwent inadvertently damaged the area related to vocalizing and language development, and also hindered his ability to verbalize the emotional Sequelae to the trauma. Hospital records indicated that Michael suffered from night terrors, incessant crying and nightmares. Michael was diagnosed with brain damage, developmental delays and emotional trauma. He manifested separation anxiety, clinging and dependent behaviors as well as withdrawal.

Upon being discharged from the hospital, Michael was placed in a Special Therapeutic Nursery Program for the Developmentally Delayed and Emotionally Disturbed Child, where he received physical, occupational and language therapy services 5 days a week. At chronological age of 2 years and 10 months, he was assessed with the Bayley Scales of Infant Development and found with a Mental Age of 29 months. Similarly, at age 4 years and 2 months he was found with the Wechsler Preschool and Primary Intelligence Scale-Revised functioning at the 3 year-5 month-old level. In his last evaluation Michael showed at age 8, Borderline Intellectual Functioning as defined by the Wechsler Intelligence Scale for Children-III, in the following areas: visual-motor coordination, non-verbal abstract thinking and capacity for new learning. In addition, he was diagnosed with a speech and communication disorder and post-traumatic stress disorder.

Michael's family was unable to sustain the stress of his trauma, and the parents later divorced. At the time of the accident, the father was overwhelmed with guilt and he withdrew emotionally from the family, unable to provide support for his wife and older son. Michael's mother also withdrew from everyone in the family, and just focused on helping Michael survive, staying with him every single day at the hospital for 6 months. Dennis, Michael's older brother, who witnessed the accident at age 4, was left with an aunt and did not receive any psychotherapy service until age 9, whereupon he began manifesting suicidal ideation at school.

Michael is currently still struggling with the complex physical and psychological Sequelae to his trauma. He continues to have difficulty walking, which hampers his ability to participate in sports or be more active; he continues to complain of headaches, dizziness, difficulty breathing and he speaks in a raspy low and slow voice, which prompts classmates to make fun of him. Michael is acutely aware he is different than other children, and lacks a positive self-image. Yet, as a result of all the varying therapeutic services he has received, and the resilience thus fostered, Michael is extremely motivated to improve his cognitive and social skills, as attested by teachers' reports. Michael has learned that in some things, "practice makes almost perfect." Encouraging Michael to identify and reinforce his areas of competence will undoubtedly improve his resilience and ability to cope, particularly as he enters pre-adolescence and socialization with peers and sports takes on a heightened significance.

Michael's parents have had difficulty accepting their son's limitations, and inadvertently have forced him to participate in activities for which he is not equipped to handle, thereby further decreasing his already low self-concept. In trying to foster resilience for his parents, the clinician recommended their participation in a support group with other parents in similar situations. The goal was for them to learn to accept their son's limitations and to set realistic goals for him, which hopefully will help him have a more positive self-concept.

Michael's case illustrates the double jeopardy of the Early Intervention Programs, which target the medically handicapped child, but at the exclusion of other family members who may need services as well. There is no doubt that Michael's life was saved by the quick and expert medical treatment given to him at a Specialized Trauma Center immediately following the accident. Further, Michael's ability to adapt to his severe trauma was clearly fostered by the comprehensive and intensive medical services as well as by the psychological services he was provided with through the auspices of the Early Intervention Programs. As a result, Michael's cognitive and intellectual functioning was safeguarded as best possible, under the circumstances. Yet, despite these safeguards, Michael's family was limited in their ability to foster more resilience for him, as they lacked the resources necessary and sufficient in themselves to do so. Thus, it is important to note that in order to foster resilience for the medically handicapped child, it is imperative that the family unit be helped in their process of coping and adapting to the multiple and varying traumas each member may be experiencing, so that they themselves may become resilient.

CLINICAL VIGNETTE 2

Kevin is a 7 year-old boy who has been diagnosed with Attention Deficit/ Hyperactivity Disorder Combined Type, and Mixed Receptive-Expressive

Language Disorder. Previously, Kevin was diagnosed with Plumbism (Lead Poisoning) at age 3, after being found with 24 micrograms of lead per deciliter of blood (24 μ/dl), which is defined as "high." Kevin was treated with iron chelation therapy and referred for a comprehensive educational evaluation. As a result of this evaluation, Kevin was placed in Special Early Education Classes receiving Speech and Language Therapy twice a week.

But as Kevin was becoming more aggressive with classmates his teacher requested a referral for a psychological evaluation. Kevin scored at the Borderline Level on the Wechsler Intelligence Scale for Children-III. He showed moderate difficulties in perceptual organizational skills, a short-attention span, poor impulse control and difficulties in receptive-expressive language skills. As Kevin was an only child, both parents doted on him and had difficulty setting limits and disciplining him. Kevin was referred to a psychiatrist, who prescribed medication, which helped decrease his distractibility and impulsivity, but increased his appetite. Kevin gained considerable weight as a result.

Kevin's parents have had difficulty understanding the extent of their son's cognitive, behavioral and emotional difficulties. The parents were encouraged to become more knowledgeable about their son's medical handicap and to acknowledge their sense of loss at not having the child they had wished for. The parents grieved, not just for their sense of loss, but also for the hardships they imagined their son would have throughout his life. The parents were also encouraged not to compare Kevin to other children, but help him keep track of his targeted areas of competence, appreciating his uniqueness and fostering a positive self-concept. In other words, they were encouraged to compare Kevin to himself, along a horizontal-developmental line and not with others on a vertical competitive plane.

This case, once again, illustrates the importance of the existence of an early intervention program on fostering resilience and maximizing adaptive coping skills to a medically handicapped child, early in life. As Kevin attended public school, he had access to special education assessment and instruction, behavior management counseling, and speech therapy. However, the school was not able to provide Kevin's parents with constructive ways to build better coping skills and foster resilience for the child and the family. School systems, already overburdened with multiple demands, typically refer the family to healthcare workers, hoping the parents will comply and receive such family counseling. Thus, it is important that the school system incorporate educational and counseling strategies and to work in tandem with the family and any corollary healthcare agencies involved in order to foster resilience for the medically handicapped child and their family.

The last two clinical vignettes demonstrated how a medically handicapped child benefited from being referred to a comprehensive intervention program, which provides medical, educational and psychological services funded by the government via school and/or community agencies. However, fostering resilience for a child not eligible to receive these services poses greater challenges for the healthcare delivery system.

SPECIAL ISSUES FOR THE NON-MEDICALLY HANDICAPPED CHILD, WHO MAY BE "AT-RISK"

The child who has not been diagnosed medically handicapped and has not been certified to be in need of special education services, may not have access to a comprehensive intervention program. No matter how "at-risk" this undiagnosed child may be, the probability is that, the undiagnosed child is provided with minimal services or, in the worst-case scenario, with no services. In these cases the financial responsibility to provide adequate care falls on the parents. If the parents have health insurance, some of the services may be partially covered. If the parents do not have health insurance and do not qualify for government assistance, the child may not receive any services.

The existence of this gap in provision of services at the level of the school care system led to the development in the early 1990's of school-based mental health services geared toward including the "non-special education child" (Ferran & Maluf, 1991). Simultaneously, intensive community-based family centered services such as Family Support Programs and Respite Programs were initiated at the state level to improve the coping skills of families with an "at risk" as well as with a medically handicapped child (State Office of Mental Health, 1990). These programs were designed to strengthen the environmental protective factors of the "at risk" and the medically handicapped child, and to foster adequate coping skills and resilience to child and family by providing a systemic intervention model integrating school and community resources.

More recently, however, as health and mental healthcare services have become less available and more expensive, parents with a child suffering from severe emotional and behavioral problems needing intensive or repeated psychiatric hospitalizations are finding it impossible to finance their child's care. In cases where the parents could finance the hospitalizations, the number of hospital beds available is limited. For example, in New York City, according to recent estimates by Officials at the Administration for Children's Services, almost "half of their intensive-care beds are filled not by abused or neglected youngsters, but by those placed there directly by their parents or through a court program for troubled youths that parents enter voluntarily" (Dewan, 2003, p. 35).

In many states, insurance companies have a maximum lifetime premium designated to reimburse for mental health care, contrary to other medical services that may not have such a limit. Once this maximum lifetime reimbursement premium for mental health is reached, parents must pay out-of-pocket for any additional mental health care needed by their child. Thus, some parents in states whose insurance does not provide mental health reimbursement equal to other medical reimbursement (Mental Health Parity), are opting to place their child temporarily in foster care in order to increase the opportunities of having their child properly treated. Since the number of beds available to children are higher in foster care, parents reason that by placing their child temporarily in foster care, they will increase their child's access to the comprehensive, yet expensive mental health services they cannot afford, and whose insurance company has denied reimbursing (Dewan, 2003).

As the non-medically handicapped or "at risk" child reaches adolescence, the chance of being classified as needing to receive special services diminishes. These chances become almost non-existent as the adolescent approaches young adulthood.

The following clinical case vignette illustrates the complexity of fostering resilience in an adolescent who is about to become a young adult and is in need of intensive care treatment. This case also highlights how the established modes of service care available were inadequate in meeting the treatment needs of the adolescent.

CLINICAL VIGNETTE 3

Donna was a 16 year-old adolescent who had been shown throughout her academic history to have mild learning problems, but had never been diagnosed to warrant any services, except for receiving tutoring in reading, which she received in school. Donna was the youngest daughter in a family of three high achieving male siblings. Her parents had divorced when she was 6 years old, and her father subsequently died when she was 11 years old. The circumstances of her father's death were questionable, and thought to possibly have been a suicide. Her male siblings reportedly had not been close to their father, a point of tension between her and her brother, whom she felt might have envied the special relationship she had with her father because she was his "little girl." Her mother had remarried when Donna was 9 years old, but reportedly she was not close to her stepfather. Donna suffered from asthma since the age of 4 and had been hospitalized for this condition numerous times.

Toward the end of her junior year in high school, Donna began to show truancy at school, staying out at night until the next morning. Her academic grades, which were always below average, worsened and she had to attend summer school. Donna barely attended summer classes and her truancy worsened, staying out for days at a time without the family knowing her whereabouts. Upon returning home, her mother would fight with her, prompting Donna to leave again. Her brothers were angry with her as well and sometimes taunted her for not being "smart."

Although Donna had some school friends, she was not close to anyone, and she felt very alone. She made her first suicide attempt by taking an overdose of an over-the-counter medication. Donna's mother took her to the hospital where her stomach was pumped and she was admitted to the in-patient unit for a two-day observation period. She was discharged from the hospital with a referral to a psychiatrist. Both Donna and her mother consulted with the psychiatrist, who recommended psychotherapy for Donna.

At the beginning of her senior year, her academic grades were so poor; she was advised she might have to repeat the year. This prompted Donna to begin to cut her arms and legs, truancy augmented and she made her second suicide attempt. This time she was hospitalized at a private psychiatric hospital paid by the mother's health insurance. Donna received pharmachotherapy as well as intensive individual, family and group therapy.

Following this initial in-patient hospital stay, Donna was referred to a Day Treatment Program at the same hospital, which she attended with the help of a bus that transported her from home to the hospital. Donna attended this program for one month, during which time she was classified as a special education student for the first time and received special education instruction at the facility. Upon discharge, Donna was referred to a treating psychiatrist affiliated with the hospital and Donna returned to school. The school placed her in regular classes and did not classify her as a student needing special education classes. Nonetheless, Donna's guidance counselor met with her twice a week in order to help her with the transition back to school from Day Treatment Program.

Donna continued having learning difficulties and problems adjusting to her classes and was advised she may not be graduating with her class. Donna became increasingly ashamed about not graduating with her peer group and this shame made her feel in turn more inadequate and incompetent. Despite being in psychiatric treatment Donna continued to cut herself and was not always compliant about taking her medications. Donna was never classified as a special education student, despite her having learning difficulties and severe emotional problems. Instead, she continued receiving tutoring and graduated, despite very low grades. Upon graduation, Donna's perspectives were more dim, as she had not been accepted at the local college, had no employable skills and her depression and asthma made it difficult to sustain a work schedule. Although she was accepted at a two-year community college, Donna's depression and suicidal tendencies made it quite difficult for her to attend regularly.

By the time Donna was 20 years old, she had made multiple suicide attempts, each time being hospitalized for short periods of time, all of which were financed by her mother's health insurance. By age 21, Donna had used the maximum benefits allowed in her mother's insurance, leaving Donna few options. Her psychiatrist recommended Donna apply to the Office of Disability Determinations in order for her to receive Supplemental Security Income (SSI) benefits and also to the State Office of Vocational and Educational Services for Individuals with Disabilities, the latter being affiliated with the State Education Department to help people with disabilities, and deemed eligible for vocational rehabilitation services, find and keep a suitable employment.

The process of applying and keeping the appropriate appointments with the specialists appointed by these institutions as well as documenting the need for intensive care was a difficult endeavor for Donna to go through without the support and back-up of an advocacy group or agency. Donna's applications to both agencies were denied and she was only able to remain temporarily employed in menial jobs for no more than 3 months at a time. Donna continued to live at home with her mother, who also provided financial assistance. She continued her psychiatric treatment and pharmachotherapy, but her depression and suicidal ideation continued unabated.

By the time she was 25 years old, Donna was referred and accepted to an intensive outpatient Day Treatment Program specializing in Borderline Personality Disorders. There she reported for the first time a history of sexual abuse perpetrated by her stepfather, starting at the age of 14. Donna's mother divorced her husband and has been supportive of her daughter's recovery, paying herself for Donna's insurance premiums and additional psychotherapy fees.

Donna continues to attend her intensive psychotherapy, struggles with her symptoms of self-mutilation, depression and suicidal ideation. However, as a result of the intensive Day Treatment care she is currently receiving, she has been able to maintain attendance at a two-year community college, and is hopeful of completing her studies.

Donna's case illustrates how precarious the school and healthcare systems are when providing for a medically handicapped youngster who may not be officially designated so, either because their handicap does not meet the established criteria for such diagnosis or the modes of services available are inadequate to their needs (Kernberg, Selzer, Koenisberg, Carr & Appelbaum, 1989). Furthermore, this case highlights how the period from adolescence to young adulthood is a critical transition period, where fostering resilience ought to be imbedded in the school and healthcare systems.

SUMMARY

In summary, the following environmental factors need to be addressed when conceiving of a model designed to promote resilience in the family of a medically handicapped or "at-risk" child. Environmental support given the medically handicapped child needs to be mediated by the parent's involvement. This involvement would allow the parents the opportunity to explore the perception of their child's handicap. Further, parental expectations need to be realistic and commensurate with their child's limitations.

As Masten (2001) has noted, it is critically important that cognition and intellectual functioning be preserved, since the research indicate that these variables are crucial for the rehabilitation of the medically handicapped child. Masten (2001) further noted that the child's self-concept, level of motivation and self-regulation skills most efficiently develop through a positive interpersonal interaction with competent and caring adults.

The medically handicapped child is often fraught with multiple or comorbid diagnostic medical and/or psychological disorders, which warrants a systemic implementation of comprehensive treatment modalities. This systemic implementation avoids compartmentalizing the disorders and provides inclusive support at the medical, academic, psychological and financial levels.

The parents of a medically handicapped child may not be able to withstand the stress of coping with the special needs of their handicapped child. Marriages are overly burdened and often dissolve, creating further stressors for the family of the handicapped child. Thus, in order to foster resilience for the medically handicapped child, it is imperative that the family unit be helped in their ability to adapt and be resilient to the multiple traumas each member of the family may be experiencing. It is also important that the school system incorporate educational and counseling strategies for working in tandem with the family and any corollary healthcare agencies involved.

When a non-medically handicapped or "at-risk" child reaches adolescence the chances of being classified as needing to receive special services diminishes, becoming almost non-existent as the adolescent reaches young adulthood. The school and healthcare systems are particularly inept when providing for a medically handicapped youngster who may not be officially designated so, either because their handicap does not meet the established criteria for treating diagnoses, or the modes of services available are inadequate to their need. Thus, the period from adolescence to young adulthood is a critical transition, where fostering resilience ought to be reinforced and imbedded as part of the school and healthcare systems.

Despite the gaps and inconsistencies existent in providing or fostering resilience, even small interventions aimed at strengthening the adapting and coping skills of a medically handicapped child, when given at developmentally critical points in a child's life, has the rippling effects necessary to help child and family survive multiple adversities. Thus, although as healthcare providers, we always aim to provide comprehensive and optimal care, the notion of fostering at least "good enough resilience" factors should motivate us to be hopeful and positive about our own ability to be resilient in coping with the myriad adversities of our own unique system of delivery of care.

REFERENCES

Albee, G.W. (1982). Preventing psychopathology and promoting human potential. *American Psychologist*, 37, 1043–1050.

American Psychiatric Association. (1994). *Diagnostic And Statistical Manual of Mental Disorders (4th ed.).* Washington, D.C.: Author.

Blosser, J.L., & DePompei, R. (1994). Planning school reintegration for a child with traumatic brain injury. In A.T. Dikengil, S. Morganstein, M.C. Smith, & M.C. Thut (Eds.), *Family articles about traumatic brain injury* (pp. 203–206). San Antonio, Texas: The Psychological Corporation.

Brooks, R., & Goldstein, S. (2002). *Nurturing resilience in our children: Answers to the most important parenting questions.* New York: McGraw-Hill.

Brooks, R., & Goldstein, S. (2001). *Raising resilient children: Fostering strength, hope and optimism in your child.* New York: McGraw-Hill.

Canino, I.A., & Spurlock, J. (1994). *Culturally diverse children and adolescents: Assessment, diagnosis, and treatment.* New York, London: The Guilford Press.

Calhoun, L.G., & Tedeschi, R.G. (1999). *Facilitating posttraumatic growth: A clinician's guide.* Mahwah, New Jersey; London, England: Lawrence Erlbaum Associates.

Chatigny, A.L. (1994). Interpersonal skill and relationships: Changes in family roles. In A.T. Dikengil, S. Morganstein, M.C. Smith, & M.C. Thut (Eds.), *Family Articles About Traumatic Brain Injury* (pp. 103–104). San Antonio, Texas: The Psychological Corporation.

Dewan, S.K. (2003). *Parents of Mentally Ill Children Trade Custody for Care.* The New York Times: February 16, 2003, pages 35 and 39.

Dikengil, A.T., Morganstein, S., Smith, M.C., & Thut, M.C. (Eds.). (1994). *Family articles about traumatic brain injury.* San Antonio, Texas: The Psychological Corporation.

Ferran, E., & Maluf, J.M. (1991). *Proposal for a mental health school-based support service to serve junior high school 56 in District I.* Manhattan Borough President's Office and Department of Psychiatry, Governeur Hospital: June 1991.

Fonagy, P., & Target, M. (2002). Early intervention and the development of self-regulation. *Psychoanalytic Inquiry, 22* (3), 307–335.

Frederick, C.J. (1985). Children traumatized by catastrophic situations. In S. Eth, & R.S. Pynoos (Eds.), *Post-Traumatic stress disorder in children* (pp. 73–99). American Psychiatric Association.

Goldston, S.E. (1977). Defining primary prevention. In G.W. Albee & J.M. Joffe (Eds.), *Primary Prevention of Psychopathology, Vol. I: The issues* (pp. 18–23). Hanover, NH: University Press of New England.

Hartshorne, T.S. (2002). Mistaking courage for denial: Family resilience after the birth of a child with severe disabilities. *Journal of Individual Psychology, 58*(3), 263–278.

Hembree, E.A., & Foa, E.B. (2000). Posttraumatic stress disorder: Psychological and psychosocial interventions. *The Journal of Clinical Psychiatry, 61* (7), 33–39.

Katz, M. (1997). *On playing a poor hand well: Insights from the lives of those who have overcome childhood risks and adversities.* New York: W.W. Norton & Co.

Kernberg, O.F., Selzer, M.A., Koenisberg, H.W., Carr, A.C. & Appelbaum, A.H. (1989). *Psychodynamic psychotherapy of borderline patients.* New York: Basic Books.

Levine, P.A. (1997). *Waking the tiger: Healing trauma.* Berkeley, California: North Atlantic Books.

Lewis, G.E. (1994). Motor learning: A primer for caregivers. In A.T. Dikengil, S. Morganstein, M.C. Smith, & M.C. Thut (Eds.), *Family articles about traumatic brain injury* (pp. 31–32). San Antonio, Texas: The Psychological Corporation.

Luthar, S.S., Cicchetti, D., & Becker, B. (2000). The construct of resilience: A critical evaluation and guidelines for future work. *Child Development, 71*(3), 543–562.

Luthar, S.S., & Cicchetti, D. (2000). The construct of resilience: Implications for interventions and social policies. *Development & Psychopathology, 12*(4), 857–885.

Masten, Ann S. (2001). Ordinary magic: Resilience processes in development. *American Psychologist, 56*(3), 227–238.

Milliren, A., & Barrett-Kruse, C. (2002). Four phases of Adlerian, counseling: Family resilience in action. *Journal of Individual Psychology, 58*(3), 225–234.

Munk, B.D., & Maluf, J.M. (1991). *A community based parent/infant therapeutic program.* Paper presented at the American Academy of Child and Adolescent Psychiatry. San Francisco, California: October 17, 1991.

Munk, B.D. (1993). Providing integrated treatment for parent/infant dyads at risk because of parental emotional and mental illness. *Zero To Three, 13*(5), 29–35.

Rutter, M. (1979). Protective factors in children's responses to stress and disadvantage. In M.W. Kent & J.E. Rolf (Eds.), *Primary prevention of psychopathology: Vol. 3. Social competence in children* (pp. 49–74). Hanover, NH: University Press of New England.

Rutter, M. (1990). Psychosocial resilience and protective mechanisms. In J. Rolf, A.S. Masten, D. Cicchetti, K.H. Nuechterlein, & S. Weintraub (Eds.), *Risk and protective factors in the development of psychopathology* (pp. 181–214). New York: Cambridge University Press.

Safer, J. (2002). *The normal one: Life with a difficult or damaged sibling.* New York: Free Press.

Safran, J.D., & Segal, Z.V. (1990). *Interpersonal process in cognitive therapy.* New York: Basic Books.

Sattler, J.M. (1992). *Assessment of children: Revised and updated (3rd Edition).* San Diego: Jerome M. Sattler, Publisher.

Sattler, J.M. (2001). *Assessment of children: Cognitive applications (4th Edition).* San Diego: Jerome M. Sattler, Publisher.

Sattler, J.M. (2002). *Assessment of children: Behavioral and clinical applications (4th Edition).* San Diego: Jerome M. Sattler, Publisher.

Stolberg, S.G. (2002). *Debating diagnosis of a sensory malady in children.* The New York Times: July 9, 2002; (Section F), page 6.

Tedeschi, R.G., & Calhoun, L.G. (1998). *Posttraumatic growth: Positive changes in the aftermath of crisis.* Mahwah, New Jersey; London, England: Lawrence Erlbaum Associates.

Tedeschi, R.G., & Calhoun, L.G. (1995). *Trauma and transformation: Growing in the aftermath of suffering.* Thousand Oaks, CA, US; London, England; New Delhi, India: Sage Publications.

Werner, E.E., & Smith, R.S. (2001). *Journeys from childhood to midlife: Risk, resilience, and recovery.* Ithaca, New York; London, England: Cornell University Press.

Wright, B.A. (1983). *Physical disability: A psychosocial approach* (2nd ed.). New York: Harper & Row.

Chapter 12

Fostering Resilience among Youth in the Juvenile Justice System

KIMBERLY T. KENDZIORA AND DAVID M. OSHER

INTRODUCTION

When one considers "resilient youth," one does not ordinarily think of young people who have become involved in the juvenile justice system. If resilience is the ability to endure adverse conditions without experiencing bad outcomes, then youth who have been arrested or detained would seem to represent the flip side of resilience—those who have succumbed to the kinds of bad choices and chances that can arise from disadvantaged situations. Yet even youth in trouble have strengths and are capable of becoming resilient (Osher, 1996). It is important to recognize that getting arrested is not just a child-driven process. Some children are differentially more likely to be arrested (such as youth with mental health challenges and youth of color), and some offenses, such as running away from an abusive home, may be a sign of personal strength.

Our current political climate favors getting tough on juvenile offenders. Despite a declining percentage of violent juvenile offenders, and in spite of the fact that incarceration is more expensive and less effective than community placements in reducing future delinquency, most U.S. states continue to incarcerate high proportions of arrested children, even for nonviolent offenses (Human Rights Watch, 1999). The task of changing the "get tough" attitude so that it is more in line with evidence-based practices is challenging. Reform must occur both within juvenile justice systems and at the intersection of justice and other child-serving systems in a community, such as mental health, child welfare, and education.

Despite the abundant challenges, pockets of reform are slowly growing in juvenile justice. The mental health prevention and treatment needs of youth in the juvenile justice system have received increasing attention in recent years after decades of neglect (Cocozza & Skowyra, 2000). For example, the federal Center for Mental Health Services has begun collecting data on what mental health services exist in juvenile justice facilities, and the Office of Juvenile Justice and Delinquency Prevention is now funding the development of a model for comprehensive mental health services in juvenile justice.

Because of these recent efforts and incipient reforms, we believe that it is not only sensible but also important and timely to address the resilience of youth in juvenile justice. In this chapter, we introduce the issue of resilience among youth in the juvenile justice system, and review both demographics and trends in juvenile offending, with special consideration of the populations of girls and youth of color in the justice system. Next, we describe the strengths of youth and suggest that the body of research on risk and prevention of problems can be recast into a positive youth development approach that recognizes not only youth strengths, but also family and community strengths. Finally, we describe how systems of care can provide the infrastructure to support the systematic recognition and use of the strengths of youth in the juvenile justice system.

Trends in Juvenile Offending

The latest available statistics on juvenile arrests are from 2000 (Snyder, 2002), when 2.4 million children (8% of the youth population) were arrested. Data based on crime victims' reports indicate that serious violence committed by juveniles was stable from 1973 to 1989, climbed markedly from 1989 to 1993, then dropped 33% between 1993 and 1997 (Snyder & Sickmund, 1999). Arrests for violent crime by juveniles followed this trend, dropping in 2000 to the lowest levels since 1988 (Snyder, 2002).

The preponderance of juvenile crime is nonviolent. In 2000, there were 309 violent crime arrests for every 100,000 youth. In the unlikely event that each of these arrests was a different person, then just 1 in every 320 youth—one-third of 1%—was arrested for a violent crime. In more than 40% of juvenile arrests, the most serious charge was larceny-theft (e.g., shoplifting), simple assault, drug abuse violation, or disorderly conduct. Only 5% of juvenile arrests were for aggravated assault, robbery, rape, or murder (Snyder & Sickmund, 1999). Juvenile property arrests have been generally stable since 1980.

Another dramatic trend in juvenile justice has been the substantial increase in the number of delinquency cases handled by juvenile courts. Between 1987 and 1996, there was a 49% increase in court caseloads, although the general population of juveniles increased only 11%. The bulk of this increase is due to more youth getting arrested, but the arrest rate increased only 35%. In the get-tough environment mentioned earlier, more youth who are arrested are referred to courts. Courts have had to adopt new procedures and programs to handle the increased loads. One trend has been to move sharply toward tougher treatment of juveniles. Between 1992 and 1997, 45 states passed laws making it easier to transfer juvenile offenders to the adult criminal justice system, 31 states increased juvenile sentencing options, and 47 states loosened confidentiality provisions for juveniles (Snyder & Sickmund, 1999).

This trend has been called the "adultification" of juvenile justice (Altschuler, 1999). As Cocozza and Skowyra (2000) indicated, this trend has also forced courts and the juvenile corrections system to address mental health-related issues for youth that had been previously restricted primarily to adults, such as the constitutional right to mental health treatment and mental competency guidelines.

Another adult trend now extending to juvenile justice is the increasing reliance on the justice system to care for individuals with mental illnesses. Just as a mental disorder can contribute to acting-out behavior, so too can a history of unmet service needs. Some youth, especially those who are poor or of color, get in trouble in part because their communities do not provide access to services to address their prior problems, such as physical and/or sexual abuse; parental drug or alcohol use; exposure to poor schools and weak teachers; poor school performance or truancy; family discord; and learning disabilities.

Mental Health Needs Among Youth in the Juvenile Justice System

Youth who have mental illnesses and who are also involved in the juvenile justice system have been referred to as the "turnstile children." They are bounced about among agencies, with mental health saying, "They're too dangerous to keep here " and juvenile justice saying, "They're too disturbed to keep here" (Fagan, 1991). In a 1997 study of 792 youth from the juvenile justice, child welfare, education, and health care sectors, researchers found that the highest rate of mental health issues was found among youth in the justice system and that staff in this system felt unprepared to address these issues (Stiffman, Chen, Elze, Dore, & Cheng, 1997). The typical result has been that these youth remain in juvenile justice placements, with their psychological needs either underestimated or denied.

Prevalence estimates of the rate of mental disorders among youth in the juvenile justice system continue to be troubled to some extent by inconsistent definitions, instruments of unproven reliability and validity, unclear or biased sampling, and over-reliance on retrospective record reviews and other weak designs (Otto, Greenstein, Johnson, & Friedman, 1992). Even with different terms, a fairly consistent picture is emerging. The Northwestern Juvenile Project (Teplin, Abram, McClelland, Dulcan, & Mericle, 2002) assessed a random, stratified sample of 1,829 youth (1,172 males and 657 females ages 10–18) who were arrested and detained in Cook County, Illinois (which includes Chicago). Researchers using a structured interview found that nearly two-thirds of males and three-quarters of females met diagnostic criteria for a mental disorder. Shelton (2001) examined rates of emotional disorder in the Maryland juvenile justice system. She selected a random, representative sample from all 15 of Maryland's juvenile facilities, and administered a validated, structured diagnostic interview to 312 committed and detained youth (ages 12–20 yrs). Fifty-three percent of youth met diagnostic criteria for a psychiatric disorder and 26% indicated a need for immediate mental health services. Two-thirds of those with any mental health diagnosis had more than one mental or substance use diagnosis, a status called comorbidity.

From these and other well-designed prevalence studies that used structured diagnostic interviewing techniques to determine diagnoses (e.g., Atkins et al., 1999; Marstellar et al., 1997; Ulzen & Hamilton, 1998), we can safely conclude that the prevalence of mental disorders among youth in juvenile justice facilities ranges from 50% to 75% in multiple well-designed studies that. Further, youth involved with the juvenile justice system frequently had more than one co-occurring mental or substance use disorder, making their diagnosis and treatment needs more complex.

Developmental Pathways to Delinquent Behavior

When considering how and when to intervene to prevent youth from entering the juvenile justice system and treat those already in the system, both those with and without mental disorders, it is important to understand how delinquency develops. It is widely recognized that there are two types of delinquents: those in which the onset of severe antisocial behavior begins in early childhood and the second in which the onset of severe antisocial behavior coincides with the onset of adolescence (Silverthorn & Frick, 1999). In fact, the diagnostic criteria for Conduct Disorder include Childhood-Onset and Adolescent-Onset subtypes (American Psychiatric Association, 1994).

In almost all cases, adult criminal behavior has a long developmental history, with the variety and intensity of early problems predicting persistence (Robins, 1966, 1978). In the Pittsburgh Youth Study (Stouthamer-Loeber & Loeber, 2002), almost half the boys who eventually became persistent serious offenders had an onset of their serious delinquent behavior by age 12, and two-thirds of the boys who came to the attention of the juvenile court already had behavior problems for at least 5 years. Among those children whose challenging behavior is extreme, the persistence of this behavior tends to be high (Moffitt, 1993). Egeland, Pianta, and Ogawa (1996) reported that 53% of children rated as having acting-out behavior problems by their teachers in kindergarten through third grade met criteria for a disruptive behavior disorder when administered a psychiatric interview at age $17\frac{1}{2}$.

According to Snyder and Sickmund (1999), 81% of male offenders and 94% of female offenders fall outside the "chronic" group, having three or fewer referrals to the juvenile justice system. Thus, the vast majority of offenders fall into the "adolescence limited" or "late starter" groups. And although early conceptualizations of this group of juvenile offenders suggested that they were not disordered and would be likely to resume normal development in adulthood without intervention (Moffitt, 1993), recent research suggests that even late starters may show long-term troubles. Moffitt, Caspi, Harrington, & Milne (2002) reported that both types of developmental patterns of delinquency predicted maladjustment at age 26. The childhood-onset group was worse off than the adolescent-onset group, with elevated mental health problems, substance dependence, financial problems, work problems, and drug-related and violent crime. The adolescent-onset delinquents at age 26 were less extreme but showed elevations in impulsive personality traits, mental-health problems, substance dependence, financial problems, and property offenses.

Early aggressive behavior is by far the most robust predictor of delinquent trajectories (see Broidy et al., 2003), but many other risk factors have been documented. Decades of research have consistently shown the following variables to be associated with serious or violent delinquency (Farrington & Loeber, 2000; Hawkins, et al., 1998; Herrenkohl, et al., 2000; Lipsey & Derzon, 1998; Loeber & Dishion, 1983; Sameroff, Bartko, Baldwin, Baldwin, & Seifer, 1998; Sameroff, Seifer, Zax, & Barocas, 1987):

- Individual factors (high impulsiveness and low intelligence)
- Family factors (parental criminality, poor supervision, harsh discipline, child maltreatment, disrupted families, large family size, and family poverty)
- School factors (academic failure, social rejection by classmates)
- Peer delinquency
- Gang membership
- Urban residence
- Living in high crime neighborhoods

Two caveats to this now-classic list of risks are in order. First, school-related risks are not limited to the individual variables studied in psychological research but rather include a number of systemic risks that have received more recent research attention. For example, Kellam, Ling, Merisca, Brown, and Ialongo (1998) showed that first-grade teachers' poor behavior management skills in the classroom were a major risk factor for aggression in middle school. Other risks in the school environment include poorly trained teachers and aides; reactive and coercive approaches to behavioral management at classroom and schoolwide levels; lack of a strong academic mission and administrative leadership; and a climate of low emotional support (Gottfredson, Sealock, & Koper, 1996; Hawkins, Catalano, & Miller, 1992; Osher, Woodruff, & Sims, 2002; Rutter, 1979).

Additionally, risk factors do not operate in isolation. Rather, they tend to function cumulatively: the more risk factors that children are exposed to, the greater the likelihood that they will experience negative outcomes, including delinquency (Masten & Wright, 1998; Rutter, 1979, 1990; Seifer & Sameroff, 1987).

Gender and Delinquency

Despite efforts over the past decade to increase the representation of girls in studies of antisocial behavior and delinquency, much remains unknown about delinquent girls. Even in very large, cross-site studies, girls' involvement in juvenile delinquency is extremely difficult to predict (Broidy et al., 2003). Despite similarities in the patterns of aggressive behavior over time, girls' absolute level of aggression is consistently much lower than that of boys (Kendziora et al., 2003). Not only are girls *less aggressive* on average (and therefore less likely to engage in antisocial and delinquent behavior), it is also true that *fewer* girls are aggressive. Moffitt and Caspi (2001) reported that boys in the life-course-persistent pattern outnumbered girls by 10 to 1, with only six girls in their sample of 1,037 fitting this developmental pattern. The authors observed that little girls were less likely than little boys to experience the early risks characteristic of the life-course-persistent pattern. In contrast, the male-to-female ratio for the adolescence-limited pattern was only 1.5:1, showing that this type of delinquent pattern was open to both genders.

However, in multiple large studies, researchers have observed a discernible group of girls who display chronic physical aggression throughout childhood. In the cross-site study of aggression and delinquency (Broidy et al., 2003), a small group of aggressive girls was more aggressive than all but the chronically aggressive group of boys. In longitudinal study of 2,451 girls, Hipwell, et al. (2002) found that the subgroup of girls who displayed a wide range of disruptive behaviors was predominantly from the most disadvantaged neighborhoods. Tiet, Wasserman, Loeber, McReynolds, and Miller (2001) found a small group of girls with pervasive conduct problems. For some domains such as stealing, lying, and relational aggression, girls showed at least as many problems as boys. Although girls in general tended to have fewer conduct problems than boys, when they *did* have such problems, the problems were *more* pervasive. This phenomenon has been called the gender paradox (Tiet, Wasserman, Loeber, McReynolds, & Miller, 2001; Loeber & Keenan, 1994).

In keeping with the notion that when girls have problems, they have big problems, Teplin Abram, McClelland, Dulcan, & Mericle (2002) showed that girls who have been detained in the justice system have higher rates of all categories of mental disorders measured. This rate is remarkable when compared with the rates of mental disorder for girls in the general population, which is lower for all disruptive behavior disorders (e.g., boys' rate of conduct disorder is 4.3%, girls' is 1.5%; Costello et al., 1996).

The complex needs of girls who are arrested, combined with increasing numbers of arrests of females, pose a special challenge to the juvenile justice system. Between 1980 and 2000, girls' arrests for all crimes had increased by 35%, whereas arrests of boys declined by 11% in the same time period. In 2000, 655,700 juvenile girls were arrested—28% of all juvenile arrests (Snyder, 2002). Most girls are arrested for non-violent, often drug-related, crimes. Although female offenders are a diverse group, many are children of color, have had significant academic difficulties, have been victims of abuse (physical, sexual, and/or emotional), come from families living in poor and unstable communities, and are substance users. Many have a sexually transmitted disease or other chronic health conditions (Office of Justice Programs, 1998).

Treatment Needs of Girls in the Juvenile Justice System

Most facilities and programs have been designed with boys in mind. Juvenile justice systems need to develop specific programs for girls that focus on building relationships, addressing victimization, and improving self-esteem.

Address Issues of Abuse and Victimization

Prescott (1997) has maintained that abuse—sexual, emotional, and physical—is the most significant underlying cause of high-risk behaviors leading to delinquency in girls. Indeed, more than 70% of incarcerated girls report a history of physical or sexual abuse (Evans, Albers, Macari, & Mason, 1996). As a result of exposure to violence, many adolescent girls in the juvenile justice system exhibit Posttraumatic Stress Disorder (PTSD), with nearly 50% meeting diagnostic criteria for the disorder. This rate surpasses both the general population rate and the rate observed among incarcerated male delinquents (Cauffman, Feldman, Waterman, & Steiner, 1998). In addition, delinquents who suffer from PTSD tend to exhibit higher levels of distress and lower levels of self-restraint (Cauffman et al., 1998).

Girls Need Mental Health Services

Given that girls in detention have higher rates of mental disorders than boys, attending to these issues is critical for remediating the offending behavior. According to the National Mental Health Association (2003a), suicide attempts and self-mutilation by girls are particular problems in juvenile facilities and are ex-acerbated by characteristics of the detention environment, such as seclusion, staff insensitivity, and loss of privacy. Many adolescent girls will not seek mental health treatment or other forms of support for themselves, instead relying on internaliza-tion, avoidance, and self-harm as coping strategies. Juvenile justice personnel and mental health professionals working with these young women must be cautious not to retraumatize girls who have been abused or victimized, while encouraging them to learn appropriate coping strategies and constructively resolve their feelings.

Girls Need Treatment for Substance Abuse

Arrests for drug abuse violations have increased markedly over the past few years for adolescent females (Snyder & Sickmund, 1999); in some cities, nearly 60% to 70% of young women tested positive for drugs at the time of arrest (National Institute of Justice, 1998). Many of these young women may be self-medicating with illegal substances in an attempt to cope with stress or mental health difficulties, such as anxiety or depression. Exposure to trauma and abuse (e.g., sexual abuse and family violence) has been consistently linked to substance use among girls (Prescott, 1997, 1998).

Youth of Color in the Juvenile Justice System

Youth of color are disproportionately represented in the juvenile justice sys-tem. Arrests for boys (but not for girls) varied systematically by race (according to self-report data from the National Longitudinal Survey of Youth; Snyder & Sickmund, 1999). White males (9%) were less likely to have ever been arrested than black males (13%) or Hispanic males (12%). Further, a greater proportion of black males (7%) and Hispanic males (6%) than White males (4%) were arrested more than once. African American youth in particular are overrepresented at all stages of the juvenile justice system (e.g., arrest, court referral, detention), espe-cially with respect to placement in secure facilities (Snyder & Sickmund, 1999). In 1997, African Americans made up 15% of the U.S. population of youth ages 10–17, but accounted for 26% of juvenile arrests, 30% of cases in juvenile court, 45% of cases involving detention, and 46% of cases transferred to adult criminal court (Snyder & Sickmund, 1999).

Although one recent analysis (Pope & Snyder, 2003) examining arrests in 17 states found no direct evidence that a juvenile offender's race affects police decisions to take juveniles into custody for particular charges, many other studies suggest that disproportionalities exist at each decision-making point (MacDonald, 2001; Pope & Feyerherm, 1991; Wordes, Bynum, & Corley, 1994). Whatever the cause, Black, Latino, and Native American youth are more likely to be treated in a manner that moves them deeper into the juvenile justice system.

Youth of color are just as likely as White youth to require mental health services (U.S. Department of Health and Human Services, 2001), but Black youth are less likely to be referred to treatment centers and more likely than their White counterparts to be referred to juvenile justice settings (Marsteller, et al., 1997; Woodruff et al., 1999). One state study found that "Blacks were three times as likely as Whites to have detention center placements rather than hospitalization although there was little difference in prevalence of presenting problems by race" (Sheppard & Benjamin-Coleman, 2001, p. 61).

When African American youth do receive mental health treatment, it is more likely to be due to a juvenile justice referral. The San Diego County Department of Mental Health Services studied 3,962 children and adolescents who received outpatient mental health services; 714 were African American (Yeh et al., 2002). They found that compared with non-Hispanic White youth, African American children and adolescents were more likely to be referred for services by juvenile justice and child welfare agencies and less likely to be referred by their schools. Attaining equity in referral for treatment is important, because once youth of color enter delinquency intervention programs, they fare just as well as White youth (Wilson, Lipsey, & Soydan, 2003).

Osher, Woodruff, and Sims (2002) have argued that the school-based risk factors as well as the failure of schools to identify and appropriately address the needs of African American children functions as a pipeline to the juvenile justice system. Teachers and school staff often respond to these children's behavior in inappropriate and potentially harmful ways. They wrote, "Many African American children with or at risk for EBD [Emotional and Behavioral Disorders] progress from a system of inadequate school-based supports, to suspension to expulsion (or dropping out), to placement into the juvenile justice system" (p. 108).

Treatment Needs of Youth of Color in the Juvenile Justice System

Cultural competence is an essential attribute of all human service systems. It involves both developing culturally appropriate assessment instruments and adequately training mental health and juvenile justice professionals in issues of cultural diversity. Because of the evidence of disparate treatment of youth of color, judges, police, prosecutors, public defenders, probation officers, and other justice staff should have access to regular training in cultural competence and individualized planning.

Because youth of color are more likely than white youth to have their mental health problems identified through the juvenile justice system, they are less likely to undergo a thorough psychological assessment and less likely to receive therapeutic treatment (National Mental Health Association, 2003b). As the Surgeon General reported, the mandate of the nation's health system is to bring services to where the people are—and for many youth of color, that means connecting services to juvenile justice (U.S. Department of Health and Human Services, 2001). Early identification and treatment must be made available to youth and families who come into contact with the juvenile justice system, with diversion into the treatment system an option whenever possible.

STRENGTHS OF YOUTH IN THE JUVENILE JUSTICE SYSTEM

One of the primary limitations of the research literature regarding delinquency has been its focus on children's deficits, with limited attention to their strengths. All children and families have individual strengths that can be identified, built on, and employed to ground effective interventions. Appropriate individualized planning for rehabilitation, which engages youth and their families, can draw out these strengths.

As Osher (1996) noted, all youth, even those involved in the juvenile justice system, search for and desire success. They wish to grow and change; they seek acceptance and want to be considered normal. They need to be valued and want to participate in decision making. These young people can learn to express their needs constructively. They have an ability to thrive when they build rapport, and they can respond positively to those who demonstrate sincere concern for them. They have values, are self-aware, and can exhibit self-control. When provided with the right support—which creates what we might call *resilient contexts* (Osher, Kendziora, VanDenBerg, & Dennis, 1999a)—young people can surpass expectations and overcome barriers. They can be confident, flexible, adaptive, and eager to learn.

In recent years, attention to youths' strengths has grown as part of a movement toward positive psychology and positive youth development. It has been argued that the behavioral sciences have been systematically biased toward negative, problem-focused frames of reference and therefore have failed to explain how most people manage to lead lives of dignity and purpose (Seligman & Csikszentmihalyi, 2000; Sheldon & King, 2001). Hope, wisdom, creativity, courage, spirituality, responsibility, and perseverance have been largely ignored.

Strengths play a central role in positive psychology, which aims not merely to fix problems but rather to identify and nurture people's strongest qualities and talents and help them find niches in which they can live out these strengths (Seligman & Csikszentmihalyi, 2000). Positive youth development rests on the notion that "problem-free is not fully prepared" (Pittman, 1991). Achieving good outcomes requires more than avoiding gangs, drugs, sex, and violence. Social, emotional, and cognitive development must be promoted.

How can social services learn from decades of deficit-oriented research to plan strengths-based interventions? Masten (2001) has argued that to some extent, it may be a matter of reframing our language. She pointed out that most risks, such as poverty, low quality of caregiving, and deviance of the peer network are actually ends on a continuum that has assets on the other side. There are some "pure" risks, such as head injury, and "pure" assets, such as a talent or a special friend. But for the most part, risks and assets are two ends of the same gradient (Kraemer et al., 1997, 1999). "Low risk on a risk gradient indicates high assets in many cases, because of the arbitrary naming of bipolar predictors" (Masten, 2001, p. 228). Some researchers (Jessor, Van Den Bos, Vanderryn, Costa, & Turbin, 1995; Stouthamer-Loeber et al., 1993) have argued that risk and protective factors are distinct and cannot be combined because they are not always related in a linear fashion. In this view, protective factors have independent effects and mediate or buffer the effects of risk on problem behaviors. The debate between these perspectives is not settled and awaits further theoretical and empirical refinement. However, the parsimonious position adopted in this chapter is to accept research grounded in the deficit-based approach as relevant to building the resilience of youth in the juvenile justice system until proven otherwise.

In support of reframing and not discarding research that originated with a deficit focus, Catalano, Berglund, Ryan, Lonczak, & Hawkins (2002) have demonstrated empirically that the same risk and protective factors that predict problem behaviors also predict positive outcomes. Using survey data from representative samples of more than 80,000 students in grades 6–12, they showed that as exposure to risk factors increase, the prevalence of problems such as drug use and crime increase. The same predictors were systematically related to the positive outcomes of academic and social competence. That both positive and problem outcomes are related to the same etiological factors suggests that programs that address these risk and protective factors are likely to enhance positive outcomes and reduce problem outcomes. Indeed, Catalano et al. (2002) generated a list of 25 effective "positive youth development" programs for the U.S. Department of Health and Human Services that were virtually all developed with problem prevention rather than health promotion in mind. The authors remarked, "We find that labeling approaches as risk focused or competence focused cuts off discussion and the possibility of transcendent solutions necessary to help children live up to their potential, both problem free and fully developed" (Catalano & Hawkins, 2002).

Strengths-Based Assessment

Adopting a strengths-based perspective requires having access to the tools for identifying youth strengths. In the intake process for most juvenile justice systems (there is significant local variation), staff must decide whether to proceed formally by filing a petition charging a youth with delinquency or informally by offering services outside the court process. When the youth and his or her family are not contesting the allegations and are willing to participate in a service plan, then strengths-based assessments can be used to construct useful plans that are acceptable and likely to be carried out.

A handful of measures assess family and youth strengths (Early, 2001), but the best-researched measure is the Behavioral and Emotional Rating Scale (BERS; Epstein, 1999). Pobanz and Furlong (2000) reported on their use of the BERS in the process of juvenile risk assessment. Risk assessment, as used in this jurisdiction, refers to the screening of first-time offenders to estimate their likelihood of becoming chronic offenders and to make referrals as appropriate. In a study with 88 youth, the researchers found that the Family Involvement scale of the BERS predicted the completion of the intervention, recidivism, and the seriousness of recidivist offenses. The other strengths factors did not predict outcomes, and the authors speculated that these specific protective factors were not mediators of delinquency.

Involving Families of Youth in the Juvenile Justice System

Families are critical to children's success. Unfortunately, the juvenile justice system has often functioned to separate families from their children and from decision making about their children. There are many reasons for this: the location of facilities, the timing of visitations, security concerns, punishment approaches that include canceling family visits, and parents being blamed for their children's behavior. Still, families frequently prevail in the most hostile circumstances, demonstrate flexibility when dealing with rigid systems, and sacrifice and struggle for their children. When they do, they provide continuity and a needed sense of culture, history, and community—a rich identity. Families are the best nurturers of children, and parents' love for their children is often a family's greatest strength. Families demonstrate an impressive range of other competencies, as well, including abilities to seek help; relate and express empathy; maintain family networks; identify their own strengths and build on them; find success despite obstacles; and realize dreams and hopes if given the tools.

When a youth encounters the juvenile justice system, it is beneficial for both the family and the system to actively involve family members (Osher & Hunt, 2002; Woodruff et al., 1999). For families, involvement can reduce anxiety, enhance self-control, reinforce treatments, coordinate multiple plans (such as an Individualized Education Plan or a child welfare plan of care), and help plan for transition. For the justice system, family involvement can improve outcomes by providing information that is critical to keeping the youth safe and stable. Successful family involvement depends on facilitating family-youth contact as well as family involvement in decision making. This includes supporting family involvement (e.g., modifying schedules or providing transportation) and providing mechanisms to give families valid and consistent information about the process, their rights and options, and what to expect (such as possibly seeing their child in handcuffs and shackles; Osher & Hunt, 2002).

Community Strengths

Another perspective that is important to consider in examining the strengths and resilience of youth in the juvenile justice system is the sociological notion that individual factors alone are insufficient to achieve success—social opportunity is also necessary (Merton, 1968). In a longitudinal study examining parenting and adolescent development in 482 urban families, Furstenberg, Cook, Eccles, Elder, and Sameroff (1999) reported that across all neighborhoods in the study, the great majority of low-income parents were competent caregivers—caring, concerned, invested, and skilled. What varied by level of material resources was parents' capacity to provide opportunities for their children, such as attending parochial or private schools, playing sports, or participating in extracurricular programs. Family success was interwoven in a system of unequal life chances. The authors wrote, "Good parenting appears to be more available than good neighborhoods, good schools, and good social services" (p. 232). Thus, addressing juvenile delinquency requires addressing not just individual but also community strengths (Osher, Kendziora, VanDenBerg, & Dennis, 1999a). Blum and Ellen (2002) wrote that the positive youth development approach is particularly receptive to interventions directed at the community because such comprehensive programs typically involve community residents, clergy, and business people rather than just health professionals.

JUVENILE JUSTICE IN SYSTEMS OF CARE: BUILDING ON YOUTH STRENGTHS

In this chapter, we have seen that although youth crime is declining, more youth are being referred to court and incarcerated (Snyder, 2002). Many of these youth have unrecognized and untreated mental health needs. Currently, the considerable strengths of these youth and their families are ignored as they are treated in an increasingly punitive fashion. However, delinquency is predictable, and many prevention and treatment programs are effective at supporting youth and building their resilience (Osher, Quinn, Poirier, & Rutherford, in press, also see Chapter 22, this volume). The challenge is to find ways to connect these programs and approaches to the youth who can benefit from them in a coordinated fashion.

The way to address delinquency and build resilience is to provide services and supports through community-based, family-focused, and prevention-oriented collaboration. To address the multiple needs of children and their families, these services must be individualized and strengths-based, and they must be available in the multiple environments in which these children live. In the past, care from different kinds of agencies has been conditional, disjointed, poorly coordinated, and agency-driven. However, coordinating and thereby strengthening the disparate services that a community already has in place has proven to be a powerful way to promote youth resilience. These coordinated, collaborative service systems are called "systems of care."

The system of care model is based on three main principles: 1) the mental health service system must be driven by the needs and the preferences of the child and family; 2) the management of services must be within a multiagency collaborative environment, grounded in a strong community base; and 3) the services offered, the agencies participating, and the programs generated must be responsive to children's different cultural backgrounds.

Recent findings from the national evaluation of a federal program to build local systems of care have addressed the issue of whether system of care development is associated with better juvenile justice outcomes. Foster, Qaseem, and Connor (2003) compared youth in the Stark County system of care with youth in Youngstown, Ohio. Using hazard modeling techniques, they found that in the system of care community, entry into the juvenile justice system was delayed or reduced, and recidivism was also reduced. These effects were largest for repeat and serious offenders. Further, Foster and Connor (2002) reported that when the phenomenon of "cost shifting" among service agencies was accounted for, expenditures for juvenile justice were lower in the system of care community than in the comparison site.

Resilient Communities

The ultimate goal in growing resilience is the creation of communities that can themselves buffer the various risks faced by all of its members and foster protective factors through building skills, providing opportunities for constructive activity, and providing opportunities for meaningful relationships. Ultimately, effective responses to youth in the juvenile justice system require progressive community development. Vera Piña, the Clinical Consultant to Wraparound Milwaukee, said,

> This is all leading us into community. Child welfare couldn't do it alone, the courts certainly can't be parents to these kids, probation can't do enough, neither can mental health. Never could. And the schools can't do it alone. So you have the systems . . . and even if all those are working together, they can't really do much without the support and commitment of the community, which is where people live, and are there for their long lives. We need the community to stay in charge of the institutions, not the other way around (quoted in Kendziora, Bruns, Osher, Pacchiano, & Mejia, 2001, p. 23).

Individual resilience alone is an insufficient target because it ignores the social context that is so important in influencing outcomes (Osher, 1998; Osher, Kendziora, VanDenBerg, & Dennis, 1999b). When both elements are combined in a vision of positive youth development, then we can imagine better lives for youth in the juvenile justice system, and better lives for us all.

REFERENCES

Altschuler, D.M. (1999). *Trends and issues in the adultification of juvenile justice.* In P. Harris (Ed.), *Research to Results: Effective Community Corrections.* Lanham, MD: American Correctional Association.

American Psychiatric Association. (1994). *Diagnostic and statistical manual of mental disorders: Fourth Edition, DSM-IV.* Washington, DC: Author.

Atkins, D.L., Pumariega, A.J., Rogers, K., Montgomery, L., Nybro, C., Jeffers, G., & Sease, F. (1999). Mental health and incarcerated youth. I: Prevalence and nature of psychopathology. *Journal of Child and Family Studies, 8,* 193–204.

Blum, R.W., & Ellen, J. (2002). Work group V: Increasing the capacity of schools, neighborhoods, and communities to improve adolescent health outcomes. *Journal of Adolescent Health, 31*(Suppl 6) 288–292.

Broidy, L.M., Nagin, D.S., Tremblay, R.E., Bates, J.E., Brame, B., Dodge, K.A., Fergusson, D., Horwood, J.L., Loeber, R., Laird, R., Lynam, D.R., Moffitt, T.E., Pettit, G.S., & Vitaro, F. (2003). Developmental trajectories of childhood disruptive behavior disorders and adolescent delinquency: A six-site, cross-national study. *Developmental Psychology, 39,* 222–245.

Catalano, R.F., & Hawkins, J.D. (2002). Response from authors to comments on "positive youth development in the United States: Research findings on evaluations of positive youth development programs." *Prevention and Treatment, 5,* Article 20. Article available online at http://journals.apa.org/prevention/volume5/toc-jun24-02.htm

Catalano, R.F., Berglund, M.L., Ryan, J.A.M., Lonczak, H.S., & Hawkins, J.D. (2002). Positive youth development in the United States: Research findings on evaluations of positive youth development programs. *Prevention and Treatment, 5,* Article 15. Article available online at *http://journals.apa.org/prevention/.*

Cauffman, E., Feldman, S.S., Waterman, J., & Steiner, H. (1998). Posttraumatic stress disorder among female juvenile offenders. *Journal of the American Academy of Child and Adolescent Psychiatry, 37,* 1209–1216.

Cocozza, J.J., & Skowyra, K. (2000). Youth with mental health disorders: Issues and emerging responses. *Juvenile Justice, 7,* 3–13. Available online at *http://www.ncjrs.org/pdffiles1/ojjdp/ 178256.pdf*

Costello, E.J., Angold, A., Burns, B.J., Stangl, D.K., Tweed, D.L., Erkanli, A., ,& Worthman, C.M. (1996). The Great Smoky Mountains Study of youth: Goals, design, methods, and the prevalence of DSM-III-R disorders. *Archives of General Psychiatry, 53,* 1129–1136.

Early, T.J. (2001). Measures for practice with families from a strengths perspective. Families in Society: *The Journal of Contemporary Human Services, 82,* 225–232.

Egeland, B., Pianta, R., & Ogawa, J. (1996). Early behavior problems: Pathways to mental disorders in adolescence. *Development and Psychopathology, 8,* 735–749.

Epstein, M.H. (1999). The development and validation of a scale to assess the emotional and behavioral strengths of children and adolescents. *Remedial and Special Education, 20,* 258–262.

Evans, W., Albers, E., Macari, D., & Mason, A. (1996). Suicide ideation, attempts, and abuse among incarcerated gang and nongang delinquents. *Child and Adolescent Social Work Journal, 13,* 115–126.

Fagan, J. (1991). Community-based treatment for mentally disordered juvenile offenders. *Journal of Clinical Child Psychology, 20,* 42–50.

Farrington, D.P., & Loeber, R. (2000). Epidemiology of juvenile violence. *Child and Adolescent Psychiatric Clinics of North America, 9,* 733–748.

Foster, E.M., & Connor, T. (2003). *The public costs of better mental health services for children and adolescents.* Manuscript submitted for publication.

Foster, E.M., Qaseem, A., & Connor, T. (2003). *Can better mental health services reduce juvenile justice involvement?* Manuscript submitted for publication.

Furstenberg, F.F., Cook, T.D., Eccles, J., Elder, G.H., & Sameroff, A. (1999). *Managing to make it: Urban families and adolescent success.* Chicago, IL: University of Chicago Press.

Gottfredson, D.C., Sealock, M.D., & Koper, C.S. (1996). Delinquency. In R.J. DiClemente (Ed), W.B. Hansen (Ed), & L.E. Ponton (Ed), *Handbook of adolescent health risk behavior* (pp. 259–288). New York, NY: Plenum Press.

Hawkins, J.D., Catalano, R.F., & Miller, J.Y. (1992). Risk and protective factors for alcohol and other drug problems in adolescence and early adulthood: Implications for substance abuse prevention. *Psychological Bulletin, 112,* 64–105.

Hawkins, J.D., Herrenkohl, T., Farrington, D.P., Brewer, D., Catalano, R.F., & Harachi, T.W. (1998). A review of predictors of youth violence. In R. Loeber & D.P. Farrington (Eds) *Serious and violent juvenile offenders: Risk factors and successful interventions* (pp. 106–146). Thousand Oaks, CA, US: Sage.

Herrenkohl, T., Maguin, E., Hill, K.G., Hawkins, J.D., Abbott, R.D., & Catalano, R.F. (2000). Developmental risk factors for youth violence. *Journal of Adolescent Health, 26,* 176–186.

Hipwell, A.E., Loeber, R., Stouthamer-Loeber, M., Keenan, K., White, H.R., & Kroneman, L. (2002). Characteristics of girls with early onset disruptive and antisocial behaviour. *Criminal Behaviour and Mental Health, 12,* 99–119.

Human Rights Watch. (1999). *World Report 1999.* New York: Author. Available online at http://www.hrw.org/worldreport99/.

Jessor, R., Van Den Bos, J., Vanderryn, J., Costa, F.M., & Turbin, M.S. (1995). Protective factors in adolescent problem behavior: Moderator effects and developmental change. *Developmental Psychology, 31,* 923–933.

Kellam, S.G., Ling, X., Merisca, R., Brown, C.H., Ialongo, N. (1998). The effect of the level of aggression in the first grade classroom on the course and malleability of aggressive behavior into middle school. *Development and Psychopathology, 10,* 165–185.

Kendziora, K.T., Bruns, E.J., Osher, D., Pacchiano, D., & Mejia, B.X. (2001). Wraparound: Stories from the field. *Systems of Care: Promising Practices in Children's Mental Health, 2001 Series, Volume 1.* Washington, DC: Center for Effective Collaboration and Practice, American Institutes for Research.

Kendziora, K.T., Greenbaum, P.E., Kellam, S.G., Brown, C.H., Vanfossen, B.E., Poduska, J.M., & Ialongo, N. (June 2003). *Gender and age differences in teacher-rated aggression: A longitudinal analysis from first grade to middle school.* Paper presented at the 11th Annual Meeting of the Society for Prevention Research, Washington, DC.

Kraemer, H.C., Kazdin, A.E., Offord, D.R., Kessler, R.C., Jensen, P.S., & Kupfer, D.J. (1997). Coming to terms with the terms of risk. *Archives of General Psychiatry, 54,* 337–343.

Kraemer, H.C., Kazdin, A.E., Offord, D.R., Kessler, R.C., Jensen, P.S., & Kupfer, D.J. (1999). Measuring the potency of risk factors for clinical or policy significance. *Psychological Methods, 4,* 257–271.

Lipsey, M.W., & Derzon, J.H. (1998). Predictors of violent and serious delinquency in adolescence and early adulthood: A synthesis of longitudinal research. In R. Loeber & D.P. Farrington (Eds.), *Serious and violent juvenile offenders: Risk factors and successful interventions* (pp. 86–105). Thousand Oaks, CA: Sage Publications.

Loeber, R., & Dishion, T.J. (1983). Early predictors of male delinquency: A review. *Psychological Bulletin, 94*, 68–99.

Loeber, R., & Keenan, K. (1994). Interaction between conduct disorder and its comorbid conditions: Effects of age and gender. *Clinical Psychology Review, 14*, 497–523.

MacDonald, J.M. (2001). Analytic methods for examining race and ethnic disparity in the juvenile courts. *Journal of Criminal Justice, 29*, 507–520.

Marsteller, F., Brogan, D., Smith, I., et al. (1997). *The prevalence of substance use disorders among juveniles admitted to regional youth detention centers operated by the Georgia Department of Children and Youth Services. Final Report.* Rockville, MD: Center for Substance Abuse Treatment.

Masten, A.S. (2001). Ordinary magic: Resilience processes in development. *American Psychologist, 56*, 227–238.

Masten, A.S., & Wright, M.O. (1998). Cumulative risk and protection models of child maltreatment. *Journal of Aggression, Maltreatment and Trauma, 2*, 7–30.

Merton, R.K. (1968). Social structure and anomie. In R.K. Merton (Ed.), *Social theory and social structure* (pp. 185–214). New York: Free Press.

Moffitt, T.E. (1993). Adolescence-Limited and Life-Course-Persistent Antisocial Behavior: A Developmental Taxonomy. *Psychological Review, 100*, 674–701.

Moffitt, T.E., & Caspi, A. (2001). Childhood predictors differentiate life-course persistent and adolescence-limited antisocial pathways among males and females. *Development and Psychopathology, 13*, 355–375.

National Institute of Justice (1998). *Arrestee Drug Abuse Monitoring Program: 1997 Annual Report.* Washington, DC: Author.

National Mental Health Association (2003a). *Mental health and adolescent girls in the justice system.* Alexandria, VA: Author. Fact sheet available online at http://www.nmha.org/children/justjuv/girlsjj.cfm.

National Mental Health Association (2003b). *Mental health and youth of color in the juvenile justice system.* Alexandria, VA: Author. Fact sheet available online at http://www.nmha.org/children/justjuv/colorjj.cfm.

Office of Justice Programs Coordination Group on Women (1998). *Women in Criminal Justice: Special Report.* Office of Justice Programs: Washington, DC.

Osher, D. (1996). Strengths-based foundations of hope. *Reaching Today's Youth, 1*, 26–29.

Osher, D. (1998). The social construction of being at risk. Introduction to R. Kronick (Ed.), *At-Risk Youth: Theory, Practice, Reform* (pp. iv–xii). New York: Garland Press.

Osher, D., Kendziora, K.T., VanDenBerg, J., & Dennis, K. (1999a). Growing resilience: Creating opportunities for resilience to thrive. *Reaching Today's Youth, 3*, 38–45.

Osher, D., Kendziora, K.T., VanDenBerg, J., & Dennis, K. (1999b). Beyond individual resilience. *Reaching Today's Youth, 3*, 2–4.

Osher, D., Quinn, M.M., Poirier, M.A., & Rutherford, R.B. (in press). Deconstructing the pipeline: Using efficacy and effectiveness data and cost-benefit analyses to reduce minority youth incarceration. *New Directions in Youth Development.*

Osher, D., Woodruff, D., & Sims, A.E. (2002). Schools make a difference: The overrepresentation of African American youth in special education and the juvenile justice system. In D. Losen & G. Orfield (Eds.), *Racial inequity in special education* (pp. 93–116). Cambridge, MA: Harvard Education Publishing Group.

Osher, T., & Hunt, P. (2002). *Involving families of youth who are in contact with the juvenile justice system.* Delmar, NY: National Center for Mental Health and Juvenile Justice. Available online at http://www.ncmhjj.com/pdfs/publications/Family.pdf.

Otto, R.K., Greenstein, J.J., Johnson, M.K., & Friedman, R.M. (1992). Prevalence of mental disorders among youth in the juvenile justice system. In J.J. Cocozza (Ed.), *Responding to the mental health needs of youth in the juvenile justice system* (pp. 7–48). Seattle, WA: National Coalition for the Mentally Ill in the Criminal Justice System.

Pittman, K.J. (1991). *Promoting youth development: Strengthening the role of youth-serving and community organizations.* Report prepared for The U.S. Department of Agriculture Extension Services. Washington, DC: Center for Youth Development and Policy Research.

Pobanz, M.S., & Furlong, M.J. (November, 2000). *Using protective factors to enhance the prediction of negative short-term outcomes of first-time juvenile offenders.* Paper presented at the TECBD Conference.

Pope, C.E, & Feyerherm, W. (1991). *Minorities in the juvenile justice system.* Washington, DC: Office of Juvenile Justice and Delinquency Prevention.

Pope, C.E., and Snyder, H.N. (April, 2003). *Race as a Factor in Juvenile Arrests.* Bulletin. Washington, DC: U.S. Department of Justice, Office of Justice Programs, Office of Juvenile Justice and Delinquency Prevention. Available online at

Prescott, L. (1997). *Adolescent girls with co-occurring disorders in the juvenile justice system.* Delmar, NY: National GAINS Center.

Prescott, L. (1998). Improving policy and practice for adolescent girls with co-occurring disorders in the juvenile justice system. Delmar, NY: National GAINS Center.

Robins, L. (1966). *Deviant children grown up.* Baltimore: Williams & Wilkins.

Robins, L.N. (1978). Sturdy childhood predictors of adult antisocial behaviour: Replications from longitudinal studies. *Psychological Medicine, 8,* 611–622.

Rutter, M. (1979). Protective factors in children's responses to stress and disadvantage. In M.W. Kent and J.E. Rolf (Eds.), *Primary prevention of psychopathology: Vol. 3. Social competence in children* (pp. 49–74). Hanover, NH: University Press of New England.

Rutter, M. (1990). Psychosocial resilience and protective mechanisms. In J.E. Rolf, A.S. Masten, D. Cicchetti, K.H. Nuechterlein, & S. Weintraub (Eds.), *Risk and protective factors in the development of psychopathology* (pp. 181–214). New York: Cambridge University Press.

Sameroff, A.J., Bartko, W.T., Baldwin, A., Baldwin, C., & Seifer, R. (1998). Family and social influences on the development of child competence. In M. Lewis (Ed) & C. Feiring (Ed), *Families, risk, and competence.* (pp. 161–185). New York, NY: Plenum Press.

Sameroff, A.J., Seifer, R., Zax, M., & Barocas, R. (1987). Early indicators of developmental risk: Rochester longitudinal study. *Schizophrenia Bulletin, 13,* 383–394.

Seifer, R., & Sameroff, A.J. (1987). Multiple determinants of risk and vulnerability. In E.J. Anthony & B.H. Cohler (Eds.), *The invulnerable child* (pp. 51–69). New York: Guilford.

Seligman, M.E.P., & Csikszentmihalyi, M. (2000). Positive psychology: An introduction. *American Psychologist, 55,* 5–14.

Sheldon, K.M., & King, L. (2001). Why positive psychology is necessary. *American Psychologist, 56,* 216–217.

Shelton, D. (2001). Emotional disorders in young offenders. *Journal of Nursing Scholarship, 33,* 259–263.

Sheppard, V.B., & Benjamin-Coleman, R. (2001). Determinants of service placements for youth with serious emotional and behavioral disturbances. *Community Mental Health Journal, 37,* 53–65.

Silverthorn, P., & Frick, P.J. (1999). Developmental pathways to antisocial behavior: The delayed-onset pathway in girls. *Development and Psychopathology, 11,* 101–126.

Snyder, H.N. (November 2002). *Juvenile Arrests 2000*. Bulletin. Washington, DC: U.S. Department of Justice, Office of Justice Programs, Office of Juvenile Justice and Delinquency Prevention. Available online through http://ojjdp.ncjrs.org/pubs/general.html.

Snyder, H. & Sickmund, M. (1999). *Juvenile offenders and victims: 1999 national report*. Washington, D.C.: Office of Juvenile Justice and Delinquency Prevention.

Stiffman, A.R., Chen, Y., Elze, D., Dore, P. & Cheng, L. (1997). Adolescents' and providers' perspectives on the need for and use of mental health services. *Journal of Adolescent Health, 21*, 335–342.

Stouthamer-Loeber, M, & Loeber, R. (2002). Lost opportunities for intervention: undetected markers for the development of serious juvenile delinquency. *Criminal Behaviour and Mental Health, 12*, 69–83.

Stouthamer-Loeber, M., Loeber, R., Farrington, D.P., Zhang, Q., Van Kammen, W.B., & Maguin, E. (1993). The double edge of protective and risk factors for delinquency: Interrelations and developmental patterns. *Development and Psychopathology, 5*, 683–701.

Teplin, L.A. Abram, K.M., McClelland, G.M., Dulcan, M.K., & Mericle, A.A. (2002). Psychiatric disorders in youth in juvenile detention. *Archives of General Psychiatry, 59*, 1133–1143.

Tiet, Q.Q., Wasserman, G.A., Loeber, R., McReynolds, L.S., & Miller, L.S. (2001). Developmental and sex differences in types of conduct problems. *Journal of Child and Family Studies, 10*, 181–197.

U.S. Department of Health and Human Services. (2001). *Mental health: culture, race, ethnicity: A supplement to mental health: A report of the Surgeon General*. Rockville, MD: U.S. Department of Health and Human Services, Public Health Service, Office of the Surgeon General.

U.S. Department of Health and Human Services. (2001). *Youth violence: A report of the Surgeon General*. Rockville, MD: U.S. Department of Health and Human Services, Centers for Disease Control and Prevention, the National Institutes of Health, and the Substance Abuse and Mental Health Services Administration.

Ulzen, Thaddeus P.M., & Hamilton, H. (1998). The nature and characteristics of psychiatric comorbidity in incarcerated adolescents. *Canadian Journal of Psychiatry, 43*, 57–63.

Wilson, S.J., Lipsey, M.W., & Soydan, H. (2003). Are mainstream programs for juvenile delinquency less effective with minority youth than majority youth? A meta-analysis of outcomes research. *Research on Social Work Practice, 13*, 3–26.

Woodruff, D., Osher, D., Hoffman, C., Gruner, A., King, M., Snow, S., & McIntire, J. (1999). The role of education in a system of care: Effectively serving children with emotional or behavioral disorders. *Systems of Care: Promising Practices in Children's Mental Health, 1998 Series, Volume III*. Washington, DC: Center for Effective Collaboration and Practice, American Institutes for Research.

Wordes, M., Bynum, T.S., & Corley, C.J. (1994). Locking up youth: The impact of race on detention decisions. *Journal of Research in Crime and Delinquency, 31*, 149–165.

Yeh, M., McCabe, K., Hurlburt, M., Hough, R., Hazen, A., Culver, S., Garland, A., & Landsverk, J. (2002). Referral sources, diagnoses, and service types of youth in public outpatient mental health care: A focus on ethnic minorities. *Journal of Behavioral Health Sciences & Research, 29*, 45–60.

Chapter 13

Clinical and Institutional Interventions and Children's Resilience and Recovery from Sexual Abuse[1]

CAROLYN MOORE NEWBERGER AND ISABELLE M. GREMY

During the past 25 years there has been an explosion of reported cases of child sexual abuse, and heightened concern about its effects on children's subsequent development. Despite this concern, our understanding of the effects of childhood sexual abuse remains limited, in part due to the methodological limitations of much research in this area. Until recently, current knowledge has rested primarily on clinically based descriptive studies and retrospective surveys of adults abused during their childhoods.

Isolated clinical impressions, retrospective interviews of adult psychiatric patients, inconsistent definitions, and surveys limited by high refusal rates and self report of past events can yield a confusing picture as to how sexual abuse affects children. Although studies are not consistent in finding links between particular abuse characteristics and predictable outcomes, most studies report significant associations between a childhood history of sexual abuse and various

[1] Research was supported by grants from the National Center on Child Abuse and Neglect (90-CA-1184), the National Institute of Justice (89-IJ-CX-0034), the National Institute of Mental Health (2T32MH 8265-09), and the William T. Grant Foundation.

deleterious outcomes in children and in adults (e.g., Dinwiddie, Heath, Dunne, Bucholz, Madden, Slutske, Bierut, Statham, & Martin, 2000; Newberger, Gremy, Waternaux, & Newberger, 1993). Longitudinal studies further support the growing evidence that sexual abuse contributes to serious emotional and behavioral problems. (e.g., Brown, Cohen, Johnson, & Smailes, 1999; Johnson, Cohen, Brown, Smailes, & Bernstein, 1999). In contrast, some investigators report few or no effects (e.g., McLeer, Deblinger, Henry, & Orvaschel, 1992).

An issue with many of the studies of sexual abuse outcomes for children lies in their reliance on maternal report. When children's self-reports rather than maternal reports of children's emotional states are used, different findings emerge. Research suggests that mothers report more severe symptoms in their children than their children report for themselves (Newberger, Gremy, Waternaux, & Newberger, 1993). When children report their own feelings, differences between sexually abused children and children in normal populations are less consistently found (Mannarino, Cohen, Smith, & Moore-Motily, 1991).

Perhaps in part due to their own distress, mothers of sexually abused children may over-report their children's emotional distress (Cohen & Mannarino, 1988; Everson, Hunter, Runyon, Edelsohn & Coulter, 1989). Alternatively, children may underreport, and mothers may be more sensitive to their children's emotional states. This interpretation is supported by the preponderance of studies using a variety of methodologies that find both shorter and longer-term emotional effects of childhood sexual abuse. Recent research also reveals that childhood abuse changes the brain in ways that may enduringly compromise emotional stability (Bremner, 2003).

Although particular aspects of victimization, such as the use of force and the relationship of the perpetrator to the child (Cosentino, 1996; Mennen, 1993), and penetration (Mannarino, Cohen, Smith, & Moore-Motily, 1991) have been associated with differences in measures of emotional symptoms, research findings remain unclear concerning the contributions of specific victimization experiences to later pathology and distress (see Beitchman, Zucker, Hood, daCosta, Akman, & Cassavia, 1992). Furthermore, children with comparable experiences have been shown to respond in very different ways (Newberger & De Vos, 1988). Broad categories of childhood stressors, including assault and victimization, appear to be associated with behavioral and emotional symptoms (Tiet, Bird, Hoven, Moore, Wu, Wicks, Jensen, Goodman, & Cohen, 2001). A major recent analysis from the National Survey of Adolescents finds that child sexual abuse is particularly associated with symptoms consistent with Post Traumatic Stress Disorder (PTSD), often accompanied by comorbid conditions (Kilpatrick, Ruggiero, Acierno, Saunders, Resnick, & Best, 2003).

The consensus of the majority of researchers and practitioners in the field is that child sexual abuse is associated with a range of short-term and long-term emotional and adjustment problems, but that not all individuals will be similarly affected (see Paolucci, Genuis, & Violato, 2001). Friedrich (1990) emphasizes that "protective factors" modulate the impact of sexual abuse. Friedrich and other investigators posit that these factors help to explain the resilience of sexual abuse survivors that do not demonstrate serious psychosocial or psychiatric difficulties. Protective factors may include supportive family environments, school success, problem solving skills and positive peer relations (Cohen & Mannarino, 1998). The conceptual framework for this study draws on such approaches to adversity and outcomes that recognize the importance of context and that seek to understand resilience as well as risk (Banyard, Williams, & Siegel, 2001).

Because characteristics of a presumably traumatizing experience provide only limited information about its impact (Garmezy, 1991; Rutter, 1987), we share a belief in the importance of an ecological perspective on the lives of child sexual abuse victims, if we are to understand the various ways that victims respond over time. Events and responses of others following a traumatic experience have important implications for children's resilience and recovery. Several investigators have identified protective and risk factors that buffer and exacerbate the effects of physical abuse on children and the interactive nature of those relationships over time (e.g., Cicchetti, & Rogosch, 2002; Kim, & Cicchetti, 2003). Events following the disclosure of sexual abuse have also been hypothesized to influence the extent to which a child will suffer enduring harm (Banyard, Williams, & Siegel, 2001). The purpose of this study is to examine the formal actions taken by professionals following sexual abuse disclosures—those interventions designed to investigate, protect, prosecute, and treat child sexual abuse and its victims. We are concerned to understand what interventions children receive, which children receive them, and how these interventions influence children's resilience and recovery during the year following children's enrollment in this study.

METHODS

Sample

The sample is comprised of children that had recently disclosed that they had been sexually abused. The disclosures of eligible children had to have been confirmed either through protective service substantiation or confession, and the children could not have major physical or mental disabilities. Forty-nine children age six through 12 and their mothers participated. Thirty-six children (73.5 percent) are White; 10 (20 percent) are African American, and 3 (6 percent) are Hispanic. Thirty-four are female (69.4 percent) and 15 (31 percent) are male, consistent with the gender distributions of other reported sexually abused samples (Finkelhor, 1990). Socioeconomic status is quite evenly distributed in the sample from levels two through five on the Hollingshead Four-factor Index of Social

Status (level 2: 26.5 percent; level 3: 22.4 percent; level 4: 20.4 percent; level 5: 30.6 percent) (Hollingshead, 1979). Please note that on the Hollingshead scale, level one represents the highest social class status; level five the lowest status. The sexual abuse disclosed by the sample appears to be quite severe. For 32 children (68 percent), digital or genital penetration of the anus or vagina occurred. Nineteen children were reported to have experienced anal or vaginal intercourse. Oral sex was imposed on 23 children (47.6 percent). Six children (12 percent) were molested by biological fathers, nine (18.4 percent) by father figures, 11 (24 percent) by other family members, and 16 (36 percent) by known but unrelated perpetrators (baby-sitters, older children, a scout master). Three children (six percent) were molested by strangers. More than half the children (53 percent) were abused by someone from within the family. Nine children were abused by more than one assailant. Duration of the abuse ranged from a single incident to five years. Thirty children (61 percent) were abused more than once, with a mean duration of seven months. Force was either threatened or used on 35 children (71 percent).

Of the forty-nine children enrolled in this study, forty-five (91.8%) participated in the 12-month follow-up. As one child did not complete the full complement of measures required for these analyses, this paper reports data from 44 subjects. Five children were unavailable: four White and one African-American; two male and three female; and one from socio-economic status (SES) level two, one from level three, and three from level five. With all five children, digital or genital penetration of the anus or vagina by a single assailant was reported (one biological father; one other relative; three known but unrelated perpetrators), with a mean duration of 6.8 months. Force was reported against three of the children. There are no significant differences in the distributions of demographic or victimization variables between the original sample and the sample of children completing the study.

Recruitment

We recruited subjects as close to disclosure as possible, but were also concerned to include only children where sexual abuse had been confirmed with reasonable certainty. In Massachusetts, the Department of Social Services (DSS) is required to investigate a report of alleged sexual abuse within 72 hours of the report's being filed and to complete the investigation within seven days. At the time of the first interview, the protective service investigation had been completed for all subjects.

Potential participants were identified from the intake records of the Emergency Department of Children's Hospital in Boston and from four prosecutors' (district attorneys') offices in the greater Boston area. In Massachusetts the DSS refers all substantiated cases of child sexual abuse by law by to the local prosecutor. Mothers of the identified children were sent letters introducing the study and were later contacted by telephone to request their participation. The initial interviews were conducted within two to four months of the children's disclosures in all but a few cases. Seventy-seven eligible families were contacted over a two-year period, and 50 (65 percent) agreed to participate. One family was dropped from the study when new evidence suggested that the child had not been abused. It is important to note that this was not a clinical sample, but a sample recruited from the community of sexually abused children. This made recruitment and follow-up particularly difficult. However, a non-clinical sample avoids a potential overstating of clinical symptoms.

Interviewing Procedures

Two female interviewers with social work, psychology, or special education backgrounds interviewed children and their mothers separately in their homes. Three interviews were administered: at recruitment, and six and 12 months following the initial interview.

Measurement

Data for this report were collected from mothers on demographic characteristics, victimization experiences, and clinical and institutional interventions received by the children and their families. Psychological symptoms experienced by the children were assessed with self-report measures. Please note that as a condition of access to the children in our sample, the district attorneys required that we use only standardized measures and not interview them about their victimization experiences.

Demographic Variables

Background information was collected on the age, gender, and ethnic status of the child, and on the socioeconomic status of the family.

Sexual Abuse Variables

Four characteristics of sexual abuse are assessed: severity of the sexual act(s), use of force, duration of the abuse, and identity of the perpetrator. A severity scale was designed for this study. An expert panel of professionals in the field assigned weights from one to ten to each of several sexual acts. The scores of each act were summed and divided by the number of raters to yield a severity score, which ranges from 0.5 to 7.5. More intrusive acts such as anal or vaginal intercourse are weighted more heavily than acts such as kissing or fondling.

Force is coded into three categories: no use of force; threat of force; and use of force. Duration is defined as the length of time between the first and last abuse incidents. The relationship of the child to the perpetrator is coded as intrafamilial or extrafamilial. Intrafamilial perpetrators include biological fathers, and father figures such as stepfathers or mothers' boyfriends, or uncles, cousins, and siblings. Extrafamilial perpetrators include unknown or known assailants with no familial relationship.

Clinical and Institutional Intervention Variables

Three types of interventions are examined: protective; criminal justice; and mental health. Only contacts in which the child participated are measured for this analysis. This information was gathered from the children's mothers. Protective intervention variables include the number of interviews with protective service social workers, the number of police interviews, and whether or not the child was placed outside the home. Criminal justice intervention variables include the number of district attorney contacts, the number of contacts with a victim witness advocate, and the number of times a child testified in deposition or in court.

Mental health intervention variables include the duration in weeks of mental health contacts (evaluation and/or treatment) between disclosure and the final interview for this study; duration in weeks of mental health contact prior to disclosure; psychiatric hospitalization; and timeliness of the initiation of contact. An onset of treatment scale was constructed with values ranging from zero to 14. A value of zero represents mental health involvement prior to disclosure, one through 12 represents months from disclosure to the first mental health contact during the year following disclosure, 13 represents contact which began later than one year after disclosure, and 14 represents no mental health interventions received. Treatment modality (individual, group, and family) is also assessed.

Children's Emotional Status

Children's psychological symptoms were assessed through two widely-used self-report measures of children's subjective feelings: the Children's Depression Inventory (CDI) (Glascoe & Ireton 1995; Kovacs, 1981); and the Revised Children's Manifest Anxiety Scale (RCMAS) (Reynolds & Richmond, 1985).

The Children's Depression Inventory (CDI) is a 27 item self-report questionnaire. Each item contains three statements, such as: "I am sad once in a while. I am sad many times. I am sad all the time." The child is asked to select the sentence from each group that best describes his or her feelings during the previous two weeks. Statements are assigned a numerical value from zero to two. The higher the numerical value, the more clinically severe the behavior being rated. The depression score is the sum of the values of the statements selected.

The Revised Children's Manifest Anxiety Scale (RCMAS) is a 37 item self-report questionnaire. The child answers yes or no to statements such as: "I worry about what is going to happen." The anxiety score is the sum of positive responses. The RCMAS has been standardized taking into account age, gender, and race. It also contains a lie scale to identify children who over-respond positively to the questions. The standardized T score was used for these analyses. Both scales also have clinical cut-off ratings established by their authors. The validity and reliability of both the CDI and the RCMAS have been extensively studied and demonstrated (Finch, Saylor, & Edwards, 1985). Twelve-month test-retest reliability on this sample is high both for the CDI ($r = .504$, $p < .000$) and for the RCMAS ($r = .406$, $p < .01$). Although maternal reports of children's feelings and behavior were also obtained for this study, these data are not used in this analysis.

Data Analysis

Paired sample t-tests are used to compare children's anxiety and depression scores at the time of the initial interview with their scores at the time of the 12-month follow-up. T-tests are also employed to compare sample means with population norms.

Change over time in children's anxiety and depression scores are measured in two ways: by subtracting scores on the 12-month follow-up from initial interview scores, yielding a change score for the 12 month interval; and by calculating the slope of change, taking into account scores from all three interviews. Because some children were not able to be located for the six-month interview, but were subsequently found in time to complete the 12-month interview, we have not done separate analyses taking into account the wave two data. The slope methodology allows us to evaluate change over time, incorporating all three data points where available, while not losing the nine subjects where only the initial and 12 month interviews were conducted. For each child, the slope of recovery is calculated by fitting a regression line to his or her scores over time (OLS linear regression). If there were no change, the slope of the line would be zero. T-tests are used to determine whether the slopes differed from zero.

Spearman correlations are used to assess the associations of demographic and victimization variables with intervention variables; to examine associations between demographic, victimization, and intervention variables and children's depression and anxiety scores on the initial and the 12-month interview; and to examine associations between demographic, victimization, and intervention variables and changes in children's depression and anxiety scores over the 12-month interval.

Regression analyses are also performed to assess the impact of interventions on depression and anxiety scores over time. Initial anxiety and depression scores are controlled in these analyses due to the correlations between scores on the initial and the twelve-month interviews. Only the 45 children who completed the study are included in analyses examining interventions, their distributions, and their consequences.

RESULTS

Emotional Responses and Recovery

Anxiety and Depression Following Disclosure

At the time of the children's initial interviews, there is evidence that both anxiety and depression are greater than would be normally expected. Although their mean anxiety t score of 52.7 (SD10.7, range: 30–71) does not differ significantly from the mean of 50 expected in a normal population (t = 1.39, p = .17), when the distribution of the scores is examined, ten children (23 percent) are found to have scores above the clinical cut-off level of 63 established by the authors of the measure. In a normal population one would expect ten percent of the children to have scores of 63 or above. Among the children in this sample, then, very high levels of anxiety are found at over twice the rate normally expected.

A similar pattern is found with the children's reported symptoms of depression. Their mean score of 9.57 (SD 6.44, range: 0–32) on the Children's Depression Inventory is not significantly different from the normal mean score of 9 found in nonpsychiatric populations (t = .61, p = .54). However, 13 of the children (27 percent) report levels of depression above the clinical cut-off level of 12, in contrast with an expected 10 percent of a normal population. Overall, 18 of the children (38 percent) report themselves as seriously anxious and/or depressed.

Neither anxiety nor depression scores are related to any of the victimization variables on this first interview. Specifically, there are no discernable relationships between our indices of emotional outcome and the identity of the perpetrator, the severity, or the duration of the abuse, or with the use of force. However, as the age of the child increases, the level of anxiety appears to increase as well (r = .30, p < .04). Additionally, a marginally significant correlation is found between socioeconomic status and depression scores, suggesting that more economically disadvantaged children may suffer greater symptoms of depression (r = .25, p < .09). Regression models combining demographic and victimization variables do not significantly contribute to the prediction of anxiety or depression scores.

Anxiety and Depression Over Time

By the 12-month interview, children were reporting significantly fewer symptoms of anxiety and depression. For example, the mean standardized anxiety score decreased from 52.15 to 44.8. A paired t test reveals that this difference is highly unlikely to have occurred by chance (t = 4.38, p < .001). The mean depression score also decreased significantly, from 9.57 to 7.2 (t = 2.68, p < .05).

When the slopes of change in anxiety and depression scores across the three interviews are calculated, clear declines are found, indicating improvement in the children's emotional states (t = -2.184, p < .04 and t = -4.131, p < .0002 respectively). Not only do both anxiety and depression scores decrease over the one-year interval, 12-month interview mean scores are below the means expected in a normal population (44 percent [SD 9.13] vs. 50 percent [SD 10] for anxiety; 7.2 [SD 5.26] vs. 9.7 [SD 7.3] for depression). On both tests, however, mean scores remain within the normal range of variation. Looking at clinical cutoffs, at the 12-month interview, only two of the children (4.5 percent) have anxiety scores above the clinical level. Depressive symptoms, on the other hand, appear to be more persistent, with seven of the children (16 percent) continuing to report symptom levels within the clinical range. It should also be noted that anxiety and depression scores are strongly intercorrelated on both the initial and the 12-month interviews (z = 2.63, p < .01; z = 3.205, p = .001, respectively), as has been found in other studies (e.g., Kovacs, 1985).

No relationships are found between children's ages, ethnic background, or socioeconomic status and recovery over time. Similarly, no clear relationships emerge between victimization experiences and changes in children's emotional status.

Interventions Following Sexual Abuse Disclosures

The Distribution of Interventions

Despite an overall pattern of improvement, there is considerable variation in children's recovery. In order better to understand this variation, the protective, criminal justice, and mental health interventions that children received are examined.

Protective Interventions. A protective service worker met at least once with a majority of the children (84 percent), averaging four encounters. Thirty-four children (77 percent) met at least once with a police officer, with a mean of two contacts. The physical custody of seven children (16 percent) changed between disclosure and the 12-month follow-up.

Children's ethnic background is strongly associated with placement outside the home (Fisher's Exact Test, p < .011). Of the twelve children of color who completed the study, five (42 percent) had been placed. In contrast, only two of the 32 White children (7 percent) were placed. This relationship remains even when controlling in regression analyses for the other demographic variables and for victimization variables. No relationships are found between protective interventions and any of the victimization variables, or initial anxiety and depression scores.

Criminal Justice Interventions. Although all children in the sample had been referred to their local district attorney's office, not all were seen by a member of the district attorney's staff or culminated in court proceedings. Thirty children (68 percent) had face-to-face meetings with an attorney, averaging three encounters and ranging from one contact to 14. A victim witness advocate, who provides guidance and support to families involved with the criminal justice system, met with twenty-two (50 percent) of the children. Fifteen (34 percent) of the children's cases involved court appearances. Eight children testified once, seven testified two or three times. Both district attorney contacts and victim witness advocacy services are associated with court appearances made by the child ($r = .576$, $p < .0002$; $r = .354$, $p < .03$, respectively).

The social status of the family is significantly related to all three criminal justice variables. Higher social status is associated with more district attorney contacts ($r = -.5$, $p < .001$), more victim witness advocacy ($r = -.386$, $p < .01$), and more court involvement ($r = -.301$, $p < .05$). These relationships remain when victimization and other demographic variables are stratified in regression analyses. Furthermore, relationships between Socioeconomic status (SES) and district attorney contacts, and between SES and victim witness advocacy remains when court testimony is partialled out. In other words, children from higher status homes received more attorney and victim witness advocacy contacts whether or not the case moved into adjudication.

Not surprisingly, age is also related to children's court involvement. Older children testified more frequently than younger children ($r = .301$, $p < .05$). Age is unrelated, however, to district attorney or victim witness advocate contacts, and no other demographic variables are related to any of the criminal justice interventions. One victimization variable is related to involvement in the criminal justice system. If force was used, children had more district attorney contacts ($r = .348$, $p < .03$) and more meetings with victim witness advocates ($r = .36$, $p < .03$). Their cases were not, however, more likely to go to court. Neither the severity of the abuse, its duration, or the child's relationship with the perpetrator appeared to influence the extent of criminal justice involvement. No relationships are found between initial anxiety scores and any of the criminal justice interventions. Initial depression scores, on the other hand, are associated with a greater number of district attorney contacts ($r = .335$, $p < .04$).

Mental Health Interventions. By the 12-month interview, most children in the sample had met at least once with someone identified by the mother as a mental health professional. Of the 44 children that completed the 12-month follow-up, 15 (34 percent) were in outpatient treatment at the time of disclosure and seven (16 percent) received some kind of mental health contact within one month of disclosure. On the other hand, six of the children (13.6 percent) were not seen until more than a year after disclosure and two children (4.6 percent) did not receive any mental health response at all. Among the children that received outpatient mental health interventions, the duration of contact ranged from a single encounter to 258 weeks (for one child who had been in treatment for four years prior to disclosure). The average length of time in treatment following disclosure was 57 weeks (SD 34). Most children were seen individually rather than in group or family therapy configurations.

Ethnic Background and Mental Health Interventions. Several relationships are found between children's ethnic backgrounds and outpatient mental health interventions. Children of color tended to wait longer for an initial contact than did White children (Mann Whitney U $z = -1.795$, $p < .07$), even when social class and severity of the abuse is stratified in regression analyses ($t = 1.918$, $p < .07$; $t = 2.25$, $p < .03$, respectively). This relationship also remains when stratifying for anxiety and depression scores on the initial interview ($t = 2.05$, $p < .05$; $t = 2.13$, $p < .04$, respectively). Children of color also received fewer weeks of treatment following disclosure than did White children (Mann Whitney U, $z = -2.004$, $p < .05$), even though there were no ethnic differences in mental health treatment prior to disclosure. The relationship between ethnic background and duration of treatment remains when controlling in regression analyses for SES ($t = 1.92$, $p < .06$), severity of the abuse ($t = 2.108$, $p < .04$), initial anxiety scores ($t = 2.131$, $p < .04$), and initial depression scores ($t = 2.26$, $p < .03$).

Children of color were also more likely to be psychiatrically hospitalized than White children. Six children were psychiatrically hospitalized at some point during the interval between disclosure and the 12-month follow-up interview. Four of the 12 children of color were hospitalized (33 percent), in contrast to only two of the 33 White children (6 percent) (Fisher's Exact Test, $p = .0385$).

Victimization Variables and Mental Health Treatment. Two victimization variables are associated with outpatient mental health contacts. Children with more severe abuse received more types of treatment ($r = .37$, $p < .02$), and victimization that endured longer is associated with a longer period of time in treatment following disclosure ($r = .459$, $p < .003$). No relationships are found between the use of force or the child's relationship to the perpetrator and any of the outpatient mental health intervention variables. For children who were not in treatment prior to disclosure, no relationship is found between anxiety or depression scores and the timing or duration of outpatient mental health intervention following disclosure. The child's initial mental health status is, however, related to receiving treatment prior to disclosure. The longer a child had been in therapy before disclosure, the less anxiety and depression reported on the initial interview ($r = -.309$, $p = .05$; $r = -.313$, $p < .05$, respectively). Children with more severe abuse were more likely to be hospitalized ($r = .39$, $p < .03$).

The Impact of Interventions on Recovery

In order to examine the impact of interventions on children's anxiety and depression scores over time, we first looked at relationships between specific interventions and children's anxiety and depression scores on the 12-month follow-up interview. Because children's mental health status on the initial interview is closely associated with their scores on each of the subsequent interviews, initial anxiety and depression scores are controlled in these analyses. Relationships are also examined between interventions and changes over time in anxiety and depression scores. Because children with initially higher scores show more decline over the course of the study, initial symptom scores are also stratified in these analyses.

Protective Interventions

The more social services contacts children received, the more anxiety they reported on the 12-month follow-up, when the influence of anxiety scores on the initial interview are partialled out (t = 1.994, p < .05). Social service contacts are also related to increases in anxiety scores over time (t = 1.994, p < .05). Neither custody changes nor police contacts are related to changes in anxiety and depression scores. Furthermore, no relationships are found between depression scores and protective interventions.

Criminal Justice Interventions

No clear relationships are found between anxiety and depression scores at the 12-month interview and contacts with either legal staff or victim-witness advocates at the district attorneys' offices. Nor are there any associations found between these contacts with criminal justice professionals and children's recovery. Of note is a lack of significant relationships between court appearances and anxiety or depression scores at the 12-month follow-up, or with anxiety or depression change over time.

Mental Health Interventions

Several relationships emerge between mental health intervention variables and improvement in both depression and anxiety scores over the duration of the study. Specifically, the earlier the initiation of mental health contact the greater the improvement in depression scores (r = .349, p < .03), and, more marginally, with anxiety scores (r = .286, p < .07). However, nearly one-third of the children in the sample were seeing a therapist at the time of disclosure. When we partial out the effects of treatment prior to disclosure, the relationships between the onset of treatment and changes in anxiety and depression scores no longer reach statistical significance.

The amount of time a child was in treatment, however, is associated with changes in depression scores. The longer a child received mental health services (counting services received both before and after disclosure), the greater the improvement in depression scores ($r = -.304$, $p < .05$). When we examine only the 34 children who were not in mental health treatment at the time of disclosure, the relationship between the duration of treatment and improvement in depression scores, although weakened, remains ($r = -.291$, $p < .07$). There is no association between treatment duration and changes in anxiety scores.

DISCUSSION

It is puzzling that on the initial interview, children's mean anxiety and depression scores were not significantly higher than published norms. This pattern has also been observed by other investigators of child sexual abuse outcomes using both maternal report and child self-report measures (e.g., Mannarino, Cohen, Smith, & Moore-Motily, 1991). When the distribution of scores is examined, however, greater than twice as many children as expected report symptoms at the higher end of the range. In contrast, there is no overrepresentation at the extremely low end. This skewing of the distribution toward the higher values suggests that with a larger sample, significant differences might have been found between sexually abused children and normal populations.

Discrepancies between our findings that sexual abuse variables do not predict depression and anxiety scores and some other studies' findings of relationships between specific sexual abuse variables and elevated symptomatology warrants further investigation. In our previous analysis comparing maternal reports of children's symptoms on the CBCL and children's self-reports of depression and anxiety, we found that, in contrast with the children's self-reports, mothers' reports of symptom severity are associated with the identity of the perpetrator and the severity of the victimization (Newberger et al., 1993). Further, we found that maternal reports of children's symptoms are associated with their own, but not with their children's, self-reports of psychological distress. This suggests the importance of the source of information when assessing children's emotional states. In studies linking specific victimization variables with maternal reports of their children's symptoms, relationships may be at least in part an artifact of maternal report.

The improvement seen in children's anxiety and depression scores over the one-year time frame of this study is a welcome finding, and is consistent with other short-term longitudinal studies (e.g., Runyan, Everson, Edelsohn, Hunter, & Coulter, 1988). The majority of longer-term studies, on the other hand, report higher levels of dysfunction among individuals with sexual abuse histories than among comparison populations (see Fergusson & Mullen, 1999). It is noteworthy that symptom improvement in our sample is not related to characteristics of the sexual abuse. This finding points to the importance of examining other factors that may contribute to risk and to resilience, including professional responses after disclosure as potential moderators of the effects of victimization experiences.

Our data suggest that several interventions influence children's anxiety and depression over time. Protective service visits, for example, are associated with higher anxiety at the 12-month follow-up. However, children who received more protective service contacts were also more likely to be placed outside the home, with its additional mental health risks (Lyon et al., 2000). With this small sample it is not possible to tease apart the emotional toll expected by placement from the affects of social worker involvement with the child and family. Mental health interventions, on the other hand, appear to be beneficial for the children in this study as well as other studies (King et al., 2000). The earlier children began treatment prior to and following disclosure and the longer they were in treatment (and evaluation), the greater the reduction in depression scores. When we examined separately the children who had not received treatment prior to disclosure, the length of time in treatment continued to predict psychological improvement.

We do not find differences in outcome as a consequence of the type of therapy received, perhaps because only a few children received family or group treatment and for all but one child these modalities supplemented individual therapy. Although mental health treatment cannot definitively be said to be a causal factor in improved outcomes, it certainly signals a more positive outcome. More troubling is the strong correlation between race and a child's chance of ever entering into therapy. Tingus and her colleagues report a comparable finding in their study of factors associated with entry into therapy for children evaluated for sexual abuse. White children between the ages of seven and 13 were most likely to receive therapy (Tingus, Heger, Foy, & Leskin, 1996).

Within the criminal justice system, not surprisingly, children whose abuse involved force and who were older were more likely to be involved in prosecution. More surprising is the finding that criminal justice involvement was also greater for children from families with higher social class status than for children from lower social class backgrounds. In part this may reflect reluctance among poorer families to become involved with a system they may not trust to help them. However, even among children whose cases were prosecuted, children from lower status families received fewer victim witness advocacy contacts, which support families through the court process. This suggests that poorer families may not be receiving the support they need to cope with and to participate more fully in bringing their children's cases to court, a process that may be beneficial (Runyan et al., 1988).

Racial differences are also noted for both protective and mental health interventions. Compared to White children, children of color were more likely to be placed outside the home, to receive later and less outpatient therapy during the time frame of this study, and were more likely to be psychiatrically hospitalized. These differences cannot be explained by other demographic variables, by initial mental health status, or by differences in victimization experiences. At the 12-month interview, the mothers whose children had not received mental health attention were asked to explain the reasons. They reported that either they had not been referred to such services or, in one case, a Latina mother could not communicate with her English-speaking social worker. An African-American mother, distraught about her daughter's deepening depression following a gang rape, asked the interviewer to help her find a therapist for her daughter. Had she not been a participant in this study, she would not have known where to turn. These troubling findings are consistent with a growing body of research revealing that children of color are over-represented in foster care (Garland, Ellis-MacLeod, Landsverk, Ganger, & Johnson, 1998), and under-represented as recipients of mental health services (U.S. Department of Health and Human Services, 2001).

One unavoidable possibility is bias in response to populations from different ethnic backgrounds (Snowden, 2003). In a recent study of caseworker assessment of parental attachment, White caseworkers gave African American mothers more negative assessments than they gave White mothers. African American caseworkers did not exhibit a similar bias (Surbeck, 2003). There is also considerable evidence that the mental health system discriminates against children of color (U.S. Department of Health and Human Services, 2001). In a study of juvenile offenders, for example, race (as well as gender and marital history of the parents) predicted whether an adolescent was placed in the juvenile justice or the mental health system, with Black adolescents overrepresented in the juvenile justice system (Westendorp, Brink, Roberson, & Ortiz, 1986). Personality/psychopathology variables, on the other hand, did not predict in which system a youth would be placed.

Another possibility is that racial groups differ in their needs for mental health and protective services. There is some support for this theory in studies reporting higher levels of depression among both Black populations (Carter, 1974) and Latino populations (Sanders-Phillips, Moisan, Wadlington, Morgan, & English, 1995) than among other population groups. However, differences in the interpretation of diagnostic criteria often result in more severe diagnoses for minorities (Wade, 1993). The more plausible difference in need is in the direction of greater, rather than less, need. About 12 percent of all children are estimated to have a diagnosable mental illness, and only about one-third of these children receive any treatment. With minority children, however, about 20 percent are estimated to be burdened with serious emotional problems, and an even smaller percentage of these children receive treatment. These findings suggest an enormous reservoir of children, and especially minority children, in need, and would argue for more, rather than less, mental health attention for children of color.

Among children at risk are those that have been sexually abused (Dinwiddie, et al., 2000; Institute of Medicine, 2003). Yet in a record review of over 200 reported cases of sexual abuse, Adams-Tucker (1984) found that only 12 percent of the children received psychiatric referrals, with Black boys least likely to be referred and White girls most likely to be referred. We believe that minority children who are sexually abused and do not receive mental health services experience a triple burden: they are at risk because they have been sexually abused; they are potentially more vulnerable to adverse mental health consequences following trauma because of higher rates of preexisting mental health problems; and they are less likely to receive mental health treatment following the disclosure of their abuse.

If there are social class and racial differences in how sexually abused children are treated, then those differences are likely to be seen in greater and greater disparities in mental health functioning between poor and privileged, and between White and minority children who share this particular risk. These findings are also of concern in light of current trends toward managed care and limitations on the amount of treatment children are permitted to receive. A national survey conducted by Consumer Reports on mental health effectiveness indicates that longer-term therapy is more beneficial than short-term treatment (Consumer Reports, 1995). This lends additional support to our findings suggesting that sexually abused children require longer-term treatment for recovery. Yet in a rationed system, children whose parents do not have the resources to purchase private services are unlikely to receive the treatment they need.

The findings of this study are of great concern. They add to the growing literature on racial and ethnic bias in the systems that purportedly serve children and families in our country. There may be many reasons for this bias, not all intentional, but bias can also be indirect, unintentional and ambivalent (Snowden, 2003). Whatever the reasons for bias, its effects are unacceptable. Our findings also offer hope, however, as the sexually abused children in our sample appear to respond positively to therapy. On both counts, children of color appear to be short-changed.

The findings reported in this study must be viewed as preliminary, for several reasons, including the relatively small sample size and lack of a normative comparison group. Furthermore, the one year follow-up period does not allow us to monitor the termination points of ongoing interventions, to identify children who receive interventions after the study is over, and to identify longer-term intervention effects. As with any longitudinal study, the possibility of regression to the mean must also be of concern. For that reason, we chose to collect data at three points in time, thereby lessening the possibility that longitudinal change could represent a regression effect. In addition, the lack of a control group and methodological limitations of correlation allow us only to suspect the causal benefits of mental health services related to outcome.

This study raises many questions for future research. Our findings of discrepancies between maternal and child reports of children's symptoms suggest how vulnerable research findings are to methodological realities. There has been to date insufficient attention to how methodology affects the conclusions drawn from sexual abuse research. An analysis of the impact on empirical research findings of particular methodological choices, such as sample sources, measurement tools, and informants would help clarify both the nature of sexual abuse outcomes and appropriate methodologies for the study of this complex phenomenon.

The content of sexually abused children's experiences only begin to be explored in this study. As described above, one condition of access to this study's sample was that the children not be interviewed about their sexual victimization. An exploration in future research of children's phenomenological experiences of victimization and the interventions that follow would provide critical new information on how children construct their experience and the relation between those constructions and child outcome. Research on the cognitive mediation of aggression suggests that it is the meaning that children make of events, rather than the events themselves, that exerts influence on the child (Dodge, Bates, & Pettit, 1990).

Another area for continued research is in the further examination of racial and social class differences in the provision and utilization of interventions for sexually abused children. Our hope is that future research will continue to explore reasons for demographic differences in interventions sexually abused children receive, such as accessibility and availability of services, acceptability of services to people from different backgrounds, and ethnic or social class biases on the part of providers toward diagnosis, parental compliance and family safety, and the value of investing resources.

Despite the limitations of this research, the issues raised by these findings are of great importance for the health and welfare of children and consequently for practice and policy, particularly at a time of major cutbacks in programs for children. We believe that it is urgently important to examine how services are delivered to children, the beneficial and harmful impacts of those services, and to ensure that all sexually abused children receive the interventions they require to enable as complete a recovery as possible.

REFERENCES

Adams-Tucker, C. (1984). The unmet psychiatric needs of sexually abused youths: Referrals from a child protection agency and clinical evaluations. *Journal of the American Academy of Child Psychiatry, 23*, 659–667.

Banyard, V.L., Williams, L.M., & Siegel, J.A. (2001). The long-term mental health consequences of child sexual abuse: an exploratory study of the impact of multiple traumas in a sample of women. *Journal of Traumatic Stress, 14*, 697–715.

Beitchman, J.H., Zucker, K.J., Hood, J.E., daCosta, G.A., Akman, D., & Cassavia, E. (1992). A review of the long-term effects of child sexual abuse. *Child Abuse and Neglect, 16*, 101–118.

Bremner, J.D. (2003). Long-term effects of childhood abuse on brain and neurobiology. *Child and Adolescent Psychiatric Clinics of North America, 12*, 271–292.

Brown, J., Cohen, P., Johnson, J.G., & Smailes, E.M. (1999). Childhood abuse and neglect: Specificity of effects on adolescent and young adult depression and suicidality. *Journal of the American Academy of Child and Adolescent Psychiatry, 38,* 1490–1496.

Carter, J.H. (1974). Recognizing psychiatric symptoms in black Americans. *Geriatrics, 29,* 95–99.

Cicchetti D., & Rogosch F.A. (2002). A developmental psychopathology perspective on adolescence. *Journal of Consulting and Clinical Psychology, 70,* 6–20.

Cohen, J.A., & Mannarino, A.P. (1988). Psychological symptoms in sexually abused girls. *Child Abuse & Neglect, 12,* 571–577.

Consumer Reports. (1995). *Mental health: Does therapy help?* November, 734–739.

Cosentino, C.E., & Collins, M. (1996). Sexual abuse of children: Prevalence, effects, and treatment. *Annals of the New York Academy of Sciences, 789,* 45–65.

Dinwiddie, S., Heath, A.C., Dunne, M.P., Bucholz, K.K., Madden, P.A., Slutske, W.S., Bierut, L.J., Statham, D.B., & Martin, N.G. (2000). Early sexual abuse and lifetime psychopathology: A co-twin-control study. *Psychological Medicine, 30,* 41–52.

Dodge, K.A., Bates, J.E., & Pettit, G.S. (1990). Mechanisms in the cycle of violence. *Science, 250,* 1678–1683.

Everson, M.D., Hunter, W.M., Runyon, D.K., Edelsohn, G.A., & Coulter, M.L. (1989). Maternal support following incest. *American Journal of Orthopsychiatry, 59,* 197–207.

Finch, A.J., Saylor, C.F., & Edwards, G.L. (1985). Children's depression inventory: Sex and grade norms for normal children. *Journal of consulting and Clinical Psychology, 53,* 424–425.

Finkelhor, D. (1990). Early and long-term effects of child sexual abuse: An update. *Professional Psychology: Research and Practice, 5,* 325–330.

Garland, A.F., Ellis-MacLeod, E., Landsverk, J.A., Ganger, W., & Johnson, I. (1998). Minority populations in the child welfare system: The visibility hypothesis reexamined. *American Journal of Orthopsychiatry, 68,* 142–146.

Garmezy, N. (1991). Resilience in children's adaptation to negative life events and stressed environments. *Pediatric Annals, 20,* 459–466.

Glascoe, F.P., & Ireton, H. (1995). Assessing children's development using parents' reports. The child development inventory. *Clinical Pediatrics, 34,* 248–255.

Hollingshead, A.B. (1979). *Four-factor Index of Social Status.* Unpublished manuscript. New Haven, CT.: Yale University.

Institute of Medicine (2003). *Unequal Treatment: Confronting Racial and Ethnic Disparities in Health Care.* Washington, D.C.: National Academy Press.

Johnson, J.G., Cohen, P., Brown, J., Smailes, E.M., & Bernstein, D.P. (1999). Childhood maltreatment increases risk for personality disorders during early adulthood. *Archives of General Psychiatry, 56,* 600–606.

Kilpatrick, D.G., Ruggiero, K.J., Acierno, R., Saunders, B.E., Resnick, H.S., & Best, C.L. (2003). Violence and risk of PTSD, major depression, substance abuse/dependence, and comorbidity: Results from the National Survey of Adolescents. *Journal Of Consulting and Clinical Psychology, 71,* 692–700.

Kim J., & Cicchetti D. (2003). Social self-efficacy and behavior problems in maltreated and nonmaltreated children. *Journal of Clinical Child and Adolescent Psychology, 32,* 106–17.

King, N.J., Tonge, B.J., Mullen, P., Myerson, N., Heyne, D., Rollings, S., Martin, R., & Ollendick, T.H. (2000). Treating sexually abused children with posttraumatic stress symptoms: a randomized clinical trial. *Journal of the American Academy of Child and Adolescent Psychiatry, 39,* 1347–55.

Kovacs, M. (1981). Rating scales to assess depression in school aged children. *Acta Paedopsychiatrica, 46, 305–315.*

Kovacs, M. (1985). The children's depression inventory. *Psychopharmacology Bulletin, 21,* 995–998.

Lyon, M.E., Benoit M., O'Donnell, R.M., Getson, P.R., Silber, T., & Walsh, T. (2000). Assessing African American adolescents' risk for suicide attempts: attachment theory. *Adolescence, 35,* 121–34.

Mannarino, A.P., Cohen, J.A., Smith, J.A., & Moore-Motily, S. (1991). Six and twelve-month follow-up of sexually abused girls. *Journal of Interpersonal Violence, 6,* 494–511.

McLeer, S.V., Deblinger, E., Henry, D., & Orvaschel, H. (1992). Sexually abused children at high risk for post-traumatic stress disorder. *Journal of the American Academy of Child and Adolescent Psychiatry, 31,* 875–879.

Mennen, F.E. (1993). Evaluation of risk factors in childhood sexual abuse. *Journal of the American Academy of Child and Adolescent Psychiatry, 32,* 934–939.

Newberger, C.M., & De Vos, E. (1988). Abuse and victimization: A life-span developmental perspective. *American Journal of Orthopsychiatry, 58,* 505–511.

Newberger, C.M., Gremy, I.M., Waternaux, C.M., & Newberger, E.H. (1993). Mothers of sexually abused children: Trauma and repair in longitudinal perspective. *American Journal of Orthopsychiatry, 63,* 92–102.

Paolucci, E., Genuis, M., & Violato, C. (2001). A meta-analysis of the published research on the effects of child sexual abuse. *Journal of Psychology, 135,* 17–36.

Reynolds, C.R. (1981). Long-term stability of scores on the Revised Children's Anxiety Scale. *Perceptual and Motor Skills, 53,* 702.

Reynolds, C.R., & Richmond, B.O. (1985). *Revised Children's Manifest Anxiety Scale (RCMAS).* Los Angeles, CA: Western Psychological Services.

Runyan, D.K., Everson, M.D., Edelsohn, G.A., Hunter, W.M., & Coulter, M.L. (1988). Impact of legal intervention on sexually abused children. *The Journal of Pediatrics, 113,* 647–653.

Rutter, M. (1987). Psychosocial resilience and protective mechanisms. *American Journal of Orthopsychiatry, 57,* 316–331.

Sanders-Phillips, K., Moisan, P.A., Wadlington, S., Morgan, S., & English, K. (1995). Ethnic differences in psychological functioning among black and Latino sexually abused girls. *Child Abuse and Neglect, 19,* 691–706.

Snowden, L.R. (2003). Bias in mental health assessment and intervention: Theory and evidence. *American Journal of Public Health, 93,* 239–243.

Surbeck, B.C. (2003). An investigation of racial partiality in child welfare assessments of attachment. *American Journal of Orthopsychiatry, 73,* 13–23.

Tiet, Q.Q., Bird, H.R., Hoven, C.W., Moore, R., Wu, P., Wicks, J., Jensen, P.S., Goodman, S., & Cohen, P. (2001). Relationship between specific adverse life events and psychiatric disorders. Journal of Abnormal Child Psychology, *29,* 153–164.

Tingus, K.D., Heger, A.H., Foy, D.W., & Leskin, G.A. (1996). Factors associated with entry into therapy in children evaluated for sexual abuse. *Child Abuse and Neglect, 20,* 63–8.

U.S. Department of Health and Human Services. (2001). *Mental Health: Culture, Race, Ethnicity—A Supplement to Mental Health: A Report of the Surgeon General.* Rockville, MD: U.S. Department of Health and Human Services, Public Health Service, Office of the Surgeon General.

Wade, J.C. (1993). Institutional racism: An analysis of the mental health system. *American Journal of Orthopsychiatry, 63,* 536–544.

Westendorp, F., Brink, K.L., Roberson, M.K., & Ortiz, I.E. (1986). Variables which differentiate placement of adolescents into juvenile justice or mental health systems. *Adolescence, 21,* 23–37.

Chapter 14

School Strategies to Prevent and Address Youth Gang Involvement

SHARON HOOVER STEPHAN, STEPHEN MATHUR,
AND CELESTE C. OWENS

The devastating nature and impact of school violence entered the nation's consciousness after the school shootings at Columbine High School in 1999. Communities have struggled to secure their high schools and their students with a renewed vigor and urgency. Many schools have taken different approaches to cope with actual and perceived threats to the safety of their students. Some have adopted "zero-tolerance" policies, installed metal detectors, toughened existing disciplinary codes, and increased security (Ashford, 2000; Kaufman et al., 2000). Additional efforts have included improving a school's ability to detect potentially violent students (Fey, Nelson, & Roberts, 2000) and instituting violence prevention programs such as conflict resolution, peer mediation, and sensitivity training programs similar to those found on college campuses (Landre, Miller, & Porter, 1997).

Each strategy has no doubt yielded positive results, but schools continue to struggle to curb school violence. Amidst the desire to profile "school shooters," to identify playground bullies, and to fortify our schools, threats to school safety persist (DeVoe et al., 2003). Gangs, in particular, pose a significant threat to our schools and communities. While certainly not a new phenomenon, gangs are flourishing in our schools (DeVoe et al., 2003). Increased media attention to the growing gang presence documents this trend, which shows no sign of reversing, with research indicating that youth gangs now exist in rural and suburban America, Europe and other foreign nations (Covey, Menard, & Franzese, 1997; Klein, 1995).

The growing influence of gangs on our youth places enormous pressure and responsibility upon our teachers, school administrators, school security staff, school boards, and most directly, the students themselves. Schools must face the possibility that greater violence may result as more of their students join gangs and gang rivalries intensify. Research indicates that gang youth are more criminally involved than other youth (Fleisher, 1998), although youth gangs only dedicate a fraction of their time to criminal activity (Klein, 1995). Despite the media portrayal of these youth as gun toting, violent criminals, other portions of their time are spent doing activities similar to other youth such as sleeping late, hanging out, and working odd jobs. Nonetheless, there is general consensus among researchers that the rate of criminal offending by gang youth is problematic, with an increase in gang membership and violent juvenile crime in the last decade (Cook & Laub, 1998).

The presence and actions of the gangs jeopardize the safety of students, schools, and communities, as well as the safety of the gang members themselves. Thus, it is critical for schools to develop competencies needed to deal with gangs and the consequences of youth gang membership. The purpose of the current chapter is to highlight important aspects of gang culture, including risk and protective factors related to youth gang membership, and to review strategies appropriate for schools to prevent and address the problem of youth gangs.

Information for this chapter is a culmination of both existing literature on gangs in schools, as well as first-hand experiences shared by the second author, who has served as a Social Studies teacher in a New York City public high school for the last nine years. In addition to teaching responsibilities, Mathur has been his high school's Peer Mediation Facilitator for its Conflict Resolution Program, enabling him to study gang life, gang rituals and culture, and gang rivalries; and to develop programs to reduce the impact of gangs in schools.

PREDICTORS OF GANG MEMBERSHIP

To address the problem of gang violence, it is critical to understand the predictors of gang formation and the factors that put youth at risk for joining gangs (Hill, Howell, Hawkins, & Battin-Pearson, 1999; Battin, Hill, Abbott, Catalano, Hawkins, 1998). The following section highlights some of the identified individual, peer, family, school and community factors associated with gang membership.

Individual Characteristics

Researchers have attempted to better understand the personal attributes that contribute to a youth's proclivity to participate in gang activity. A primary question addressed in the literature is whether gang youth are substantially different from non-gang youth. Esbensen, Huizinga, and Weiher (1993) examined the differences between gang youth, juvenile delinquents not involved in gangs and non-delinquent youth, and found that non-delinquent youth preferred to associate with youth similar to themselves, had lower tolerance for deviance, and lower levels of social isolation than delinquent youth and gang youth. In an extension of this study, Deschenes and Esbensen (1997) reported findings from a study of eighth grade students divided into four groups: non-delinquent, minor delinquent, serious delinquent, and gang member. Gang youth differed significantly from all other groups, especially those youth labeled as non-delinquent, such that they were less committed to school, more impulsive, reported less communication with parents, and engaged in more risky behaviors.

Other research has documented particular attitudinal characteristics that predict gang involvement including deviant attitudes (Esbensen, Huizinga, & Weiher, 1993) and a proclivity for trouble and excitement (Pennell, Evans, Melton, & Henson, 1994). Behavioral correlates of gang involvement include prior delinquency (Bjerregard & Smith, 1993; Curry & Spergel, 1992), aggression (Sanchez-Jankowski, 1991), alcohol and drug use (Bjerregaard & Smith, 1993; Curry & Spergel, 1992; Esbensen, Huizinga, & Weiher, 1993), and drug trafficking (Fagan, 1990; Thornberry, Krohn, Lizotte, & Chard-Wierschem, 1993). Early or precocious sexual activity, particularly among females, has also been identified as a predictor for gang involvement (Kosterman, et al., 1996; Bjerregaard & Smith, 1993).

Peer Group Influences

Peer group factors serve as a primary influence on adolescent behavior and propensity toward gang involvement (Esbensen, 2000). Curry and Spergel (1992) identified several peer group factors that are associated with youth gang involvement including having friends who use or distribute drugs or who are gang members, and simply having gang members in one's class. Youth who have a high commitment to delinquent peers and low commitment to positive peers are also at greater risk for becoming affiliated with a gang (Esbensen, Huizinga, & Weiher, 1993). Even interaction with delinquent peers places a youth at greater risk of later gang activity (Kosterman et al., 1996).

Family

Family disorganization, including broken homes, poor family management, and parental drug/alcohol abuse, has been identified as a key risk factor for gang involvement (Bjerregaard & Smith, 1993; Kosterman et al., 1996). Other family troubles have been identified as contributing to youth gang activity including incest, family violence, and drug addiction (Moore, 1991). A lack of adult male role models or parental models in a family and low parental attachment to children has also been shown to contribute to gang involvement (Thornberry, 1998; Wang, 1995; Vigil, 1988). Youth whose family members have been in gangs in prior generations are also at greater risk for gang involvement (Curry & Spergel, 1992; Landre et al., 1997).

School

Several indicators relevant to the school environment have been identified as risk factors for youth gang membership. Academic failure is a common risk factor for youth involved in gangs (Bjerregaard & Smith, 1993; Curry & Spergel, 1992; Kosterman et al., 1996). Related factors such as educational frustration, low educational aspirations (especially among females), and trouble at school all place youth at greater risk for becoming involved with gangs (Bjerregaard & Smith, 1993; Kosterman et al., 1996). Additionally, students with low achievement test scores and those identified as learning disabled are more vulnerable to gang membership (Hill et al., 1999). Hill and colleagues (1999) have documented an association between gang activity and youth's low commitment to school and low school attachment. Ebensen and colleagues (1993a, 1993b) also note that negative labeling by teachers is a risk factor for youth gang involvement.

Community

Communities that are disorganized and maintain low levels of social integration put youth at heightened risk for gang involvement (Curry & Spergel, 1988). Other community risk factors for youth gang activity include: barriers to and lack of social and economic opportunities (Moore, 1991); the availability of firearms (Lizotte, Tesorio, Thornberry, & Krohn, 1994; Miller, 1992), and the presence of drugs and gangs in a neighborhood (Curry & Spergel, 1992). Youth who feel unsafe in their neighborhood, or who live in neighborhoods with high crime rates are also at greater risk of joining a gang (Kosterman, et al., 1996).

GANG CULTURE

A comprehensive discussion of the intricacies of gang culture is beyond the scope of the current chapter; therefore, the following section provides only a brief overview of common features of gangs and gang membership.

Levels of Gang Membership

There are many different levels of gang membership, ranging from imitators who do not necessarily associate with gang members but may admire the gang life and gang members, to the hard core members who are totally committed to the gang and the gang's values. In between these two extremes are, in ascending order of involvement, the "wannabes," "associates" and regular gang members (National Youth Gang Suppression and Intervention Program, 1990). While not officially gang members, wannabes and associates contribute to the glorification of gang life and gang membership. They may also serve as fertile ground for sprouting future gang members as they consider gangs and related activities as normal and acceptable (Landre, et al., 1997). Thus, gang members have a built-in audience of peers who may admire, respect, and support gang activity. However, the regular and hard core members are the ones who actively perpetrate much of the violence and crime associated with gangs (Spergel et al., 1994). Adhering to a complete gang lifestyle and gang values, they represent the most serious threats to school and public safety as they reject completely or in part anyone or any value systems other than the gangs (National Youth Gang Suppression and Intervention Program, 1990).

Compounding the problem of identifying gang members and the levels of involvement is the fact that informal youth gangs have emerged, adding to the perception of an increasing gang presence in schools. Known as "crews," "sets," "blocks," and "cliques," these informal youth groups exhibit the characteristics of formal gangs (Landre, et al., 1997). While they lack the structure and membership size of formal gangs, these informal gangs often mimic gang activities and gang member behaviors. On many occasions, members of these informal groups stick together because they live in the same neighborhood or on the same block. They could also be a group of friends who decide to wear similar clothing and hang out together. However, for the purposes of identification, gang membership means more than wearing "colors," and "throwing signs." Gangs typically reinforce anti-social values and behaviors, with members sometimes engaging in criminal and other illegal activities including violent offenses (Decker & van Winkle, 1996). It is not unusual for hard core gang members to delegate criminal acts to other regular or associated members, and/or to pressure other youth to get involved in criminal activity (Bjerregaard & Smith, 1993; Landre et al., 1997).

Gang Recruitment and Initiation

Gangs recruit their members in many different ways. While some use peer pressure and their gangs' established reputations to convince youths to join their ranks (e.g. coercion), others use a more formal application process. Affiliating with gang members may place youth at greater risk for joining gangs. If gang leadership approves of the "candidate," the candidate usually goes through an initiation process, a ritual that binds the individual to the gang and demonstrates commitment to their new family (Curry & Decker, 1998). One gang may require that a candidate victimize a stranger, while another gang may "jump in" the candidate, which means that the gang members kick and punch the initiate for a brief period of time (Trump, 1998). Female candidates can be "sexed in," where they are expected to perform sex acts with members of the gang in order to be initiated (Decker & van Wickle, 1996).

These initiation rites may also include learning about the gang's history and development, its codes of conduct and rules, its customs and rituals, and its philosophies, beliefs, and values. More recent studies of gang rituals and practices have concluded that modern gangs make less use of symbols, including clothing and traditional initiation rites, than gangs of the past (Howell, 2000).

Attire and Tattoos

Gangs often employ a variety of visible indicators that establish membership and also serve as warnings to rival gang members and the general public (Trump, 1998). Some of the more common visible indicators are the clothes, hats, and bandannas (also known as "flags") in the gang's specified colors. Gangs may wear the traditional baseball cap of a specific team with markings from a permanent marker in the gang's specified color under the brim (e.g. the Bloods would have a red marking; Landre et al., 1997). Gang members sometimes sport beaded necklaces or bracelets with specific colors and patterns, which can signify the gang member's rank or status. Among the Latin Kings, for example, members wear five black beads alternating with five gold beads, while the executive members wear five black beads with two gold beads. Members responsible for being the trigger person wear all black beads (Landre, et al., 1997).

Tattoos are a common method of nonverbal used to publicize membership and commitment to a particular gang (Howell & Lynch, 2000). Tattoos are used to bind members together and symbolize a lifelong commitment to the gang. They are also used to prevent members from joining rival gangs. Tattoos are often in conspicuous parts of the body such as the fingers, neck, and forehead in the shapes of teardrops, weapons, and chains (Jackson, 1998).

Hand Signals

The hand gestures and signals that gang members flash to one another range from subtle and difficult to detect to obvious two-hand configurations (Landre et al., 1997). Used as greetings and means of brief communication, these "signs" act as codes that only members of the gang know and use. When these signs are flashed to a fellow gang member they are considered an expression of unity and bonding; however, in the presence of a rival, it is considered a gesture of gross disrespect (Jackson, 1998).

Language

Gangs create their own vocabulary and jargon, and nicknames. As part of the initiation process new members are given a nickname that symbolizes some aspect of his/her physical or psychological makeup. Some examples include: El Loco, Little Patches, 8-ball, Glockmaster, and N-sane (Jackson, 1998). They also have unique vocabularies that help to bond members and provide a barrier from interference by outsiders (Landre, et al., 1997).

Graffiti

Aside from the visible indicators that gang members often possess or utilize, graffiti represents a prevalent mode of gang identification and communication in schools and communities. Whether scrawled on desktops, hallways, or on buildings, graffiti serves numerous purposes for gangs (Trump, 1998). The graffiti, sometimes referred to as "tags," can be used to mark turf and to relay information or orders to other gang members. Some common graffiti abbreviations include: AOK (Always Out Killing); ATC (Addicted To Crime); LTK (Live to Kill/License to Kill); 187 (California Penal Code Number for Murder); 916/415 (Telephone Area Codes used by gangs to show where they are from) (Landre et al., 1997). Extensive gang graffiti in a location, such as in a section of the school cafeteria or on a certain neighborhood block, provides a gang with a sense of territorial claim (Curry & Decker, 1998).

IMPACT ON SCHOOLS

Student Performance and Attendance

Delinquency and gang involvement are associated with academic failure and truancy, both having a negative impact on the school environment (Dryfoos, 1990; Landre et al., 1997). An investigation of risk factors for sustained (multiple-year) gang membership indicated that low academic achievement and learning disabilities each strongly predicted sustained membership versus non-membership in gangs (Battin-Pearson, Guo, Hill, Abbott, & Hawkins, 1999). In addition to associations with academic performance, gang involvement is associated with truancy among gang members and overall attendance fluctuations in the student body. Landre and colleagues (1997) note that changes in student attendance, including habitual tardiness and sudden drops in attendance may indicate the avoidance of either impending gang violence or pressure to be involved in gangs. Both truancy and academic performance may be linked with another factor shown to be correlated with gang membership, low school commitment. Several researchers have demonstrated a link between youths' gang involvement and low commitment to their school (Bjerregard & Smith, 1993; Ebensen & Deschenes, 1998; Hill et al., 1999; Maxson, Whitlock, & Klein, 1998).

School Property

As noted previously, a hallmark characteristic of gang activity is graffiti, with schools often being the target of such destruction. The prominence of such graffiti rewards the gang with greater public recognition, which may send the message that the gangs have "taken over" a school or that they are so deeply entrenched that the school can do little to stop their influence. In addition to the inherent destruction of property caused by graffiti in schools, graffiti symbolizes both a perceived and real deterioration of school safety.

School property might also be a target of other types of vandalism by gang members, in part due to their convenient locale (Landre et al., 1997). Initiation rituals might require gang members to commit vandalism against school property, again with the gang's intention being to establish itself as a force within the school and community.

School Safety

In addition to the impact of gangs on school participation and property, probably the most concerning effect of youth gang involvement with regard to schools pertains to student and staff safety. Gang rivalries, in particular, pose an immediate and consistent threat to school safety. Simmering tensions among rival gangs or groups explode into full-scale fights that can jeopardize the safety of all students and staff. The slightest provocation among rival gangs can set a fight in motion: an "accidental" bump in the halls, a stare that lasts too long (commonly known as "grilling"), a rumor, or a verbal challenge or threat. Other indications of growing gang rivalries include verbal altercations among gang members, crossed out gang tags and graffiti by rival gang members, and reports of intensified arguments and confrontations over territory, girlfriends, and disrespect (Landre et al., 1997). Knowledgeable school staff members may also see an increase in the number of students wearing or displaying gang identifiers. Once a fight occurs, retaliation become more likely, as gang violence begets more gang violence.

The outbreak of gang violence may originate in classrooms and cafeterias, and spill out into the neighborhood. Gang rivalries are just as likely to start off campus and reach their boiling points at school. Many schools attempt to mitigate gang violence and gang rivalries by instituting zero-tolerance policies the prohibit students from displaying or wearing gang regalia, though there is little documentation available to support the effectiveness of these strategies.

SCHOOL STRATEGIES TO ADDRESS GANG INVOLVEMENT

In addition to having the direct impact of gang culture, schools also serve as one of the most appropriate sites for addressing the problem of youth gang involvement. Due to the direct impact of gang activity on schools, school staff may be inherently motivated to reduce youth gang involvement in order to avoid associated school failure, truancy, and dropout, school vandalism, and to improve student and staff safety. In addition, schools serve as a universal, natural setting to spearhead gang intervention efforts given that they hold the greatest time and programmatic responsibility for school-age children second to families. Although many youth involved in gangs are dropouts with little to no connection to their school, a significant proportion of gang members are still active students. Therefore, not only can schools serve as a site for preventive interventions targeting a broader school population, they can also direct efforts toward reducing ongoing gang activity and encouraging students' disengagement from gang involvement. In the final section of this chapter, school-based strategies for addressing gangs are described, with mention of some specific programs that have been evaluated and identified as promising practice in the area of gang prevention and intervention.

Prevention

Prior to a discussion of identifying and addressing *ongoing* gang activity in a school, our focus will turn to programs targeting the prevention of gang establishment and at the promotion of resilience in youth in order to avoid gang membership. Several promising gang prevention programs have been developed and evaluated for use in schools to prevent students from becoming involved in gangs. Some are discussed below. (For a comprehensive summary of gang prevention program evaluation, see Howell, 1998).

The High/Scope Perry Preschool Project

The High/Scope Perry Preschool Project (Schweinhart, Barnes, & Weikart, 1993) utilized family involvement as a means of promoting resilience in youth at-risk for gang involvement. Specifically, poor 3- and 4-year-old African American preschoolers were enrolled in preschool, and their teachers conducted home visits to promote parental involvement in their children's educational experiences. During home visits, parents were also informed about their child's activities in school.

Long-term follow-ups of the program showed it to be effective in reducing severe and chronic delinquency among the youth, placing them at less risk for adolescent gang involvement.

The Montreal Preventive Treatment Program

The Montreal Preventive Treatment Program (Tremblay, Masse, Pagan, & Vitano, 1996) was designed to address early childhood risk and protective factors for gang involvement among boys of low socioeconomic status who displayed disruptive behaviors in kindergarten. Individual social skills training for boys ages 7 to 9 was combined with parent training that focused on monitoring children's behavior, reinforcing prosocial behavior, using effective punishment, and managing family crises. Seventeen parent training sessions and 19 individual training sessions were offered to participants. The boys received training in small groups, containing both non-disruptive and disruptive youth, and used peer modeling, self-instruction, and reinforcement contingencies to build pro-social skills and self-control among the boys. A longitudinal program evaluation indicated positive short- and long-term gains, including less substance use, delinquency, and gang involvement at age 15 (Tremblay et al., 1996).

Se Puede

The Se Puede ("You Can") program works to prevent gang involvement, gun violence, and drug use and to improve academic performance among at-risk middle school youth in a Tri-city area (Alamo, Pharr, and San Juan) of Puerto Rico where approximately 5,000 gang members reside (Office of Juvenile Justice and Delinquency Prevention, 1999). Program activities include: individual and group counseling; a voluntary one-year positive alternative and role model program; a curriculum component that introduces substance abuse and violence prevention skills; and, monthly weekend camping experiences promoting survival skills and relationship development with participants and mentors. Despite an increase in gang presence in the Tri-city area throughout the duration of the project, Se Puede participants showed a decrease in gang and crime involvement, as well as improvements in school performance and individual skills (Office of Juvenile Justice and Delinquency Prevention, 1999).

Gang Resistance Education and Training Program

The Gang Resistance Education and Training (GREAT) Program, developed by the Bureau of Alcohol, Tobacco, and Firearms (ATF), utilizes a classroom-based educational approach to discourage children and young adolescents from joining gangs. Uniformed law enforcement officers teach a 9-week course to middle school students in which students learn about how crime, cultural differences, and drugs impact their neighborhood and school (Esbensen & Osgood, 1997). Students are also taught skills to resolve conflicts and to meet their basic social needs without resorting to gang membership. Finally, participants are encouraged to establish short- and long-term personal goals in order to avoid the trap of gang membership. Though effects are relatively modest, compared to control subjects, participants in the GREAT Program reported lower levels of gang affiliation and delinquency, including drug use, property crimes, and crimes against persons at 12- and 18-month follow-ups (Esbensen & Osgood, 1997, 1999). In addition, relative to the control group, participants in the GREAT Program reported more negative attitudes about gangs, fewer delinquent friends, more friends involved in prosocial activities, greater commitment to school success, greater attachment to parents, and less likelihood of impulsive behavior.

Beyond Prevention: The School's Role in Addressing Gang Activity

While schools clearly have the potential to impact gang involvement through the implementation of prevention activities, the school's role in addressing ongoing gang activity is less obvious. In fact, research suggests that a comprehensive, multi-system approach is necessary to combat the problem of youth gangs in communities (Spergel & Grossman, 1997; Spergel, Grossman, & Wa, 1998). In the Office of Juvenile Justice and Delinquency Prevention (OJJDP) report on Youth Gang Programs and Strategies (Howell, 2000), Howell reiterates this message: "A more comprehensive approach, combining program elements such as social services, crisis intervention, gang suppression, and community involvement, might be more effective than a one-dimensional approach" (p. 34). Therefore, it is unrealistic, and probably unhelpful, for schools to attempt to address the problem of gang violence in isolation. Rather, schools can productively facilitate the process of gang prevention, intervention, and suppression by: a) working toward reducing risk factors and enhancing protective factors in youth to prevent them from gang affiliation; b) developing an approach to identify gang activity in schools in order to alert school- and community-based professionals to potential problems and to facilitate intervention; c) establishing a school climate to combat gang activity via rules and procedures as well as physical environment; and d) developing a school crisis teams to assist students in dealing with the violence and destruction that may result if gang activity occurs in schools.

Gang Identification

A critical, but often difficult component of addressing gang violence in schools is the process of actually identifying the presence of gang activity. Although many gangs would prefer to go unnoticed by school officials, school personnel can utilize knowledge and awareness of gang culture to measure the severity of a gang problem and the level of student involvement. It should be noted that identifying gang membership and aspects of gang culture is not an exact science. In the quest to discover the nature and types of gangs in a school, concerned school stakeholders use newly acquired information about gangs, hand signals, and tags to investigate their students, to decipher graffiti, and to determine if incidents of school violence are somehow gang related. These well-intentioned individuals may jump to conclusions about their students, unfairly profiling them as gang members, simply because some students wear certain colors and clothing that are associated with a particular gang. Unless completely obvious to even the untrained eye, it takes more than using one or two common gang identifiers to implicate a student. Nonetheless, there are some common identifiers that school personnel can utilize as part of the assessment process to expose gang activity within the school. A Gang Assessment Tool was developed by the National School Safety Center for use by community leaders and school administrators to evaluate the level of gang activity in their locale.

A potential resource for accomplishing the task of gang identification is a School Safety Team (SST), or other similar school-based committee designed to monitor school safety conditions, report on school violence, and review school safety policies and procedures. Ideally, many school constituencies should be represented on the SST, including school security personnel, school administrators, teachers, guidance counselors, and social workers. Meeting monthly or weekly, the SST can effectively share information about violent incidents, school conflict trends, and gang activities. In addition, the SST can mobilize its resources, and involve community affiliates, to provide gang intervention services for identified students who are in gangs and may need assistance.

School Climate

Rules and Procedures

Although there is limited research evidence documenting the effectiveness of instituting rules and procedures and establishing a physical environment to counter gang activity, experts in the area of community- and school-based approaches to gang violence often recommend these approaches as a means of combating gang activity (Wiener, 1999; Landre et al., 1997). Landre and colleagues (1997) recommend a number of rules and procedures to schools including: a) clearly explaining and obtaining student acknowledgement of school rules regarding gang activity, drugs, weapons, and the consequences for violations; b) instituting restitution-based punishment (e.g., students found guilty of vandalism are made responsible for cleanup and repair) in conjunction with local courts, if possible; c) punish individuals rather than groups for violations of school rules; d) establish a clear and easily interpreted dress code policy with the involvement and consensus of parents, students, and staff in its development; and, e) report crimes that occur in school to the police.

Physical Environment

Wiener (1999) emphasizes the importance of establishing a physical environment in schools that promotes safety and prohibits gang activity. Suggestions for promoting a safe physical environment include implementing metal detectors, eliminating lockers, providing quality lighting, rapidly removing graffiti, and offering on-site policing (Wiener, 1999). Additional suggestions include controlling access to campus by limiting and supervising the entry, movement, and exit of persons within school buildings and on school grounds, keeping rival gang members (especially leaders) separated through controlled scheduling, and reducing crowds where possible (e.g., via staggering lunch periods and release times).

In the establishment of school rules and policies, we recommend the involvement of local law enforcement officials. Schools may consider inviting local law enforcement officers to conduct "walkarounds" of the school grounds. If possible, an officer of a police department gang intelligence unit should conduct the walkaround. A knowledgeable law enforcement officer can point out possible gang members, detect gang identifiers, and decipher the significance of tags and graffiti. With information from walkarounds and gang intelligence officers, school safety officers and the local police department can collaboratively design gang prevention programs with school officials and devise appropriate anti-gang policies for schools.

School Crisis Teams

Given the potential for violence and destruction as a result of gang activity, a critical component in addressing gangs in schools involves the establishment of school crisis teams. In the aftermath of serious violence and threats to school safety, school crisis teams provide students and staff members with guidance and services to help them cope with the fallout from emergencies. School crisis teams mobilize to react to these dangers in order to secure students and staff. To perform the various functions needed during an emergency, school crisis teams should be composed of key school stakeholders. Important members may include administrators, teachers, security agents, guidance counselors, school psychologists and social workers. Although it is difficult to anticipate a crisis, frequent meetings of a school crisis team enhance a school's response to emergencies and situations that jeopardize the well being of students and faculty. After a severe violent incident or trauma that affects a school, a school crisis team meets to gather information about the event, discuss its potential impact on the students and school, and determine how best to respond to the situation. An excellent resource guide for advance preparation and early response to school crises is Brock, Sandoval, and Lewis' (2001) text, *Preparing for Crises in the Schools: A Manual for Building School Crisis Response Teams: Second Edition.*

CONCLUSION

In response to the increase in gang activity across communities, schools have a growing responsibility to prevent gang involvement among their youth and to protect students from the risks associated with gangs. As noted in this chapter, several programs have been developed to discourage children and adolescents from joining gangs, resulting in some promising outcomes among participating youth. However, given the diversity of the prevalence and nature of gang activity across communities, it is essential that schools and communities adapt programs and solutions to suit their particular needs. In doing so, it is ideal for schools to function within a multi-system approach to combating youth gang activity (i.e., a community-based approach involving multiple stakeholders). In the absence of a well-integrated, community-based approach, (or even as part of such a program), there are several steps that individual schools can take to positively address the problem of gangs and to promote resilience among students in order to assist them in avoiding gang involvement. For instance, given the research documenting the link between several school-related factors and youths' affiliation with gangs (e.g., low commitment to school, educational frustration), school personnel might consider methods of identifying these risk factors in youth and promoting positive change in these areas. In addition, schools can work toward developing a school climate that counters the impact of gang activity via the implementation of rules, procedures, and a safe physical environment. Finally, schools serve a critical role in addressing gang activity by engaging in effective crisis response planning to assist students in coping with gang-related incidents (e.g., violence) should they occur.

REFERENCES

Ashford, R. (2000). *Can zero-tolerance keep our schools safe?* Principal, 80(2), 28–30.

Battin-Pearson, S.R., Guo, J., Hill, K.G., Abbott, R.D., & Hawkins, J.D. (1999). *Early predictors of sustained adolescent gang membership.* Unpublished manuscript. Seattle, WA: University of Washington, School of Social Work, Social Development Research Group.

Bjerregaard, B., & Smith, C. (1993). Gender differences in gang participation, delinquency, and substance use. *Journal of Quantitative Criminology,* 9(4): 329–355.

Cook, P.J., & Laub, J.H. (1998). *The unprecedented epidemic in youth violence.* In *Youth Violence,* edited by M. Tonry and M.H. Moore. Chicago, IL: University of Chicago Press, pp. 27–64.

Covey, H.C., Menard, S., & Franzese, R.J. (1997). *Juvenile Gangs,* 2nd Ed. Springfield, IL: Charles C. Thomas.

Curry, G.D., & Decker, S.H. (1998). *Confronting gangs: Crime and community.* Los Angeles: CA: Roxbury Publishing Company.

Curry, G.D. & Spergel, I.A. (1988). Gang homicide, delinquency, and community. *Criminology, 26,* 381–405.

Curry, G.D. & Spergel, I.A. (1992). Gang involvement and delinquency among Hispanic and African-American adolescent males. *Journal of Research in Crime and Delinquency, 29,* 273–291.

Decker, S.H., & van Winkle, B. (1996). *Life in the gang: Family, friends, and violence.* New York, NY: Cambridge University Press.

DeVoe, J.F., Peter, K., Kaufman, P., Ruddy, S.A., Miller, A.K., Planty, M., Snyder, T.D., & Rand, M.R. (2003). *Indicators of School Crime and Safety, 2003.* NCSE 2004-004/NCJ 201257. U.S. Departments of Education and Justice. Washington DC.

Deschenes, E.P., & Esbensen, F. (1997). *Saints, delinquents, and gang members: Differences in attitudes and behavior.* Paper presented at the American Society of Criminology Annual Meeting, San Diego, CA.

Dryfoos, J.G. (1990). *Adolescents at risk: Prevalence and prevention.* New York: Oxford University Press.

Esbensen, F. (2000). Preventing adolescent gang involvement. *Juvenile Justice Bulletin.* September 2000. U.S. Department of Justice, Office of Juvenile Justice and Delinquency Prevention.

Esbensen, F. & Huizinga, D. (1993a). Gangs, drugs, and delinquency in a survey of urban youth. *Criminology, 31(4),* 565–589.

Esbensen, F., Huizinga, D., & Weiher, A.W. (1993b). Gang and non-gang youth: Differences in explanatory factors. *Journal of Contemporary Criminal Justice, 9(2),* 94–116.

Esbensen, F. & Osgood, D.W. (1997). *National Evaluation of G.R.E.A.T.* Research in Brief. Washington, DC: U. S. Department of Justice, Office of Justice Programs, National Institute of Justice.

Esbensen, F., & Osgood, D.W. (1999). Gang Resistance Education and Training (GREAT): Results from the national evaluation. *Journal of Research in Crime and Delinquency, 36(2),* 194–225.

Fey, G., Nelson J., & Roberts, M. (February, 2000). *The perils of profiling.* School Administrator, Web Edition. http://www.aasa.org/publications/sa/2000_02/fey.htm.

Fleisher, M. (1998). *Dead end kids.* Madison, WI: University of Wisconsin Press.

Hill, K.G., Howell, J.C., Hawkins, J.D., & Battin-Pearson, S.R. (1999). Childhood risk factors for adolescent gang membership: Results from the Seattle Social Development Project. *Journal of Research in Crime and Delinquency, 36(3),* 300–322.

Howell, J.C. (1998). Promising programs for youth gang violence prevention and intervention. In R. Loeber & D.P. Farrington (Eds.). *Serious and Violent Juvenile Offenders: Risk Factors and Successful Interventions* (pp. 284–312). Thousand Oaks, CA: Sage Publications.

Howell, J.C. (2000). *Youth gang programs and strategies.* National Youth Gang Center, Institute for Intergovernmental Research, Office of Juvenile Justice and Delinquency Prevention, U.S. Department of Justice, Washington, D.C.

Howell, J.C., & Lynch, J.P. (2000). Youth gangs in schools. *Juvenile Justice Bulletin.* August 2000. U.S. Department of Justice, Office of Juvenile Justice and Delinquency Prevention.

Jackson, L. (1998). *Gangbusters: Strategies for prevention and intervention.* American Correctional Association, Lanham, MD.

Kaufman, P., Chen, X., Choy, S.P., Ruddy, S.A., Miller, A.K., Fleury, J.K., Chandler, K.A., Rand, M.R., Klaus, P., & Planty, M. (2000). *Indicators of School Crime and Safety, 2000.* NCSE 2001-017/NCJ-184176. Washington D.C.: U.S. Departments of Education and Justice.

Klein, M.W. (1995). *The American street gang.* New York, NY: Oxford University Press.

Kosterman, R., Hawkins, J.D., Hill, K.G., Abbott, R.D., Catalano, R.F., & Guo, J. (1996). *The developmental dynamics of gang initiation: When and why young people join gangs.* Paper presented at the annual meeting of the American Society of Criminology, Chicago, IL.

Landre, R., Miller, M., & Porter, D. (1997). *Gangs: A handbook for community awareness.* New York: Checkmark Books.

Lizotte, A.J., Tesorio, J.M., Thornberry, T.P., & Krohn, M.D. (1994). Patterns of adolescent firearms ownership and use. *Justice Quarterly, 11,* 51–74.

Maxson, C.L., Whitlock, M.L., & Klein, M.W. (1998). Vulnerability to street gang membership: Implications for practice. *Social Service Review, 72:* 70–91.

Moffitt, T. (1993). Adolescence-limited and life-course-persistent antisocial behavior: A developmental taxonomy. *Psychological Review 100*(4):674–701.

Moore, J.W. (1991). *Going down to the barrio: Homeboys and homegirls in change.* Philadelphia, PA: Temple University Press.

The National Youth Gang Suppression and Intervention Program (1990). *Youth Gangs: Problem and response.* University of Chicago, 14.

Office of Juvenile Justice and Delinquency Prevention (1999). *Promising strategies to reduce gun violence.* Report. Washington, DC: U. S. Department of Justice, Office of Justice Programs, Office of Juvenile Justice and Delinquency Prevention, Supplement to vol. 12.

Pennell, S., Evans, E., Melton, R., & Hinson, S. (1994). *Down for the set: Describing and defining gangs in San Diego.* San Diego, CA: Criminal Justice Research Division, Association of Governments.

Spergel, I.A. & Grossman, S.F. (1997). The Little Village Project: A community approach to the gang problem. *Social Work, 42,* 456–470.

Spergel, I.A., Grossman, S.F., & Wa, K.M. (1998). *The Little Village Gang Violence Reduction Program: A three year evaluation.* Unpublished report. Chicago, IL: University of Chicago, School of Social Service Administration.

Spergel, I.A., Curry, D., Chance, R., Kane, C., Ross, R., Alexander, A., Simmons, E., & Oh, S. (1994). *Gang suppression and intervention: Problem and Res*ponse. Publication, Office of Juvenile and Delinquency Prevention, October 1994. Retrieved from: http://www.ncjrs.org/pdffiles/gangprob.pdf

Thornberry, T.P., Krohn, M.D. Lizotte, A.J. & Chard-Wierschem, D. (1993). The role of juvenile gangs in facilitating delinquent behavior. *Journal of Research in Crime and Delinquency, 30,* 55–87.

Tremblay, R.E., Masse, L., Pagani, L., & Vitaro, F. (1996). From childhood physical aggression to adolescent maladjustment: The Montreal Prevention Experiment. In R. D. Peters & R. J. McMahon (Eds.) *Preventing Childhood Disorders, Substance Abuse, and Delinquency,* (pp. 268–298). Thousand Oaks, CA: sage Publications, Inc.

Trump, K.S. (1998). *Practical school security: basic guidelines for safe and secure schools.* Thousand Oaks, CA: Corwin Press/Sage Publications, Inc.

Vigil, J.D. (1988). *Barrio gangs: Street life and identity in Southern California.* Austin, TX: University of Texas Press.

Wang, Z. (1995). Gang affiliation among Asian-American high school students: A path analysis of a social developmental model. *Journal of Gang Research, 2,* 1–13.

Weiner, V. (1999). *Winning the war against youth gangs: A guide for teens, families, and communities.* Westport, CT: Greenwood Press.

Chapter 15

Promoting Resilience in Military Children and Adolescents[1]

MICHAEL E. FARAN, MARK D. WEIST, DIANE A. FARAN,
AND STEPHEN M. MORRIS

Children and adolescents of military families (military children) face numerous challenges that their civilian counterparts do not experience. Stressors are particularly intense now related to sustained military deployments in Afghanistan and Iraq. These stressors including the frequent deployments of parents, the associated fear of losing a parent, the move of remaining family members "closer to home" while the active duty parent is deployed, and the financial stress of only having one person work with no second job, all test the resilience of the military child and his or her family. With a much smaller military than the United States (U.S.) has had in the past, the onus of protecting the nation falls to highly trained and effective but less numerous forces. This translates into more frequent deployments for many.

Other common stressors that are a constant even during times of peace for soldiers and their families are moves on average every three years, often to other countries and/or remote places such as Alaska and Hawaii, being isolated from their support system (e.g., extended family) and transitioning into new cultures. Children may be required to learn new languages, which while beneficial, is still

---

[1] The views expressed in this manuscript are those of the authors and do not reflect the official policy or position of the Department of the Army, Department of Defense, or the U.S. Government.

stressful. For single parent families or families where both parents are active duty, the military requires a "care plan" designating who will care for the children in the event of parental deployment. This forces families to deal with the reality of separation in a very tangible manner.

Because of the moves and periodic deployments, children are faced with the loss of friends and familiar surroundings and must meet the challenge of forming new relationships when they change schools. This can be particularly stressful for some, but also may contribute to building resilience in others. While many civilian families must contend with a parent who travels, when an active duty parent goes on a "business trip" there are major differences. The service member is often placed in imminent danger, and most school age children understand that their parent is in a potentially dangerous place. The children must cope with the knowledge that their parents may be harmed or killed as well as the uncertainty of how long the parent will be gone. Communication with the parent is unpredictable. In addition to missing key family events, such as birthdays and holidays, the active duty parent may return to find a child at a different developmental stage. In the case of children with ongoing mental health problems, the child may also be in a different place therapeutically. For example, one of us (MEF) recently treated an 11-year-old girl with Bipolar Disorder whose father had been deployed to Korea for one year. When the father returned he said he did not recognize his daughter, and while she was doing better therapeutically, he missed the aggressive, moody and oppositional girl that he left behind.

Given public awareness and media coverage, the nondeployed parent may find it very difficult to shield children from the frightening realities of combat conditions where their dad or mom is stationed. For many families who are stationed overseas, when the active duty parent is deployed, the remaining family returns to the U.S. mainland to be closer to home and their extended family and friends. Although this may improve day-to-day functioning of the family, it is highly disruptive to the children's school lives. For the recent deployment of troops from the 25th Infantry Division at Schofield Barracks, Hawaii, many of the remaining families are taking their children out of school and returning to their "homes" on the mainland.

When children are being constantly challenged as described above, resilience becomes a requirement for healthy functioning. In this military system children and families must be flexible and adaptable, capable of coping with stressors most families do not have to endure. Resilience in both parents and children directly contributes to "soldier readiness" and ultimately has an impact on how well a military unit is able to accomplish its mission. Those that have difficulty coping are often referred for support services. If a family member is having significant problems, particularly externalizing behaviors, this member may be sent back to their home of record.

BACKGROUND

The military plays an important role in the lives of its families and provides a wide range of family support (Jensen, Lewis, & Xenasis, 1986). Most of the early research concerning military children was centered on observational data, clinic based studies, anecdotal evidence and hypotheses. Only within the last twenty years have there been good cross-sectional controlled studies. Though it is helpful to look at the work done by these early researchers, it is important to keep in mind that today's military family is very different than those originally studied. Currently, there is no draft, the military is a downsized force, there are more active duty women, and more single parent military families. The military is invested in promoting resilient families and providing resources for families' emotional health.

Cantwell (1974) wrote on the prevalence of psychiatric disorders in military children ages 8–11 seen in a pediatric clinic. He used a semi-structured interview with the parents, a behavior questionnaire with teachers and a diagnostic play interview of the child. He found that 35% of the children had a psychiatric disorder. In 1978, LaGrone described what he coined the "Military Family Syndrome" based on a review of clinic records of 792 children and adolescents seen in a military mental health clinic. He stated: "the greatest number of behavioral disorders, nearly 93%, came from the authoritarian families" (p. 1042). He described a system where children had higher rates of mental disorders than their civilian counterparts, fathers were autocratic and controlling, scapegoating of family members was common, and the children suffered as a result of the paranoid system.

Morrison (1981) first challenged the "Military Family Syndrome" in a prospective clinic based study of 140 military children and adolescents and 234 nonmilitary patients. The only difference he found between the two samples was that the nonmilitary children had a higher prevalence of schizophrenia and schizophreniform disorder. Jensen, Xenasis, Wolf, and Bain (1991) reexamined the "Military Family Syndrome" by surveying 213 military families and compared their results to national norms. Parents and teachers rated the children's behavior using established measures of internalizing and externalizing behavior, children completed measures of depression and anxiety, and parents reported on their life stress and depression and anxiety. Based on the use of established and commonly used measures of psychosocial functioning, Jensen et al. (1991) concluded that rates of psychopathology in military children, aged 6 to 12 years old were not different from national normative data. However, they did find that mothers rated a greater proportion of the children as presenting clinically significant levels of emotional and behavioral problems than did fathers or teachers. Jensen et al. (1991) attributed the higher ratings of child emotional/behavioral problems by mothers as reflecting the higher stress they were experiencing in maintaining the household as the nondeployed parent. This is an important finding for treatment efforts with military families; that is that reported child behavioral problems may signal problems in parental, particularly maternal coping. Finally, Jensen et al. (1991) found no evidence of a "Military Family Syndrome."

In 1995, Jensen et al., assessed the prevalence of mental disorders in a sample of 294 six to seventeen year-old military children, using a similar measurement approach to that used in the Jensen et al. (1991) study, with the addition of structured diagnostic interviewing using the NIMH Diagnostic Interview Schedule for Children (Shaffer et al., 1996). The military parents were 70.1% enlisted (median rank Staff Sergeant E-6) and 29.9% officer (median rank Major O-4) with median incomes of $25,000–$30,000 a year. Structured diagnostic interviewing identified the following prevalence rates of disorders in the 294 children: 25.2% with any anxiety disorder, 4.3% with Major Depressive Disorder (MDD) and Dysthymic Disorder, 20.0% with Attention Deficit/Hyperactivity Disorder (ADHD) and 5.2% with Oppositional Defiant Disorder (ODD). The total prevalence was 40.8% of children with any disorder (many children qualified for more than one disorder with mean number of disorders being 1.3), which is lower than the rate seen in the U.S. civilian population as described in the Methodology for Epidemiology in Children and Adolescents (MECA) study of 48.5% for subjects 9–17 years of age (Shaffer et al., 1996). When these rates were further restricted by the requirement of diagnosis-related impairment and "need for services/use" the prevalence rates decreased to 11.4% for any anxiety disorder, 0.6% for MDD/Dysthymia, 2.7% for ADHD and 3.3% for ODD. The rates of ADHD were higher than seen in the MECA study, but the levels of ODD and conduct disorder were lower. In summary, Jensen et al. (1995) found lower rates of psychopathology in the military children than found in the civilian population, again discounting the "Military Family Syndrome."

DEPLOYMENT

A few reports have looked at how children and families experience deployment at different times during the deployment cycle. Logan (1987), writing about Navy wives whose husbands routinely went out to sea, listed seven stages of deployment broken into the three phases of Pre-Deployment, Deployment and Post-Deployment. Pre-Deployment consists of Stage 1—Anticipation of Loss, occurring one to six weeks prior to deployment and Stage 2—Detachment, which happens during the last week before deployment. Deployment itself includes Stages 3–5, and consists of Emotional Disorganization, Recovery and Stabilization, and Anticipation of Homecoming, respectively. Post-deployment consists of Stages 6 and 7, Renegotiation of Marriage Contract and Reintegration and Stabilization.

Nice (1983) studied the course of depressive affect in Navy wives whose husbands were deployed as compared to those wives whose husbands remained at home using a depression questionnaire that was completed on a biweekly basis beginning six weeks prior to deployment and ending two weeks after return (a seven-months period). He found that the wives of the deployed group reported significantly more depression than the wives of the nondeployed group and that their mood improved to baseline within two weeks of their husbands' return. Age correlated with depressive symptoms, with younger wives reporting more symptoms than older ones.

Pincus, House, Christenson, and Adler (2001) modified the deployment cycle of Logan to five stages: Pre-Deployment (preparation for leaving), Deployment (leaving), Sustainment (on assignment away from the home base), Re-Deployment (preparing to return home) and Post-Deployment (back at home base). This model was based on the authors' observations of families during deployment and based on our experience, appears to provide a better fit to what actually occurs. Pincus et al. (2001) emphasized the potentially large emotional impact deployment may have on children and spouses. They reported: "Each stage is characterized both by a time frame and specific emotional challenges, which must be dealt with and mastered by each of the family members" (p. 15). According to Pincus et al. (2001), Pre-Deployment is a highly stressful period when numerous crucial tasks need to be accomplished to get ready for deployment. During the Deployment and Sustainment stages, the remaining spouse becomes a "married single parent." She or he must take on full responsibility for the children and household, then relinquish it when the deployed spouse returns home. The role of head of household takes on a "revolving door" quality in many military families.

Pincus et al. (2001) found that a child's response to the deployment of a parent is variable and listed some of the "negative changes" seen in children. For ages 1 through 12 the behaviors reported were "cries, tantrums, clingy, potty accidents, whining and body aches with irritable sad moods" (p. 19). For adolescents 12–18 of age, behaviors listed were "isolates, uses drugs with mood changes of anger and apathy" (p. 19).

In a study of Army children's response to parents (90.8% fathers) being deployed for Desert Shield/Storm in 1990/1991, Rosen and Teitlebaum (1993) assessed parent-rated emotional and behavioral problems in 1,798 children, and depression and anxiety in the nondeployed spouse. The following were found to be significant predictors of children's symptoms: symptoms of mother and other siblings, history of counseling, history of poor school performance, history of being on medication for hyperactivity, health problems, learning disabilities, younger age and male gender. For example, high depression and/or anxiety in the mother was correlated with more symptoms in the children, such as eating problems, nightmares, sadness, and "perceived need for counseling."

In a study of Army wives during the Operation Desert Shield/Storm deployment of their husbands, Rosen and Teitelbaum (1994) reported that in general, younger spouses had more difficulty coping with deployment and utilized more medical resources than older spouses. In an earlier study (Rosen & Moghadam, 1991) of Army wives, the strongest predictor of general well being (e.g., marriage, friendship, financial satisfaction, military life stress, role satisfaction) was previous general well being. Predictability of husband's schedule, marital satisfaction, financial satisfaction, and experiencing a sense of "mastery" over their lives and obligations was predictive of wives' well being.

In 1989, Jensen, Grogan, Xenakis, and Bain studied the effects of an Army father's absence on his children's and wife's psychopathology. Families whose father was gone greater than one month in the last year were compared to families in which the father was gone less than a month. Children for whom father was gone more than a month had significantly more depressive and anxiety symptoms than children whose fathers were gone less than a month. Mothers' report of child behavior problems correlated with the amount of stress experienced by the mother and the level of her self-reported psychiatric symptoms. Jensen et al. (1989) suggested that children's difficulties as a result of father's absence were related to family stresses and the level of emotional/behavioral problems experienced by the mother.

Jensen, Martin and Watanabe (1996) examined children's response to parents being deployed during Operation Desert Storm, specifically looking at children prior to deployment and after with respect to age and gender. Three hundred eighty-three children ages 4 to 17 and their parents were examined using a measurement approach similar to Jensen et al. (1991) as well as measures of coping and social resources. Findings from the study showed that children of deployed parents reported significantly more depressive symptoms than children whose parents were not deployed. Boys of a deployed parent reported significantly more depressive symptoms than control boys and significantly more than either girls with a deployed or nondeployed parent. The caretaking spouses of deployed soldiers also had more depressive symptoms and more reported stress than controls, but no differences with nondeployed spouses in marital adjustment, social supports, or coping were shown. The lower the military rank the greater the symptoms in the nondeployed parent. Previously, Nice (1983) reported the same pattern of increased depressive symptoms in Navy wives and children, with more depressive symptoms during fathers' deployments, returning to baseline after their return. These findings support the notion that in military children having problems it is likely that the caretaking parent also has elevated levels of stress and depression. We have also found this to be true in our clinical experience.

Kelley et al. (2001) studied internalizing and externalizing behaviors in very young children (mean age of 3.1) of enlisted Navy mothers who were deployed and compared these behaviors to children of nondeployed Navy mothers and civilian controls. Eighty-three percent of the deployed women were separated from their children for 5 or 6 months. When the three groups were compared, 12% of children of deployed mothers presented clinically significant levels of internalizing behaviors as compared to 1% of children of nondeployed mothers, and 3% of civilian control children. No significant differences were found for externalizing behavior between groups, although children of deployed Navy moms had slightly higher scores. Kelley et al. (2001) summarized that for deployed mothers their very young children may be susceptible to anxiety and sadness during deployment periods similar to results found in previous studies of deployed fathers even though the effects are small and not suggestive of higher psychopathology.

RISK AND PROTECTIVE FACTORS IN MILITARY CHILDREN

As shown in the above literature review, the concept of the "Military Family Syndrome" has been repeatedly debunked. Military children, if anything, exhibit less psychopathology than their civilian counterparts. This is remarkable given the additional challenges of growing up in a military family that moves every three years on average, in which one parent may be absent for prolonged periods on a regular basis. There have been no controlled studies that we know of that have specifically examined protective factors in military children. Some military-related protective factors that have been hypothesized are lower divorce rates in military families; relative job security; screening of the active duty member for criminal history or significant history of psychopathology; free medical, behavioral health, legal and recreational services; and more family support from allied agencies such as Family Advocacy, Alcohol and Substance Abuse Program, and the Exceptional Family Member Program. These latter organizations are specifically designed to assist families with problems, whether it is family violence, substance abuse, or a family member with a chronic illness or mental disorder. Undoubtedly these programs have benefit and, in some instances, greatly improve the lives of families, which we have witnessed on numerous occasions.

As we have demonstrated, deployment is a notable risk factor for emotional/behavioral problems in military children, and nondeployed spouses (usually mothers; e.g., Jensen et al., 1989, 1991, 1996; Kelly et al., 2001; Rosen & Teitelbaum, 1994). Other risk factors for the development of emotional/behavioral problems in military children have been suggested. These include: lower rank of the soldier parent, isolation from extended family and friends, frequent moves and school changes, dual active duty parents, single active duty parent, frequent parental deployments, and history of emotional/behavioral problems. Other risk factors are the same as those experienced by civilian families, such as family discord and divorce, parental substance abuse, younger age of the child, male gender (particularly for father's absence), illness, and sibling position. (Jensen et al., 1996). Lower rank families' susceptibility to more stress and emotional/behavioral problems may be explained by a combination of factors, such as greater financial stress, less time and experience with the military, and younger age of parents (see Jensen et al., 1996). Regarding frequent moves, in a review article, Jensen et al. (1986) wrote that the difficulties with moves "are probably time-limited" and "may actually represent growth opportunities and increase coping capacities for most military families . . . (p. 230)." More pronounced problems may occur in a small proportion of families, with negative attitudes about moving associated with dysfunction.

PROMOTING RESILIENCE IN MILITARY CHILDREN AND ADOLESCENTS IN 2004

Operations tempo (OPTEMPO) is loosely defined as the rate of military actions or missions to include training exercises, garrison duties and deployments affecting the unit, the soldier and the family. Since the Iraqi War the OPTEMPO in the Military has greatly increased to a level most soldiers have not experienced in their military lives. The military and civilian populations are at heightened alert, and a great number of active duty personnel are in harm's way. The reasons for this are many. Since 1990 the military has downsized from 2,043,705 to 1,411,634 (Department of Defense [DOD] statistics, web1.whs.osd.mil/mmid/military/miltop.htm, September, 2003). The Army's numbers have decreased from 732,403 to 499,301 active duty soldiers during the same period (DOD statistics, September, 2003). Combined with the greatly increased OPTEMPO, the likelihood of a soldier being deployed is much higher and the probability of more frequent deployments, greater.

Also, military technology has drastically improved over the last decade requiring more training and experience. The individual soldier's life is growing in complexity. A soldier must be capable of functioning for prolonged periods of time, under any environmental conditions in dangerous places, and be highly effective 24 hours a day. In addition, performance of duty has become more public as was the case when reporters were embedded within units fighting in Afghanistan. Soldiers themselves must be very physically fit and emotionally resilient.

Military demographics have also undergone considerable changes. In a review of the demographics of Army active duty and families members, data from 1990 to 2001 show that family members outnumber the actual number of active duty military, comprising 57.9% of the total military population in 2001 (Military Family Resource Center, www.mfrc-dodqol.org/, 2002). There were 1,221,951 military children and adolescents under the age of 18 (in 2003), of which 497,843 (41%) were 5 years old and younger, 426,151 (35%) were 6 to 11 years old, and 297,957 (24%) were 12 through 17 years old. The percentage of females on active duty has also dramatically increased from 1.4% in 1970 to 14.9% on 30 July 2003 (Women in the Military www.gendercenter.org/military.htm, multiple sources listed). Currently there are about 33,913 dual-military marriages and 87,475 single parent active duty families (Navy having 7.8 %, Army 7.5%, Air Force 5.0% and Marine Corps 3.2%).

Even though the military has expanded the types of behavioral health services available to families, there are still problems of stigma in seeing a military mental health care provider, "stove piping" (i.e., separate silos with their own bureaucracies) of services and shortages in certain specialties, such as child psychiatrists that are actually seeing children. The stigma about seeing a mental health provider is not unique to the military, but is probably amplified by the fear that military commanders might discover that a soldier or sailor, for instance, seeks help and this might in some way affect their career. Confidentiality issues remain a concern for the active duty military, even though in most circumstances confidentiality in seeing a provider is closely maintained. Because of the recognized concern that soldiers and/or family members might not seek assistance when needed, the Army instituted a new program called "Army One Source" that began in August 2003 (www4.army.mil/ocpa/read.php?story_id_key=5183). This program provides 24/7 telephone access for information/counseling and referral, if requested, from a social worker or psychologist. The program offers six sessions from a civilian social worker that is free of charge and completely confidential. It is hoped that individuals and families that would not otherwise seek help within the system will take this opportunity to get assistance.

SCHOOL MENTAL HEALTH AS A VEHICLE TO PROMOTE RESILIENCE IN MILITARY CHILDREN

The movement toward more comprehensive school mental health approaches, involving school-community partnerships to provide a full continuum of mental health promotion and intervention (see Weist, Evans, & Lever, 2003) is beginning to develop in military schools. Faran et al. (2003) described the first such comprehensive program—the Hawaii Wellness for Education Program (HWEP) on a military installation that included prevention, early identification and treatment of students within the school environment. In this partnership between Tripler Army Medical Center (TAMC) and the Hawaii Department of Education, child psychiatry fellows and a group of allied mental health trainees and professionals are providing a full continuum of mental health promotion, early intervention and treatment to youth and families in one elementary schools (Solomon) on Schofield Barracks and is expanding to two others (Hale Kula and Wheeler Elementary Schools on military bases in Oahu, Hawaii). Preliminary analyses of data indicate that the project is having a positive impact on the students and teachers from the participating schools. Over a period of $2\frac{1}{2}$ years at Solomon Elementary School on Schofield Barracks, 123 students have been treated. Of these students referred for emotional/behavioral problems only 1 was referred to special education (SPED), which contrasts with the rest of the Central Oahu District schools where about 25% of referrals to SPED are for emotional/behavioral problems. Parent satisfaction data at Solomon and school climate data at Wheeler Elementary School also strongly support the positive impact HWEP is having.

Importantly, the HWEP program is building interventions for students and families based on reducing the impact of risk/stress factors and on enhancing protective factors. Currently, Schofield Barracks, Hawaii is getting ready for the deployment of soldiers to Afghanistan and Iraq. The goal is to prepare students as best as possible for a parent being sent into a dangerous environment for a period of a year or more. This is a daunting task. It is remarkable that military families, in general, function so well in coping with profound stressors such as this. Fortunately there are several other Army agencies involved in the process of preparing families, such as Army Community Services (ACS), Community Mental Health Services, Family Readiness Groups, and Behavioral Health at Tripler Army Medical Center. At present, HWEP staff are holding "teach the teacher" sessions with teachers, childcare providers and child recreational staff on how to communicate with kids about the deployment of a parent. Within the school, in-class sessions with the children discussing deployment of their parents are also planned. Numerous other activities are being planned or are in progress that involve all the above agencies listed. At present the response to the coming deployment is fluid and attempts to adapt to the needs of the community.

In addition to the major focus on preventing and addressing deployment related stresses, HWEP is seeking to build interventions in each of the three elementary schools to reduce unique stressors on military families and to enhance protective factors. For example, working collaboratively with Army Community Services, a family outreach initiative is taking shape, whereby families are trained in positive mental health (including relevant stress and protective factors, and information on coping with deployment), and in turn reach out to and support other families, and help to connect them to needed resources, such as the HWEP program. Protocols are being developed to assist in identifying families who might be at particular risk (e.g., younger families, lower rank, evidence that nondeployed spouse is highly stressed).

The HWEP program is attempting to expand resources through connections with training programs in Hawaii for psychologists and social workers, and through the development of research grants. As staff in HWEP expand a training agenda is beginning to be developed in provided guided readings and training programs on reducing stress and risk and enhancing protective factors in military children and families. For example, the training program will include segments on: unique stressors of military families (e.g., deployment, risk, moves, isolation); transitioning to new communities/cultures; developing relationships in new communities; improving parent-child communication; controlling access to negative media; avoiding school disruptions; stress reduction; promoting positive family management, rituals and routines; sound financial management; promoting healthy marriage; and helping families connect to available Army resources. This training program is being developed based on the literature reviewed in this chapter.

AREAS OF NEED AND FUTURE RESEARCH

Our involvement in practice and research in child and adolescent mental health and school-based mental health for military children and families supports a number of realities. As confirmed in this chapter, there is limited literature on factors that place military children and families at risk for problems, and a limited literature on factors that may help them promote resilience. But there are many gaps in the literature. First, there is evidence that deployment is a major stressor for military children and families, but there is little empirical evidence on child and family functioning during other periods (e.g., pre and post deployment). There is a strong need to study the impact of Operation Enduring Freedom (operations in Afghanistan and Iraq) on military children and families, as was done in the past during Desert Storm. Importantly, our literature search failed to identify any comprehensive approach to assist families in coping with deployment, and similarly there was no literature on strategies to promote positive functioning during other deployment phases. There are clear needs for the future development of programs and connected research agendas related to assisting military children, families and soldiers in coping with and showing resilience during all phases of pre-deployment, deployment, sustainment, re-deployment, and post-deployment.

There are many other related research agendas ready to be pursued, such as exploring protective factors that operate for military children, understanding relationships between family well being and systems negotiation within the military, understanding negative and resilience promoting aspects of military culture, evaluating the impact of programs to support nondeployed parents, strategies to train school-based staff in reducing stress and enhancing protective factors (as beginning to be done in HWEP), and methods to promote family routines and rituals, and to promote communication (within the family and with the deployed spouse).

Similarly, our literature review highlighted problems in traditional clinic based mental health services for military children and families, and identified only a few innovative approaches to bringing needed mental health promotion and intervention services to them. One of these innovative approaches is expanded school mental health (ESMH) for military families, and we are fortunate to be a part of a leading ESMH-military school program in the Hawaii and the U.S. (see Faran et al., 2003). But again, the literature and research here is extremely limited. There is much mutual advantage to school-military partnerships. For schools that serve high percentages of military families, partnering with the military mental health community brings a high level of expertise and resources into the school, makes military officers (e.g., medical personnel with ranks of Captain or higher) human and accessible to school staff and families, and as shown by the HWEP experience, leads to outcomes valued by the families and the schools. For the military, well done ESMH provides needed care for military children and families, enhances support to them, and contributes to soldier readiness.

In spite of these advantages the reality is that there are very few ESMH programs in military schools, and the research literature on effectiveness within them is very limited. There is a tremendous opportunity to advance an interconnected program development and research agenda related to ESMH in military schools, consistent with the field's national development (see Weist, Evans, & Lever, 2003).

It is also noteworthy that nationwide there is a critical shortage of child and adolescent psychiatrists. Kim (2003) analyzed data from the American Physician Masterfile for 2000, and found that there were about 6,300 child and adolescent psychiatrists in the U.S., which correlates to a national average of 1 psychiatrist per 15,000 youths under the age of 18. He stated, "if a child and adolescent psychiatrist is to take care of the most severely impaired children and adolescents (5% of the population), each one has to carry a case load of 750 severely disturbed children and adolescents at any given time."

In the Army there is also a shortage of child and adolescent psychiatrists, although not as severe in Hawaii. There are 57 Army active duty child and adolescent psychiatrists of which only 8–12 (15–20%) are serving in full-time child and adolescent psychiatry positions (Colonel William S. Evans, personal communication, December 12, 2003). If it is assumed that there are 12 practicing child and adolescent psychiatrists, then this translates into one provider per 38,659 children and adolescents under the age of 18 (total population of 463,903). The remaining child and adolescent psychiatrists in the Army are practicing predominately adult psychiatry, although many of those (40–50%) see children on a space available basis.

These data are comparable with previous reports. Jensen et al. (1986) stated that of the 45 child and adolescent psychiatrists in the Army at that time, less than 20 "were actually serving in child psychiatry positions" given an estimated population of 630,000 children. The reason for this is there is also a shortage of psychiatrists in the Army and many child and adolescent psychiatrist are needed to care for active duty soldiers. The military has relied predominately on the TRICARE, U.S. Department of Defense (DOD) Military Health System (primarily a civilian system), to provide the additional services necessary to provide care, although there are DOD civilian psychiatrists at certain installations. For those who are referred to TRICARE providers, again the civilian system is greatly strained, in addition to the fact that in some geographic areas, TRICARE's payment rates for child and adolescent psychiatrists are below the norm for that region of the country. We found in a review of patients referred to the TRICARE network on the island of Oahu, Hawaii, only about 50% of the children were ever seen by any mental health provider.

Thus, on the one hand HWEP provides an important example of the potential for child psychiatry and ESMH, but shortages of child psychiatrists generally and in the military, are a factor that will mitigate against such involvement. This underscores the need for interdisciplinary approaches involving child psychiatry, psychology, social work and education working closely together to develop plans to promote student mental health and assist youth in need (Weist, Prodente, Ambrose, Proescher, & Waxman, 2001). It also underscores a need for advocacy within the military regarding the need for (e.g., to promote resilience in the face of deployment) and benefit (e.g., to promote soldier readiness) of enhancing involvement of child mental health professionals in interacting with students and families, such as the schools, as in the expanded school mental health approach. Clearly, an outcomes focus, as begun in the HWEP project on the impacts of ESMH in military schools, will propel further research, the growth of resources, and the advancement of the field.

ACKNOWLEDGEMENTS

We would like to sincerely thank Dr. Albert Saito for allowing us to incorporate data from a project he organized into this chapter. We also want to recognize the leadership and support we have received from the Hui E Malama Project, particularly from Gary Griffiths, Oahu Central District School Superintendent and Linda Yoshikami, Principal, Solomon Elementary School. We also want to thank Colonel William Evans, MD, Consultant for Child and Adolescent Psychiatry to the Army Surgeon General, for providing information on Army active duty child and adolescent psychiatrists.

REFERENCES

Army Public Affairs (2003). Army One Source gives around the clock human touch. www4.army.mil/ocpa/read.php?story_id_key=5183, 30 Nov 2003.

Evans, William S. (December 12, 2003). Personal communication.

Faran, M.E., Weist, M.D., Saito, A.Y., Yoshikami, L., Weiser, J.W., & Kaer, B. (2003). School-based mental health on a United States Army installation. In M.D. Weist, S.W. Evans, & N.A. Lever

(Eds.), *Handbook of school mental health: Advancing practice and research* (pp. 191–202). New York, NY: Kluwer Academic/Plenum Publishers.

Jensen, P.S., Grogan, D., Xenakis, S.N., & Bain, M.W. (1989). Father absence: Effects on child and maternal psychopathology, *Journal of the American Academy of Child and Adolescent Psychiatry, 28*(2), 171–175.

Jensen, P.S., Lewis, R.L., & Xenakis, S.N. (1986). The military family in review: Context, risk, and prevention, *Journal of the American Academy of Child and Adolescent Psychiatry, 25*(2), 225–234.

Jensen, P.S., Martin, D., & Watanabe, H. (1996). Children's response to parental separation during operation desert Storm, *Journal of the American Academy of Child and Adolescent Psychiatry, 35*(4), 433–441.

Jensen, P.S., Watanabe, H., Richters, J.E., Cortes, R., Roper, M., & Liu, S. (1995). Prevalence of mental disorder in military children and adolescents from two-stage community survey, *Journal of the American Academy of Child and Adolescent Psychiatry, 34*(11), 1514–1524.

Jensen, P.S., Xenakis, S.N., Wolf, P., & Bain, M.W. (1991). The "Military Family Syndrome" revisited: "By the Numbers", *The Journal of Nervous and Mental Disease, 179*(2), 102–107.

Kelley, M.L., Hock, E., Smith, K.M., Jarvis, M.S., Bonney, J.F., & Gaffney, M.A. (2001). Internalizing and externalizing behavior of children with enlisted navy mothers experiencing military-induced separation. *Journal of the American Academy of Child and Adolescent Psychiatry, 40*(4), 464–471.

Lagrone, D.M. (1978). The military family syndrome. *American Journal of Psychiatry, 135*(9), 1040–1043.

Logan, K.V. (1987). The emotional cycle of deployment. *Proceedings*, February 1987, 43–47.

Morrison, J. (1981). Rethinking the military family syndrome, *American Journal of Psychiatry, 138*(3), 354–357.

Nice, D.S. (1983). The course of depressive affect in navy wives during family separation, *Military Medicine, 148*, 341–343.

Pincus, S.H., House, R., Christenson, J., & Adler, L.E. (2001). The emotional cycle of deployment: A military family perspective. *US Army Medical Department Journal*, PB 8-01, 15–23.

Rosen, L.N., & Teitelbaum, J.M. (1993). Children's reactions to the desert storm deployment: Initial findings from a survey of army families, *Military Medicine, 158*, 465–469.

Shaffer, D., Fisher, P., Dulcan, M.K., Davies, M., Piacentini, J., Schwab-Stone, M.E., Lahey, B.B., Bourdon, K., Jensen, P.S., Bird, H.R., Canino, G., & Regier, D.A. (1996). The NIMH Diagnostic Interview Schedule for Children Version 2.3 (DISC-2.3): Description, acceptability, prevalence rates, and performance in the MECA study. Methods for the Epidemiology of Child and Adolescent Mental Disorders Study. *Journal of the American Academy of Child and Adolescent Psychiatry, 35*, 865–877.

Weist, M.D., Evans, S.W., & Lever, N.A. (2003). Advancing mental health practice and research in schools. In M.D. Weist, S.W. Evans, & N.A. Lever (Eds.), *Handbook of school mental health: Advancing practice and research* (pp. 1–8). New York, NY: Kluwer Academic/Plenum Publishers.

Weist, M.D., Prodente, C., Ambrose, M.G., Proescher, E., & Waxman, R.P. (2001). Mental health, health, and education staff working together in schools. *Child and Adolescent Psychiatry Clinics of North America, 10*, 33–43.

Part 4

Promising Resilience-Promoting Developments

Chapter 16

Applying Research on Resilience to Enhance School-Based Prevention

The Promoting Resilient Children Initiative

PETER A. WYMAN, WENDI CROSS, AND JASON BARRY

What has research taught us about processes that promote resilience among children facing significant challenges to healthy development? How can that knowledge be applied to enhance interventions and contribute to prevention of children's mental health problems and promotion of positive social and educational outcomes? This chapter responds to those questions in two ways. First, we summarize key research findings from a 15-year project investigating competence and resilience among urban children and families in adversity, the Rochester Child Resilience Project (e.g., Wyman, 2003; Wyman et al., 1999). Second, we describe how we have applied research findings from Rochester Child Resilience Project to develop the Promoting Resilient Children Initiative (PRCI). The PRCI is a school-based intervention designed to prevent children's conduct and emotional problems and promote positive educational attainment. PRCI builds on components of the widely disseminated Primary Mental Health Project model (Cowen, Hightower, Pedro-Carroll, Work, & Wyman, 1996) to create a second-generation prevention program.

It is timely to apply research findings from studies of risk and resilience to enhance community interventions. In response to widespread interest in the construct of resilience, there has been a burgeoning of research studies investigating that topic (e.g., Luthar, 2003; Masten & Coatsworth, 1998). For example, many studies have reported on predictors of positive social and mental health outcomes among youths in distressed urban or rural communities (e.g., Furstenberg, Cook, Eccles, Elder, & Sameroff, 1999; Masten et al., 1999; Werner & Smith, 1982). Several projects originally designed to study the etiology and course of antisocial behavior have focused on identifying predictors of positive conduct and lower risk for antisocial problems (e.g., Fergusson & Lynskey, 1996). Other researchers have studied competence among children of parents with major psychiatric disorders (e.g., Beardslee & Podorefsky, 1988) and predictors of increased functioning among maltreated children (Cicchetti & Rogosch, 1997).

Another reason to focus on transferring knowledge about resilience to communities is the growing consensus that an effective public health-mental health policy must include various intervention approaches, including programs that proactively strengthen families and children (National Institute of Mental Health, 1998; Prinz, 2002). Knowledge from studies of risk and resilience has the potential to enhance the efficacy and ecological validity of preventive interventions in several ways. By identifying diverse resources and protective factors (e.g., qualities of family environments, schools, communities) that predict positive adaptation for at-risk youths, studies of resilience point to opportunities for proactively strengthening systems of children's development to achieve prevention objectives (Wyman, Sandler, Wolchik, & Nelson, 2000). Finally, researchers of risk and resilience have enhanced understanding of processes that reduce the escalation of risk factors for disorders, which is another potential focus for interventions to avert emerging problems. Studies of risk and resilience have also clarified a number of processes that open up opportunities for at-risk children to draw on new social resources that enhance functioning (e.g., adult mentors) or acquire new skills that initiate shifts in developmental trajectories from disorder towards competence (e.g., Quinton, Pickles, Maughan, & Rutter, 1993). By applying this information to design linkages between systems (e.g., between families and schools), interventions may be able to facilitate children's "turning points" in adaptation.

GOALS OF THIS CHAPTER

Under the organizing structure of the Rochester Child Resilience Project, we have conducted a series of studies with urban families and children designed to identify predictors of competence in adversity and to clarify some component processes that contribute to resilience (e.g., Cowen et al., 1991; Hoyt-Meyers et al., 1995; Wyman, 2003). Our research questions have focused on identifying potentially "actionable" variables linked to children's resilience, which may be modifiable within interventions (e.g., children's social-cognitive skills, family access to school and community resources). Recently, we have focused on applying core research findings into creating and implementing the Promoting Resilient Children Initiative (PRCI) using a sustainable school-based intervention delivery system, the Primary Mental Health Project model (Cowen et al., 1996).

Part one of this chapter introduces the Primary Mental Health Project (PMHP) model, which provided an intervention framework upon which the expanded, "second-generation" Promoting Resilient Children Initiative was built. In the second part of this chapter we outline the Rochester Child Resilience Project samples, several research methodologies employed and principal aims of the project. Next, we summarize key research findings from the 15-year Rochester Child Resilience Project and our application of those findings towards developing intervention components and strategies for the second-generation Promoting Resilient Children Initiative (PRCI). This chapter is selective in several respects. We summarize only a portion of our research findings from the Rochester Child Resilience Project, and this summary does not include an analysis of many conceptual issues (e.g., the distinction between resource variables identified as compensatory factors vs. protective factors) that would be appropriate for a detailed research report. In addition, this chapter does not describe all sources that contributed to the PRCI intervention. For example, several social-emotional skill development components from the second author's manualized group psychotherapy programs for children (Cross & Bhutwala, 2000; Cross & Jewell, 1998; Cross & Newkirk, 1999) were incorporated into the PRCI activity components. In addition, we drew on strategies from several other evidence-based prevention models (e.g., Greenberg, Domitrovich, & Bumbarger, 2001; Wasik & Bryant, 2001) in designing PRCI components.

PRIMARY MENTAL HEALTH PROJECT (PMHP) MODEL: A STRUCTURE FOR DELIVERING SCHOOL-BASED PREVENTION SERVICES

The Promoting Resilient Children Initiative uses structural features of the Primary Mental Health Project (PMHP) model (Cowen et al., 1996) to deliver prevention services to children and families through elementary schools. The PMHP program was one of the first school-based prevention programs implemented in the United States (Cowen et al., 1963). A chief innovation of PMHP was the introduction into schools of trained paraprofessionals to address young children's behavioral and social-emotional needs. PMHP is an "indicated" prevention program, which means that the intervention targets a population showing early signs of problems. The PMHP target population is young (kindergarten—3rd grade) children showing emerging signs of behavioral and/or social-emotional problems identified in the school setting.

PMHP Components

The Primary Mental Health Project model is based on three core components:

Standardized Procedures for Early Detection of Children's Adjustment Problems

Schools implementing the PMHP model use standardized, multi-step screening procedures to identify the target population of children. Teachers in K—3rd grade classrooms complete a brief screening measure for all children in their classroom to identify those showing elevations in: aggressive, disruptive behavior; peer-social problems; and/or anxious-withdrawn behaviors. The rationale for using a standardized classroom-wide screening measure is to reduce the potential for bias in referral of targeted children. Additional screening information is provided by school mental health professionals, school records, or child self-report measures (e.g., self-report depression or anxiety). By identifying young children early in the onset of disordered development, PMHP aims to intervene in order to reduce the occurrence of serious, difficult to modify problems.

School-Based Paraprofessionals: Social-Learning Intervention

The PMHP program places trained paraprofessionals in schools to provide intervention to targeted children. The intervention consists of a non-directive, play interaction sequence designed to provide children with a supportive adult relationships in the school setting. The intervention model is based on: (1) a social-learning framework that emphasizes a child's learning of social competence through interaction and observation, and (2) attachment principles which emphasize the importance of a nurturing relationship with an adult in helping a child establish a secure base within the school. Each referred child is assigned to a paraprofessional adult, who meets individually with that child (typically weekly for one school year). Paraprofessionals are trained in skills of active listening and strategies for encouraging a child's verbalization of feelings through nondirective play. The PMHP program seeks qualified adults for the paraprofessional role from within the local school community.

Expansion of School Mental Health Professional Role

PMHP paraprofessionals work under the supervision of the school-site mental health professionals. School mental health professionals in many sites also provide consultation to teachers of referred children.

Strengths of the PMHP Model: Ecological Validity and Transportability

The PMHP program has proven to be an ecologically valid model through its transportability and sustainability in a variety of school settings (urban, rural sites). The use of a school-based intervention team supervised by school-site mental health professionals promotes integration of the project within a school setting. In turn, high integration within the school structure is associated with program "buy-in" by administrators and teachers and successful referral of targeted children. Due to those factors promoting ecological validity and sustainability, the PMHP program has been widely disseminated and is being implemented in approximately 1,400 school sites across the United States.

Evidence from several decades of program evaluation suggests that a child's participation in the PMHP program is associated with short-term gains in classroom adjustment (e.g., Chandler Weissberg, Cowen, & Guare, 1984; Weissberg, Cowen, Lotyczewski, & Gesten, 1983; Winer-Elkin, Weissberg, & Cowen, 1988). Although most PMHP evaluation studies have used comparison group designs (e.g., non-random within-school control groups, alternate school-sites), random-assignment studies have documented small to moderate reductions in aggressive-disruptive behavior and enhanced peer-social competence (e.g., Kafpaktitis & Perlmutter, 1998).

PMHP Components Used to Deliver PRCI Intervention

The Promoting Resilient Children Initiative uses structural features that have made the first-generation PMHP model an ecologically valid and sustainable school-based preventive intervention. The PRCI intervention also targets kindergarten—3rd grade children showing elevated (sub-clinical) behavioral and social-emotional problems (e.g., classroom aggression, social isolation, anxious-withdrawn behavior) identified through standardized classroom screening. This "indicated" prevention approach of the PMHP model was retained in the PRCI because this approach efficiently uses resources by focusing intervention on a group of children likely to develop later mental health problems or have poor social and educational outcomes (Offord, 1996). In addition, PRCI uses trained school-based paraprofessional teams to deliver intervention services and collaborates with school-based mental health professionals to train and supervise paraprofessionals. However, the PRCI requires additional training and ongoing supervision components for school-based teams, which are necessary to deliver the expanded intervention objectives.

Need for Expanded Intervention Goals and Strategies in the PMHP Model

One limitation of the PMHP model is the focus of intervention services on individual children without well-defined strategies for strengthening children's families or classroom environments. To address this limitation, the Promoting Resilient Children Initiative was developed with intervention components targeting an individual at-risk child as well as that child's family and school environments. Another limitation of the non-directive PMHP intervention is that few goal-directed intervention strategies are used and the intervention does not focus on standardized skill-development activities, which are important components of other evidence-based interventions (Kazdin & Weisz, 1998). To build opportunities for children to transfer skills from the intervention to other settings, the Promoting Resilient Children Intervention extensively incorporates strategies for emotional and social-cognitive skill building (see below). In addition, since the PMHP model was first developed there has been an expansion of information about resources and processes of resilience that promote positive developmental trajectories for at-risk children (e.g., Masten & Coatsworth, 1998; Wyman, Sandler, Wolchik, & Nelson, 2000). We have drawn on that knowledge in targeting specific resources and competencies for focus within the Promoting Resilient Children Initiative. For example, in PRCI children are introduced to the concept of "solvable" and "unsolvable" problems and assisted in applying this concept to challenges they face. In studies of urban children as young as 7–9 years old, the ability to distinguish between solvable from unsolvable problems was identified as a predictor of competence in adversity.

In the sections to follow, we first introduce the Rochester Child Resilience Project design and objectives. Next, we summarize selected findings from the Rochester Child Resilience Project and the contribution of those findings to the second-generation Promoting Resilient Children Initiative (PRCI).

ROCHESTER CHILD RESILIENCE PROJECT: DESIGN AND STUDY SAMPLES

Since 1987, the Rochester Child Resilience Project (RCRP) has conducted a series of studies with urban families and children (e.g., Cowen et al., 1991; Parker, Cowen, Work & Wyman, 1990; Wyman et al., 1999). The RCRP has focused principally on African American and Hispanic families (but also includes a proportion of White families) because increased knowledge of positive adaptation and resilience among minority youths is an important public health priority. Diverse racial/ethnic groups are at increased risk for many adverse health and mental health outcomes and have disparately low access to health services (U.S. Department of Health & Human Services, 1999). Therefore, the RCRP focused on attaining information about naturally embedded resources and protective factors for youth of color because this information can contribute to developing culturally valid prevention initiatives.

RCRP Cohorts: Urban Families and Children

Nearly 1,400 urban families and children (ranging from early school age—mid-adolescence) have enrolled in the RCRP since 1987. Most RCRP studies have focused on two cohorts. The first cohort of 10–12 year old children was selected from urban elementary schools (Rochester City School District) from 1987–1989. A portion of those Cohort 1 youths and families participated in a $1\frac{1}{2}$–2 year follow-up evaluation (e.g., Wyman, Cowen, Work, & Kerley, 1993). A second cohort of younger children (7–9 year olds) was enrolled from 1991–1993. By enrolling younger children, we sought an opportunity to both replicate findings from the Cohort 1 sample and test developmentally-oriented questions (e.g., whether social-cognitive skills linked to resilience among 10–12 year old children could be reliably assessed in younger children to determine their emergence within children's cognitive development). That sample, now in mid-adolescence, is the focus of an ongoing 8-year follow-up evaluation (Wyman et al., 2003).

Defining at-Risk Status in RCRP Cohorts: Family Psychosocial Adversities

There is general consensus that studies of resilience require: (a) evidence of positive adaptation (e.g., a child's social-emotional competence, recovery from disorder), co-occurring with (b) the presence of a defined risk factor(s) that poses a threat to healthy functioning and development (Masten et al., 1999). Within the RCRP cohorts, threat to development was defined by cumulative, lifetime exposure to four or more psychosocial adversities (birth—enrollment). That criterion was selected based on evidence that the likelihood of a child developing a behavioral and/or emotional disorder increases markedly with multiple risk factors during childhood (Seifer & Sameroff, 1987).

In the RCRP, three constellations of psychosocial adversities have been assessed in participating families to define high-risk status (Kilmer, Cowen, Wyman, Work, & Magnus, 1998): (1) Family poverty and/or deficiencies in the physical environment, which included parent unemployment, family income below the federally-defined poverty line, and frequent changes in residence. (2) Functional impairment of a child's parent or guardian, e.g., substance use problems, psychiatric problems, or chronic physical illness. (3) Family discord and violence. Other risk factors used to define RCRP samples include a child's exposure to neighborhood violence and death of a parent or other close family member. In our cohort 2 sample, 43% of children had a family member in their home with an alcohol/drug problem; 29% had a family member in their home arrested or in jail; and 20% had a family member with a serious emotional problem. At ages 13–15 (6-year follow-up), 24% of sample youths reported that a member of their family had been murdered.

RCRP Methodologies and Study Designs

Selection criterion for youths to enroll in the RCRP included lifetime exposure to multiple psychosocial adversities. Multiple adversities among all participants represented a "shared risk factor" for poor developmental outcomes and/or psychopathology (Seifer & Sameroff, 1987). In the context of that shared risk, youths demonstrated wide variation in competence and levels of problems: whereas a substantial proportion of youths in both RCRP cohorts demonstrated high levels of behavioral and social competence relative to similar age peers, others showed significant problems of adaptation including aggressive and disruptive behavior problems (Parker, Cowen, Work, & Wyman, 1990; Hoyt-Meyers et al., 1995). Although a portion of the variation in youths' functioning was undoubtedly due to differences in the severity and/or chronicity of risk factors, differences in youth and family resources were also expected to account for a portion of variation in youths' functioning, and identification of those resources was a principal objective. Many RCRP studies have employed a "person-centered" methodology (Cairns & Cairns, 1994) designed to test differences in predictors (e.g., children's attributes, family processes) between children demonstrating resilience (i.e., high competence- low problems despite multiple family risks) with youths demonstrating problems of adaptation. In other studies we have tested multivariate models to identify resources that predicted variation in youths' positive behavioral or social-emotional functioning over time (e.g., Cowen et al., 1991; Wyman et al., 1993). Several recent studies have also sought to identify factors in families and communities that reduce youths' level of exposure to risk factors (e.g., Barry & Wyman, 2003).

APPLYING RESEARCH ON RESILIENCE TO PREVENTION: PROMOTING RESILIENT CHILDREN INITIATIVE

Findings from the Rochester Child Resilience Project studies point to several conclusions about processes of resilience initiated by children and families, and in their transactions with communities. Those conclusions are summarized below in three sections. Each section is followed by a description of how the information contributed to new intervention objectives and components for the second-generation Promoting Resilient Children Initiative, which builds on the first-generation PMHP model. It is important to note that the RCRP research findings used to formulate our conclusions are generally congruent with findings reported by other investigators of risk and resilience (e.g., Luthar, 2003; Masten & Coatsworth, 1998). We used this congruence as a gauge of generalizability and for selecting findings to apply in intervention development.

Children's Social-Cognitive and Emotional Competencies: Contribution to Establishing Trajectories of Positive Adaptation

One broad conclusion from RCRP studies is that a child's acquisition of competencies in interpreting social relationships, regulating emotions, and personal self-efficacy contribute to mastery of adverse experiences and towards establishing a trajectory of positive adaptation (e.g., Cowen et al., 1991; Hoyt-Meyers et al., 1995; Parker et al., 1990). Our findings suggest that competence within those domains assist children in forming more accurate interpretations of family problems, managing emotional responses to distressing events, and in accessing social resources for support (Wyman, 2003).

For example, one early goal of the RCRP was to determine the degree to which 10–12 year old children differentiated between their ability to influence challenges that are generally outside of children's control (e.g., parent substance use) from challenges that children typically can influence (e.g., whether they get in trouble in school). We hypothesized that children who made realistic distinctions in their control attributions (i.e., low expectations for control of family problems coupled with high expectations for control child problems) would experience lower distress and be better able to direct their attention to achievable goals (Wannon, 1990). Indeed, a substantial proportion of the sample of 10–12 year olds made realistic distinctions between controllable and uncontrollable challenges, and that capacity predicted behavioral and social-emotional competence based on teacher and parent ratings (Parker et al., 1990).

Subsequent research with the second, younger RCRP cohort (7–9 year olds) found that many children at that younger age also differentiated between controllable and uncontrollable challenges in their lives and that capacity predicted higher levels of classroom behavior competence and positive social-emotional functioning (Hoyt-Meyers et al., 1995). However, realistic control attribution was, as expected, a less articulated skill in younger compared to older children. Those findings suggested that early school years is a period when children's capacity to distinguish between controllable and uncontrollable challenges undergoes significant modification and differentiation, indicating that this age-period may be appropriate for enhancing this skill.

Other domains of children's competence that predicted children's positive adaptation and lower levels of problems in RCRP cohorts included: emotional and behavioral self-control skills (e.g., teacher ratings of children's positive frustration tolerance), positive social attributions (e.g., empathy for other children), and perceptions of self-efficacy (Cowen et al., 1991; Wyman et al., 1992). In addition, findings from longitudinal studies established continuity between children's early competencies and positive behavioral and social-emotional functioning several years later, over and above the effects of cumulative risk factors (e.g., Kerley, 1997; Wyman et al., 1993).

Another conclusion from the RCRP is that young children's social and emotional competencies assist them in drawing on school and community resources in later phases of development. In a 6-year follow-up of cohort 2, Wyman et al., (2003) found that competent children were more likely as adolescents to be involved in youth development activities (e.g., organized clubs, sports, artistic activities), which in turn predicted lower levels of antisocial behavior, including reduced delinquency and substance use.

PRCI Child-Focused Skill Component

One way the Promoting Resilient Children Initiative (PRCI) augments the PMHP model is through the addition of a skill-development component for participating children. The skill component focuses on enhancing each child's emotional-regulation skills, accurate attributions for coping with life challenges, and problem-solving skills. Figure 1 summarizes the intervention conceptual model for the Promoting Resilient Children Initiative.

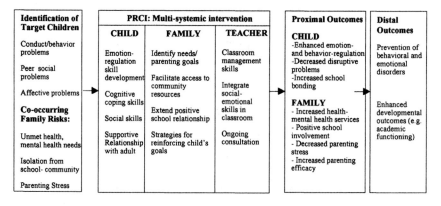

Figure 1. Conceptual Model for Promoting Resilient Children Initiative

Following classroom-wide screening to identify targeted children, each referred child (following parent consent) is assigned to an adult paraprofessional who meets weekly with that child for 12–14 weeks in the first year of the intervention. Each child's experience in the program is designed to address his/her behavioral needs and promote identified competencies, in three phases: (a) establishing a supportive relationship between paraprofessional mentor and child; (b) promoting affect and social-cognitive competencies including identifying and labeling feelings, identifying controllable aspects of challenging experiences; (c) coping and mastery, including developing individual strategies for behavior control and for social relationships.

In order to implement the child competence component of the PRCI intervention, paraprofessionals receive extensive training in how to incorporate skill-building exercises within their supportive interactions with children and their work is guided by a "toolbox" of exercises (Cross & Wyman, 2002). For each targeted child, facilitating a supportive relationship with an engaged, competent adult within the school setting is itself a focal objective and is designed to build a "secure base" for learning new skills. Through generalizing that positive relationship to other relationships within the school setting (e.g., teachers), the objective is to increase a child's school bonding.

PRCI Classroom Component

The PRCI also incorporates a teacher-consultation component (see Figure 1) designed to assist teachers in reinforcing and extending a child's work on developing effective coping and behavioral strategies. The PRCI teacher consultation component provides information to teachers about: (a) effective behavior management techniques, and (b) the program model that emphasizes children's emotional competence as a building block to effective behavior control and interpersonal relationships. An additional goal is that these teacher skills will generalize to other children in the classroom not specifically targeted by the intervention. Ongoing consultation among teacher, paraprofessional and mental health professional is used to promote consistency of strategies in working with each child. We are continuing to develop and refine the teacher consultation component of the PRCI. However, preliminary process evaluations comparing PRCI implementation at different sites suggest that a lead teacher consultant within each school who can work with the PRCI team in assessing teachers' needs is an essential component for success.

Effective Family Systems: Role in Competence Promotion and Risk Protection

Several RCRP studies point to another broad-band conclusion: family systems with one or more competent caregivers exert a strong protective effect for most children in reducing harm from psychosocial risk factors (Kilmer, Cowen, & Wyman, 2001; Wyman et al., 1991, 1999). In RCRP cohorts, a large proportion of children within family contexts that provided them with a competent caregiver (i.e., emotionally engaged with the child and provided age-appropriate structure) demonstrated high levels of functioning and few demonstrated emerging problems, despite many psychosocial adversities. Further, emotionally-responsive parent-child relationships appeared to play an important role in a child's acquisition of competence in emotional and behavioral self-regulation, upon which children could build further skills for coping and adaptation. In addition to parenting practices, another feature of family competence was the capacity of adult caregivers to draw on extended family and community resources (Wyman et al., 1991, 1999).

Our studies also suggest that effective parenting may reduce youths' exposure to some community risk factors, which can be considered another process of resilience. Specifically, Barry and Wyman (2003) in follow-up evaluations of cohort 2 youths into adolescence (six and eight years after enrollment) found that higher levels of parent monitoring of children's behavior predicted less exposure to community violence. In addition, higher parent monitoring of behavior at ages 13–15 predicted reduced violence exposure two years later, above and beyond the effects of SES and cumulative family risk factors, suggesting some protective effects of effective parenting are enduring.

RCRP findings also underscored how many family risk processes extend across long phases of children's development if not successfully addressed. For example, a six-year follow-up evaluation of cohort 2 families found that nearly 70% of families reporting a parent substance use problem at enrollment reported a family substance use problem six years later (Wyman et al., 2003). Continuity of family risk factors had significant implications for children's development over time: children in families with high levels of ongoing psychosocial adversities were more likely to develop significant antisocial problems as adolescents, show academic failure, and emerging problems of anxiety and depression.

PRCI Family Component

The Promoting Resilient Children Initiative adds to the PMHP model a family component directed towards enhancing the capacity of each participating child's parent or guardian to achieve parenting goals and to draw effectively on community resources to address needs they identify (see Figure 1).

In the PRCI family component, contacts are made to each family (usually through a home visit, other times at school) to achieve several specific objectives: introduce the program; assess family needs and competencies; facilitate family access to identified community services to address needs and goals; extend a positive home-school relationship; and develop with the parent strategies for reinforcing a child's program goals. Family home visits are made by the paraprofessional accompanied by the supervising mental health professional or senior (mentor) paraprofessional. A minimum of two family contacts is the goal for the first 14-week intervention phase. An extended, more intensive family contact component (6–8 contacts) is made for families requiring more services. Paraprofessionals receive training in the goals and objectives for family contacts, and in identifying and accessing community resources (Cross & Wyman, 2002). Following the first parent contact, a goal-setting conference is held with the prevention team and child's classroom teacher (to which parents are invited) to establish specific goals for each child. Practices are designed to deliver culturally competent services to families. For example, Spanish translations of many project materials have been made to enhance access for Latino families. Similarly, in one school with a high Latino family population, lists of resources for parents showing family health services include information about bilingual services. Further, paraprofessionals are encouraged to assess differences in family structure and in values about help-seeking and family-community contacts.

Differences in Pathways of Risk and Resilience

Recent RCRP studies point to meaningful variations in how children and families use resources to promote competence and resilience depending on individual differences and social contexts (Wyman, 2003). As a case in point, our early studies found that children's tendency to report positive future expectations predicted classroom behavioral and social competence for 10–12 year olds youths because those views appeared to reflect engagement in active striving and optimism (Wyman et al., 1993). However, a recent study with cohort 2 adolescents found that positive future expectations were not adaptive for all youths. For a subgroup of youths with histories of elevated antisocial behaviors, there was an inverse relationship between positive future expectations and effective school conduct and engagement (Wyman & Forbes-Jones, 2001). For those conduct problem youths, positive expectations appeared to reflect a "bravado" and lack of ability to tolerate frustration. Thus, whereas some children may benefit from facilitated creative exploration of their future goals, other children may benefit more from developing skills for considering the consequences of behavior and assistance in developing realistic, achievable goals. This is just one instance of how interventions to develop skills and competencies must take into account a child's individual context and existing cognitive and behavioral functioning.

Another recent study based on follow-up of cohort 2 children in adolescence found that positive bonding to family predicted behavioral competence for the sample as a whole, but not for all groups of youths. For a group of youths from low functioning families, enhanced behavior functioning in adolescence was associated with low bonding to parents, suggesting that resources promoting adaptation for this group were not based in the parent-child relationship but in other resources (Wyman et al., 2003). In the aggregate, these findings suggest that resilience represents a diverse set of processes that vary in effectiveness for children depending on the particular challenges they face, opportunities available to them, and capacity to effectively use those resources (Wyman, 2003).

PRCI: Individual Goal-Setting and Multiple Systems Focus

We have developed the Promoting Resilient Children Initiative mindful that children face different risk factors and that there are individual differences in how children and families use resources to promote positive adaptation. First, the PRCI is designed to reduce risks and enhance resources at several levels of a child's developmental context (i.e., individual child resources, family, and classroom). One reason is because strategies for reducing some risk factors (e.g., reducing unintentional reinforcement of children's coercive behavior) are more effective if instituted across settings. However, an additional reason for targeting multiple systems simultaneously is because this approach provides more opportunities for children to draw on resources according to individual differences. For example, whereas some children may draw effectively on the PRCI paraprofessional mentors as a resource to help them master challenges and experience support, other children may focus on teachers or other adults and the intervention is designed to increase those multiple opportunities.

The PRCI also incorporates individual goal setting with each child and family at multiple points during the intervention. The intervention is designed to establish for each targeted child one or more specific behavioral goals based on information from the screening (e.g., levels of classroom aggression, peer-social problems), from the child's classroom teacher, and, whenever possible, from parents. A child's (and his/her family's) participation in a second year of the PRCI is also designed to match intervention components and goals to ongoing needs and risks. During the second year of PRCI participation, a child re-establishes the relationship with the adult paraprofessional mentor and continues skill development activities tailored to his/her needs. The PRCI year 2 program also includes opportunities for children to enhance skills for developing and maintaining friendships within small "friendship groups."

SUMMARY AND FUTURE DIRECTIONS

We have applied findings from a program of research investigating competence and resilience to develop the Promoting Resilient Children Initiative, a second-generation preventive intervention that builds on components of the school-based PMHP model. The expanded intervention components of the Promoting Resilient Children Initiative include: (1) Introduction of a skill-development component designed to enhance children's social-cognitive and emotion-regulation competencies as they work with an engaged, responsive adult paraprofessional in their school. Findings from our research suggest that those skills can both address immediate problem areas for children (e.g., assist children in reducing impulsivity) and also prepare them to better negotiate future challenges, including family adversities and peer influences. (2) We have introduced a family component into the PRCI intervention, designed to enhance a family's opportunities to identify and meet parenting goals and family needs through school and community resources. A major impetus for this goal was our finding that resilience often occurs through a family's capacity to access and use a variety of community resources. (3) We have also introduced into the new PRCI model a teacher-consultation component. Combined with the opportunity for children to form a positive, secure relationship with an adult paraprofessional, these components are designed to increase children's school bonding and assist them in generalizing positive relationships in early elementary years to future effective relationships within schools. That goal is based on our research findings that underscored the importance of school relationships and resources in helping children to establish trajectories of competence and educational success.

We have begun program evaluation of the new PRCI intervention within urban elementary schools. Our preliminary findings (Cross, Wyman, & Hightower, 2002) suggest that the intervention is effective in reducing children's classroom behavior problems, including lowering rates of children's formal disciplinary problems, and increasing children's peer-social functioning. Our findings also suggest that the PRCI model has a larger "effect size" in reducing children's behavior problems compared to the first-generation PMHP model (Wyman et al., 2003). In our initial implementations, the PRCI intervention successfully engaged most targeted children, and the PRCI program has been retained within implementing schools, suggesting that the PRCI intervention retains the ecological validity of the first-generation PMHP program. However, we have also identified numerous challenges for further program development. A substantial proportion of families did not complete their participation in the PRCI family component, suggesting that we must formulate new and creative ways to successfully engage parents of children served by PRCI. Moreover, the PRCI intervention requires substantial training for school-based prevention teams and mental health professionals. Although we found most paraprofessionals and mental health professionals enjoyed this training, it is time-consuming and requires resources. Establishing cost-effective and transportable training methods will be a challenge for larger scale dissemination of PRCI. However, those challenges are worthy of the collective efforts by researchers and communities as we strive to promote resilience and reduce the burden of mental health problems in children.

ACKNOWLEDGMENT

We thank the William T. Grant Foundation for its generous support of our research conducted under the Rochester Child Resilience Project. We also wish to acknowledge the assistance of a grant from the Center for Mental Health Services (SAMHSA) to implement the initial evaluation trials of the Promoting Resilient Children Initiative.

REFERENCES

Barry, J., & Wyman, P.A. (2003). Family system predictors of violence exposure among urban high-risk adolescents. Submitted.

Beardslee, W.R., & Podorefsky, D. (1988). Resilient adolescents whose parents have serious affective and other psychiatric disorders: Importance of self-understanding and relationships. *American Journal of Psychiatry, 145*(1), 63–69.

Cairns, R.B., & Cairns, B. (1994). *Lifelines and risks: Pathways of youth in our time.* New York: Cambridge University Press.

Chandler, C., Weissberg, R.P., Cowen, E.L., & Guare, J. (1984). The long-term effects of a school-based secondary prevention program for young maladapting children. *Journal of Consulting and Clinical Psychology, 52,* 165–170.

Cicchetti, D., & Rogosch, F.A. (1997). The role of self-organization in the promotion of resilience in maltreated children. *Development and Psychopathology, 9,* 797–815.

Cowen, E.L., Hightower, A.D., Pedro-Carroll, J.L., Work, W.C., & Wyman, P.A. (1996). *School based prevention for children at risk: The Primary Mental Health Project.* Washington, DC: American Psychological Association.

Cowen, E.L., Izzo, L.D., Miles, H., Telschow, E.F., Trost, M.A., & Zax, M. (1963). A preventive mental health program in the school setting: Description and evaluation. *Journal of Psychology, 56,* 307–356.

Cowen, E.L., Work, W.C., Hightower, A.D., Wyman, P.A., Parker, G.R., & Lotyczewski, B.S. (1991). Toward the development of a measure of perceived self-efficacy in children. *Journal of Clinical Child Psychology, 20,* 169–178.

Cross, W., & Bhutwala, S. (2000). *A social skills group for girls 7–9 years old.* Unpublished manual.

Cross, W., & Jewell, H. (1998). *All about friends and feelings: A social skills group for 8–10 year old boys.* Unpublished manual.

Cross, W., & Newkirk, J. (1999). *Coping with death, grief and loss: A group for school-aged children.* Unpublished manual.

Cross, W., & Wyman, P.A. (2002). *Promoting Resilient Children Initiative: A manual of child, teacher, and parent program components.* Unpublished manual.

Cross, W., Wyman, P.A., & Hightower, A.D. (2002, October). *Preliminary evaluation of a school-based 'indicated' prevention program.* Poster session presented at the 49th Annual Meeting of the American Academy of Child & Adolescent Psychiatry, San Francisco, CA.

Fergusson, D.M., & Lynskey, M.T. (1996). Adolescent resiliency to family adversity. *Journal of Child Psychology and Psychiatry, 38,* 899–908.

Furstenberg, F.F., Cook, T.D., Eccles, J., Elder, G.H., Jr., & Sameroff, A. (1999). *Managing to make it: Urban families and adolescent success.* Chicago: University of Chicago Press.

Greenberg, M.T., Domitrovich, C., & Bumbarger, B. (2001). The prevention of mental disorders in school-aged children: Current State of the field. *Prevention and Treatment, 4,* 1–59.

Hoyt-Meyers, L.A., Cowen, E.L., Work, W.C., Wyman, P.A., Magnus, K.B., Fagen, D.B., & Lotyczewski, B.S. (1995). Test correlates of resilient outcomes among highly stressed 2nd and 3rd grade urban children. *Journal of Community Psychology, 23,* 326–338.

Kafpaktitis, M., & Perlmutter, B.F. (1998). School-based early mental health intervention with at-risk students. *School Psychology Review, 27,* 420–432.

Kazdin, A.E., & Weisz, J.R. (1998). Identifying and developing empirically supported child and adolescent treatments. *Journal of Consulting and Clinical Psychology, 66,* 19–36.

Kerley, J.A. (1997). *Social competence and life stress as predictors of school adjustment in urban early adolescents: A prospective-longitudinal study.* Unpublished Ph.D. dissertation, The Fielding Institute.

Kilmer, R.P., Cowen, E.L., & Wyman, P.A. (2001). A micro-level analysis of developmental, parenting, and family milieu variables that differentiate stress-resilient and stress-affected children. *Journal of Community Psychology, 29,* 391–416.

Kilmer, R.P. Cowen, E.L., Wyman, P.A., Work, W.C., & Magnus, K.B. (1998). Differences in stressors experienced by urban African-American, White and Hispanic children. *Journal of Community Psychology, 26,* 415–428.

Luthar, S. (Ed.) (2003). *Resilience and vulnerability: Adaptation in the context of childhood adversity.* New York: Cambridge University Press.

Masten, A.S., & Coatsworth, J.D. (1998). The development of competence in favorable and unfavorable environments: Lessons from research on successful children. *American Psychologist, 53,* 205–220.

Masten, A.S., Hubbard, J.J., Gest, S.D., Tellegen, A., Garmezy, N., & Ramirez, M. (1999). Competence in the context of adversity: Pathways to resilience and maladaptation from childhood to late adolescence. *Development & Psychopathology. Vol 11(1), 143–169.*

National Institute of Mental Health. (1998). *Priorities for prevention research.* (NIH Publication No. 98–4321 ed.). Washington, DC: U.S. Department of Health and Human Services.

Offord, D.R. (1996). The state of prevention and early intervention. In R. Peters & R. McMahon (Eds.), *Preventing childhood disorders, substance abuse, and delinquency* (pp. 329–244). Thousand Oaks, CA: Sage.

Parker, G.R., Cowen, E.L., Work, W.C., & Wyman, P.A. (1990). Test correlates of stress resilience among urban school children. *Journal of Primary Prevention, 11,* 19–35.

Prinz, R.J. (2002). The Fast Track Project: A seminal intervention efficacy trial. *Journal of Abnormal Child Psychology, 30,* 61–64.

Quinton, D., Pickles, A., Maughan, B., & Rutter, M. (1993). Partners, peers, and pathways: Assortative pairing and continuities in conduct disorder. *Development & Psychopathology, 5* (4), 763–783.

Seifer, R., & Sameroff, A.J. (1987). In E.J. Anthony & B.J. Cohler (Eds). *The invulnerable child. The Guilford psychiatry series.* (pp. 51–69). xiv, 432 pp.

U.S. Department of Health and Human Services. (1999). *Mental Health: A report of the Surgeon General.* Rockville, MD: U.S. Department of Health and Human Services, Substance Abuse and Mental Health Services Administration, Center for Mental Health Services, National Institutes of Health, National Institute of Mental Health.

Wannon, M. (1990). Children's control beliefs about controllable and uncontrollable events: Their relationship to stress resilience and psychosocial adjustment. Unpublished Ph.D. dissertation, University of Rochester, Rochester, NY.

Wasik, B.H., & Bryant, D.M. (2001). *Home visiting.* (2nd Edition). Thousand Oaks, CA: Sage.

Weissberg, R.P., Cowen, E.L., Lotyczewski, B.S., & Gesten, E.L. (1983). The Primary Mental Health Project: Seven consecutive years of program outcome research. *Journal of Consulting and Clinical Psychology, 51,* 100–107

Winer-Elkin, J.I., Weissberg, R.P., & Cowen, E.L. (1988). Evaluation of a planned short-term intervention for school children with focal adjustment problems. *Journal of Clinical Child Psychology, 17,* 106–115.

Werner, E.E., & Smith, R.S. (1982). *Vulnerable but invincible: A study of resilient children.* New York: McGraw-Hill.

Wyman, P.A. (2003). Emerging perspectives on context-specificity of children's adaptation and resilience: Evidence from a decade of research with urban children in adversity. In S. Luthar (Ed.), *Resilience and vulnerability: Adaptation in the context of childhood adversity* (pp. 293–317). New York: Cambridge University Press.

Wyman, P.A., Cowen, E.L., Work, W.C., Hoyt-Meyers, L.A., Magnus, K.B., & Fagen, D.B. (1999). Caregiving and developmental factors differentiating young at-risk urban children showing resilient versus stress-affected outcomes: A replication and extension. *Child Development, 70,* 645–659.

Wyman, P.A., Cowen, E.L., Work, W.C., & Parker, G.R. (1991). Developmental and family milieu correlates of resilience in urban children who have experienced major life-stress. *American Journal of Community Psychology, 19,* 405–426.

Wyman, P.A., Cowen, E.L., Work, W.C., & Kerley, J.H. (1993). The role of children's future expectations in self-system functioning and adjustment to life-stress. *Development and Psychopathology, 5,* 649–661.

Wyman, P.A., Cowen, E.L., Work, W.C., Raoof, A., Gribble, P.A., Parker, G.R., & Wannon, M. (1992). Interviews with children who experienced major life stress: Family and child attributes that predict resilient outcomes. *Journal of the American Academy of Child and Adolescent Psychiatry, 31,* 904–910.

Wyman, P.A., Cross, W., Hightower, A.D., Barry, J., & Montes, G. (2003). Promoting Resilient Children Initiative: Results of two randomized trials of a school-based prevention program. Submitted.

Wyman, P.A., Forbes-Jones. E.L., Cowen, E.L., Lotyczewski, B.S., Kilmer, R.P., Kaufmann, D., Barry, J., & Spomer, M. (2003). Which resilient children maintain competence vs. transition to antisocial problems? Contributions of social resources, poverty, and violence from childhood to adolescence. Submitted.

Wyman, P.A., Sandler, I.N., Wolchik, S., & Nelson, K. (2000). Resilience as cumulative competence promotion and stress protection: Theory and intervention. In D. Cicchetti, J. Rappaport, I.N. Sandler & R.P. Weissberg (Eds.), *The promotion of wellness in children and adolescents* (pp. 133–184). Thousand Oaks, CA: Sage Publications.

Chapter 17

Educational Resilience in Life's Second Decade
The Centrality of Student Engagement

RICHARD DE LISI

INTRODUCTION

This chapter provides a review of the recent literature on *educational resilience,* a sub area within the larger field of resilience. Resilience refers to a process by which good outcomes occur despite previous or ongoing adversity that threatens development (Luthar, Cicchetti, & Becker, 2000a; Masten, 2001). Resilience is typically studied in the context of major life tasks or domains of competence (Masten & Coatsworth, 1998). In western cultures, *academic performance* (Masten et al., 1995) is clearly one such domain that has a long and rich history of investigation in both developmental psychology and educational psychology. The past century's worth of research in these two fields has led to a rich corpus of knowledge about predictors and correlates of academic performance such as: intelligence as measured by Intelligence Quotient (IQ) tests, prior academic performance, disability status, socio-emotional functioning including peer relationships, behavioral conduct, motivation to achieve in school, cognitive self regulation abilities, self concept and confidence in one's ability to learn, socioeconomic status, parent variables including childrearing styles, demographic variables (ethnic/language/gender/racial categories), school variables including grade transitions, teacher variables including expectations for students, curriculum area (reading, mathematics, science, etc.), and assessment format. This list is far from complete. See Berliner and Calfee's (1994) *Handbook of Educational Psychology* for summary reviews.

Although this body of work on academic achievement has served as a foundation, the area of educational resilience suffers from the same problems that plague the field of resilience (Luthar et al., 2000a; Masten, 2001). Definitions and measurement approaches to educational resilience vary on the assessment of academic risk and on the criteria for academic performance that need to be present in order for a student to be classified as resilient. The field is shifting from viewing educational resilience as an individual trait to an unfolding process that is both context and time specific. Finally, there is not yet a unified model or theory that explains educational resilience, especially when viewed as a developmental process (Noam & Hermann, 2002; Richardson, 2002).

Due to limitations of space, this review is highly selective and limited in the following three ways. (1) Publications from 1994 to 2002 that self-identified as pertaining to resilience in educational contexts were included. (2) Research on educational resilience in students in the late elementary school years through college graduation was reviewed. (3) The focus (but with some exceptions) is on research in which academic performance itself was initially an area of measured risk and subsequently an area of measured competence. This is a fairly new focus in resiliency research. It is important to examine evidence of educational resilience in the second decade of life, especially when this entails recovery from previous academic deficiencies. The larger literature in educational psychology has consistently found that students who fall behind in school and perform below grade-level targets tend to stay behind for the rest of their academic careers. Therefore, recent work that views academic performance itself to be a risk factor that some students can overcome and turn into an area of competence is important. This work also provides a foundation for intervention efforts after the early childhood years.

With these restrictions, two broad types of studies are reviewed in this chapter. The first is recent qualitative work in which students give "voice" to their experiences in academic settings. These studies are designed to clarify what factors are responsible for good academic outcomes despite prior threats to development. The students' views provide an important addition to quantitative findings reported since the 1970's. An overview summary of studies using interviews and surveys to measure educational resilience is presented in Table 1. Note that in only about half of these studies is initially poor academic performance used as the defining risk factor (see column 2 of Table 1). In the other half of the studies, more distal factors such as social address are used as the defining risk factor. The second body of work reviewed in this chapter consists of quantitatively focused studies that seek to explain resilient versus nonresilient outcomes using regression or modeling analytic techniques. An overview of these studies can be found in Table 2. Note that in all but one of these studies, poor academic performance was used to define risk or adversity (see column 2 of Table 2). The chapter concludes with a brief discussion

Table 1. Overview of Interview/Survey Studies Pertaining to Educational Resilience (1998–2002)

Reference	Target Group	Competence Criteria	Participants	Method/Analysis	Major Finding
Howard & Johnson (2000)	Poor, urban students in Australia.	None listed.	125 9–12 yr olds 25 teachers.	Interview: Why do some make it despite tough life?	Students > teachers in importance of school achievement.
Kenny et al. (2002, Study 2)	Urban, ethnic minorities. Lower GPA/higher depressive symptoms.	College preparation Saturday program. Higher GPA/lower depressive symptoms.	16 HS Seniors with 4 years in special program.	Interview & questionnaires.	Peer support a protective factor; lack of stress in resilient subgroup.
Miller (2002)	Learning Disability; Major GPA < B+.	Major GPA of B+ = resilient.	10 Undergraduates, State University.	Interview: recall school experiences.	7 areas of difference for resilience.
Montgomery et al. (2000)	Native Americans, traditional rearing.	College Graduation (near or attained).	9 females, 5 males aged 21–52.	Interview: interest and persistence.	Culture-education integration needed.
Morrison et al. (2002)	Low SES Latinos.	Self-report change in antisocial behaviors.	115 fifth/six graders; boys/girls.	Surveys in November and May.	School engagement is protective.
O'Connor (1998)	Poor, urban African American students.	School achievement.	24 female, 22 male HS sophomores.	Interviews: race & school experiences.	Role-model—optimism—school engagement linkage.
Weinstein (2002)	Classrooms that accentuate achievement differences.	Students labeled as high or low achievers.	Various grade school & college students.	Interviews & surveys about school experiences.	Expectations vary with classroom "cultures."

Table 2. Overview of Quantitative Studies Pertaining to Educational Resilience (1994–2002)

Reference	Target Group	Competence Criteria	Participants	Method/Analysis	Major Finding
Cappella & Weinstein (2001).	Low Grade 8 reading level.	Grade 12 reading level.	NELS-88 national sample ($n = 1362$).	Mediational regression analyses.	Student race, gender, LOC, & curriculum predicted resilience.
Catterall (1998).	Low Grade 8 academic commitment & GPA < "C" in English (grades 6–8).	Increased academic commitment and grades in English at grade 10.	NELS-88 national sample (4,000–7,000 at risk in grade 8.	Regression analysis for total sample and by student subgroups.	Family support, school safety, resp., student participation predict resilience.
Connell et al. (1994)	Low SES, African American students.	High attendance, high test scores, grades.	3 Independent samples of 10–16 yr. olds.	Path Model with distal & proximal predictors.	Student engagement predicted school performance/adjust.
Finn & Rock (1997).	Low GPA in Grades 8, 10; reading/math. test scores. Grade 12 drop out.	G 8. 10 average GPA; test scores; complete G 12.	NELS-88: two minority subgroups ($n = 1,803$).	MANOVA's: resilient vs. 2 types of nonresilient.	Student engagement key to academic resilience.
Jimerson et al. (1999)	Negative achievement trajectories Grades 1–6 and G 1- age 16.	Positive achieve. trajectories G 1–6 and G 1- age 16.	Longitudinal study of 174 children at risk due to poverty.	Correlations & hierarchical regressions.	SES, home envir., & parental involvement predicted achievement & growth.
Kenny et al. (2002, Study 1)	Urban, ethnic minority students.	College preparation Saturday program.	100 G 9, 10, 12 HS Students.	Correlations.	Maternal attachment-GPA correlation.
Turner & Schallert (2001).	Self-reported shame following midterm coupled with no improvement in test scores.	Self-reported shame following midterm coupled with improvement in test scores.	84 undergraduates in upper-level course for majors.	Correlations, hierarchical regression, t-tests.	Shame induced resilience (> effort) when important future goals viewed as threatened.

of the impact that high stakes achievement testing will have on theory, research, and practices pertaining to educational resilience.

VOICES OF STUDENTS JUDGED TO BE EDUCATIONALLY RESILIENT

Elementary School Students

Howard and Johnson (2002) visited five primary schools in an economically depressed urban area in South Australia and interviewed 125 randomly selected 9–12 year old children in groups of 2–5 and also individually interviewed 25 teachers. Both the children and teachers were asked: (a) "what they thought a 'tough life' was; (b) why 'some kids have a tough life and don't do O.K.', and (c) why 'some kids have a tough life but do O.K'" (p. 324). Children's and teachers' perspectives on what makes the difference were grouped in terms of three contexts: family, school, and community. Both children and teachers viewed loving relationships within families as important. Teachers also mentioned the need for parents to encourage independence and maturity in children and the fact that parents can provide role models for children living in difficult circumstances. The children stressed the importance of parents helping them (the children) to succeed in school and to become competent. With respect to the role of the school, teachers and students had different views. Teachers emphasized the importance of social skills training and making the child feel comfortable in school. The students said schools that made a difference help the child to overcome learning difficulties. The students viewed school failures as causing a tough life; the teachers viewed a tough life as causing school failures. Both groups had the least to say about the role of community in making a difference. Teachers mentioned the importance of clubs and extra-school learning and recreation centers. The children saw clubs as places to learn new skills, places to see friends, and said the community agencies needed to protect them from bullies. The authors concluded that teachers of students from these poor, urban neighborhoods need to view academic achievement as playing as important a role in making a child resilient as the children themselves did.

Morrison, Robertson, Laurie, and Kelly (2002) surveyed 115 fifth- and six-grade (primarily) Latino youth who were identified as being at risk for substance abuse by their teachers. About 70% of the students in participating schools qualified for the free or reduced lunch program. Other risk factors included frequent school absences and low academic achievement, as well as other indices. The students were surveyed about their engagement in antisocial behaviors and about various individual and social protective factors. Both students and teachers also rated the students' classroom behavioral participation. These surveys were done in the

Fall and Spring of the school year, so that Spring level of antisocial behavior was the dependent variable of interest. Significant predictors of higher Spring levels of antisocial behavior were Fall levels of antisocial behavior, being a boy, student perception of low social support, low classroom participation, and student report of high parental supervision. (The authors speculated that the latter variable probably followed, rather than preceded, increased levels of problem behaviors.) The authors stress the importance of perceived social support from family and friends, and the importance of student engagement in everyday classroom life (i.e., paying attention, completing assignments) as critical protective factors leading to decreases in antisocial behaviors prior to the either middle or junior high school for these youth.

Weinstein (2002) reports on a body of work demonstrating that elementary school students perceive that teachers provide differential opportunities for learning and for classroom engagement for high versus low achievers. These differences are especially pronounced in teacher-shaped classroom cultures that are teacher-directed, consist of rigid ability groupings with differentiated curricula in which individual performance differences are accentuated as is the performance aspect of learning. Weinstein (2002) summarizes interviews with high and low achieving African American students in classrooms that vary in terms of the "focus on achievement culture." These fourth graders perceived that low achieving children had little chance of being successful learners if teachers treated students differently based on ability levels. Weinstein's (2002) work shows the importance of teacher expectations as a critical variable that influences students' classroom engagement in academic learning tasks.

High School Students

O'Connor (1998) interviewed 46 African American high school sophomores from two Chicago public schools located in areas characterized by poverty, low employment and heavy reliance on public assistance. The students were approximately equally divided by gender and academic achievement. They were asked numerous questions about their perceptions of the role of race and social class in shaping their future academic and occupational attainment. O'Connor (1998) found other persons played a significant role in distinguishing between those students who were and were not optimistic about the future in terms of believing that their own agency and ability would matter (e.g., overcoming racial and social class prejudice and discrimination). Those students with optimistic voices had role models who had "made it," they had parents and teachers who supported them and made them feel worthwhile by providing structure and having high expectations. O'Connor (1998) concluded that student engagement, or the willingness to accommodate to school norms and expectations, needs to be understood in the context of the significant structural limitations that the students in her study face on a daily basis. If students had reasons to be optimistic about the future, they were more likely to be engaged in school tasks.

College Students

Miller (2002) conducted open-ended, two-hour, individual interviews with college students with learning disabilities at a Midwestern state university. Six of the ten students were designated as resilient for data analytic purposes because their major grade point average (GPA) was B+ or better, and their disability predicted a lower level of achievement. Four participants were designated as not resilient because their GPA's were not at this level. Miller (2002) found that resilient students were more likely than nonresilient students to recall or discuss each of the following in their previous academic histories: (i) identifiable success experiences, (ii) particular areas of strength, (iii) self-determination and self-drive, (iv) distinctive turning points, (v) special friendships, (vi) encouraging teacher, and (vii) acknowledgement of the learning disability.

Montgomery, Miville, Winterowd, Jeffries, and Baysden (2000) interviewed 14 Native American college students (or recent graduates) who, on average, self identified as being raised in their traditional culture. They were asked to describe how/why they were able to succeed in college. Internal factors emerged as important in the pursuit of higher education, especially "traditional self-talk" which "refers to an internal dialogue of encouragement and empowerment in dealing with daily experiences of life" (Montgomery et al., 2000, p. 390); much of which came from family or tribal lore/wisdom. The students cited the importance of learning via mentoring, observation, and direct experience. The students thought it was crucial to be able to merge their cultural identities with the academic system. Finally, the students mentioned social support from family and from tribal members/elders as a factor in their academic success.

Comments on Interview/Survey Studies of Educational Resilience

It is difficult to reach definitive conclusions from these studies as they varied in terms of student background characteristics (age/grade level, gender, race/ethnicity); criteria for educational resilience, and methodology (interview/survey; analytic tool used). In some cases, subgroups of resilient/nonresilient students were quite small, so that caution concerning the reliability and generalizability of results is warranted at this time. The findings are not without merit, however. The importance of support from family, friends, and teachers emerged as a theme in most of these studies, confirming findings from previous work that used distal measures of risk coupled with success in academic settings as an index of resilience. These studies also found that resilient students were optimistic about their own chances for success despite awareness of adversity (due to a learning disability, racism, or cultural mismatch). In each case, the resilient students were well aware of limiting factors, but were able to integrate them into a self-system in a motivating-engaging fashion, rather than a disengaging fashion. A history of prior, personally relevant (either self or role model) success emerged as a key factor in these feelings of optimism despite awareness/acknowledgment of adversity in resilient students. Finally, the studies of African American and Native American students show the importance of building in variables such as racism, segregation, and adaptive culture to account for outcomes in minority students (García Coll et al., 1996).

QUANTITATIVE STUDIES PREDICTING OR MODELING EDUCATIONAL RESILIENCE

Most of the studies summarized in Table 2 had specific criteria for educational risk and subsequent educational competence that served to identify a group of resilient versus nonresilient students. Given a common risk status, these studies identified significant correlates/predictors of subsequent academic competence, or looked for significant differences between students grouped as resilient or nonresilient.

Educational Resilience in Nationally Representative Samples: Three NELS-88 Studies

Three of the studies used the U.S. Department of Education's National Longitudinal Study of 1988 (NELS-88). This study obtained a nationally representative sample of eighth grade students from 800 public and 200 private schools and obtained several background measures and measures of student academic performance at grades 8, 10, and 12. Finn and Rock (1997) studied 1,803 African American and Hispanic-origin students who were in public schools and in the lower half of the entire NELS-88 SES distribution. They classified students as resilient ($n = 332$), nonresilient completers ($n = 1301$), or nonresilient dropouts ($n = 170$) based on reading and mathematics test scores and composite GPA's in grades 8 and 10, and based on whether or not the student was still in school at grade 12. The major finding of this study was that resilient students differed from nonresilient students in terms of several measures of student engagement, even when differences in background and psychological characteristics such as self esteem and locus of control, were statistically controlled.

Catterall (1998) identified two subgroups of NELS-88 eighth graders who were at risk. One group indicated that they were not confident they would complete high school ($n = 4,000$ or about 18% of the sample). The other group considered to be at risk, self-reported grades in English classes of mostly "C's" or lower in grades 6–8 ($n = 7,000$ or about 26% of the sample). Catterall (1998) classified these at risk students as having "commitment resilience" (i.e., their commitment to an objective or goal helped them persevere and overcome obstacles) if at tenth grade they were still in school and reported confidence in finishing high school. Students were classified as academically resilient if their tenth grade English teachers now reported that they received grades higher than "C." For the entire sample, commitment resilience was predicted by student socioeconomic status (SES) academic test scores, grades, family conditions conducive to schoolwork, student reports of greater involvement in school-based and extracurricular activities, and higher student-reports of greater teacher responsiveness to students, and descriptions of schools as having fair discipline systems. Not all of these predictors were significant when subgroups such as African American students and Hispanic students were analyzed separately. For example, SES was not a significant predictor for these groups of students. For the entire sample, academic resilience was predicted by many of the same variables: SES, family supports, school responsiveness, and student engagement in school activities. In addition, homes with rules governing television viewing, and a pattern of lower English but higher math grades in eighth grade were associated with greater academic resilience. Once again, patterns differed slightly for subgroups of students. Catterall (1998), like Finn and Rock (1997) concluded that these findings showed that large numbers of students doing poorly in grade 8, could improve by grade 10 due to environmental and contextual factors.

Cappella and Weinstein (2001) used NELS-88 grade 8 reading proficiency Level 0 (not proficient) as an index of risk ($n = 1362$) and grade 12 reading proficiency Level 0 (not proficient, $n = 1161$) as an index of nonresilience, and grade 12 reading proficiency Levels 2–3 (intermediate and advanced proficiency, $n = 201$) as an index of academic competence and resilience. The reading tests and proficiency levels were developed by experts from Educational Testing Service for NELS—88. Cappella and Weinsten (2001) found SES (higher), ethnic background (being Caucasian), and gender (being female) to be predictors of resilience. Resilience was also predicted by grade 8 locus of control and future expectation scores, grade 10 extracurricular activities, and level of the academic curriculum reported on the student's transcript. Exposure to academic courses increased a student's chances of improving their reading ability by grade 12. Mediational regression analyses revealed that SES and grade 8 aspirations were no longer significant when these other variables were taken into account.

Educational Resilience in Diverse Groups of Students

Using a cross-sectional design, and distal indices or risk (being poor and African American), Connell, Spencer, and Aber (1994) tested a model that used contextual, self, and action variables to predict either negative or positive educational outcomes in three different samples of youth enrolled in grades 5–9. Distal, demographic variables (gender, family economic risk, female-headed household, and neighborhood risk) were also tested as predictors of educational outcomes. Educational outcomes were assessed as negative or positive based on composite scoring systems that considered attendance, school suspension, age relative to classmates, standardized test scores, and GPA's. The general model held in all three samples based on path analytic results. The action variables that assessed students' emotional and behavioral engagement in school were recursive predictors of positive and negative educational outcomes, and nonrecursive predictors of perceived parental involvement. Thus, students who reported greater engagement did better in school and reported greater parental involvement in their lives. Student engagement, in turn, was predicted by locus of control for school success, feelings of self worth, and emotional security with others. Each of these model variables was significant when more distal, demographic variables were statistically controlled. The authors state that student engagement is the most proximal point of entry for intervention efforts.

Jimerson, Egeland and Teo (1999) used data from a 20 year longitudinal study of 174 children deemed to be at risk due to family poverty and low maternal educational attainment. Eighty percent of the mothers were White, 13% African American, and 7% Native American or Hispanic. Academic measures were examined for grades 1 and 6, and when the students were 16 years old. Standardized reading and mathematics achievement test scores were used as measures to create either positive or negative achievement trajectories. Variables used to predict these trajectories were SES, quality of the home environment at grade 1, parent involvement in the child's education as reported by teachers in grades 1, 2, 3, and 6, teacher reports of students' socioemotional and behavioral functioning in these same elementary grades, and number of years in special education. Jimerson et al. (1999) found that despite the restricted range, SES was the most consistent predictor of both positive and negative achievement trajectories. Quality of the home environment measured at grade 1 also predicted positive reading and math achievement trajectories at grade 6 and also positive growth in reading at age 16. Parental involvement in grades 1–3 predicted growth in math at grade 6. Number of years in special education in grades 1–3 predicted negative deflections in reading at grade 6. Behavior problems in elementary grades predicted downward achievement trends.

Kenny, Gallagher, Alvarez-Salvat, and Silsby (2002) studied 100 high school students who participated in a high school-university collaborative program designed to prepare urban public school students for college admission/success. Students were drawn from two ethnically and culturally diverse urban high schools in which the majority of students were African American and Latino. The authors examined relationships between parental attachment, psychological distress, and academic achievement. Adolescents' reports of secure maternal attachment, especially the affective quality of attachment, were significant predictors of (higher) GPA. Adolescents' reports of secure paternal attachment, especially the affective quality of attachment, were significant predictors of reports of fewer depressive symptoms. The authors conclude that these associations between affective quality of maternal and paternal attachment and measures of academic and emotional functioning are consistent with previous findings but merit further investigation.

Shame and Resilience in an Advanced Undergraduate Course

Turner and Schallert (2001) studied 84 undergraduates enrolled in an upper division undergraduate psychopharmacology course. Students' expectancies and values were assessed in the first week of class. After obtaining feedback on their course midterm, their emotional reactions were assessed. Prior to taking all course exams, students' reported their study efforts and their grade goals for the exam. Of the students who reported shame based on their midterm grade, the authors formed two groups. The resilient group was able to increase subsequent exam scores by 8 points or more; the nonresilient group was not able to increase their subsequent exam grades. Several expectancy, value, and motivational differences distinguished the shame-induced resilient versus nonresilient students: certainty of ability; importance of class grade for future academic success; the importance of class content information for future career success; study effort for subsequent exams; and scores on exam 2. Based on these and other findings, these authors (Turner, Husman, & Schallert, 2002) present a comprehensive model that "demonstrate[s] how students' self-regulatory and goal-attainment processes are imbued with emotion" (p. 87).

Comments on Quantitative Studies Predicting/Modeling Educational Resilience

As was the case with the interview/survey studies, it is difficult to reach firm conclusions from this set of studies because of differences in sampling, measures of risk/protective factors, definitions of academic risk, and definitions of academic competence. For example, undergraduates in an advanced course who feel shame due to feedback that their midterm was lower than expected, are not exposed to the same degree of academic risk as eighth graders whose reading proficiency levels are poor. Similarly, as Cappella and Weinstein (2001) point out, Catterall's (1998) measure of academic resilience—recovery of English grades from "C" or lower in grades 6–8 to better than this in grade 10 is problematic because it does not control for the academic level of the course over time. Students may be getting better grades in high school because they have been placed in less rigorous courses than in grades 6–8.

A positive methodological feature of some of these studies was use of longitudinal methods. Since all these studies use correlational techniques, it is helpful to have measures at earlier points in time (in grade 8, for example) predict resilient or nonresilient outcomes at later points in time (in grade 10 or 12, for example). Although other variables, not measured, might underlie these associations or account for greater variability in resilient outcomes, the direction of causality is not in question in these cases. Despite this considerable heterogeneity in theory and method, the present review finds *student engagement* to be an essential component of educational resilience. Specifically, various risk and protective factors and processes predict level of student engagement; and level of student engagement in turn, predicts achievement levels and trajectories. The present work on educational resilience has gone beyond global associations between "distal" measures of risk such as demographic characteristics and either negative (nonresilient) or positive (resilient) outcomes. Instead, these distal variables have been linked to home (e.g., perceived parental support and involvement), school (e.g., perceived teacher support), and individual subject (e.g., locus of control, student optimism) variables that are linked to student engagement (e.g., pay attention in class, complete assignments on time). Finally, several studies found level of student engagement to be a significant, proximal predictor of academic achievement. Many recent educational intervention programs for middle school and high school students are based on these findings concerning educational resilience. These interventions seek to enhance student engagement by providing significant mentors or counselors who seek to develop supportive relationships for students in order to promote present and subsequent school success (see McClendon, Nettles & Wigfield's, 2000 description of the PASS program; Noam & Hermann's, 2002 description of RALLY and Waller, Okamoto, Hankerson, Hibbeler, Hibbeler, McIntyre, & McAllen-Walker's, 2002 description of the "Hoop of Learning" for three representative examples of school-based interventions).

Looking Forward: Educational Resilience in the Context of High-Stakes Testing

Despite theoretical eclecticism, most work in the area of resilience recognizes the importance of studying risk and protective factors and processes in multiple and nested contexts that include families, schools, and communities (Luthar et al., 2000). This type of ecological approach points to the potential harm that arises from an exclusive focus on child and family "risk factors," especially in the case of minority and poor youth (Franklin, 2000). As we look to what schools and communities can do to help as many students as possible achieve educational resilience, I think it is important to acknowledge that these institutions are themselves enmeshed in a larger, societal context. In particular, students in the United

States are now being educated in schools and communities that are subject to the new federal law called, *No Child Left Behind*. This law says that every racial and demographic group in each school must score higher on standardized tests every year; if any group fails to advance for two consecutive years, a school is labeled 'needing improvement.' A school that does not shed the label by improving students' scores may have its principal and teachers replaced and face other sanctions, including closing (Dillon, 2003). This new law, however well intentioned, is already starting to have a chilling effect in real schools. Two recent reports by Dillon (2003) and Winerip (2003) describe elementary schools that are viewed as highly successful by the school's administration, teaching staff, parents, and community. However, due to quirks in the law, the schools are in danger of being labeled 'needing improvement.' For example, if a subgroup of students made significant improvements in reading comprehension from 2001 to 2002 but then in 2003 had a test average in between these two numbers, the school is viewed by the law as going in the wrong direction. The law does not distinguish between schools that miss the mark by small versus large amounts. Although scores on standardized test are an important part of the educational assessment process, very few would argue that a child's educational attainment should be measured by a single test score. Yet test scores, aggregated by racial, ethnic, and language groupings, are becoming a major focus at the state and local administrative levels due to this new federal mandate. At the time of this writing, the impact of this legislation on the classroom teaching-learning process is not known. Strategic efforts to foster student engagement in the United States need to acknowledge that assessment of academic progress is increasingly being accomplished via high stakes achievement testing. The effect of this larger contextual factor on efforts to increase student engagement for those judged to be at risk in academic settings needs to be acknowledged by both researchers and practitioners.

REFERENCES

Berliner, D., & Calfee, R.C. (Eds.) (1994). *Handbook of educational psychology.* New York: Macmillan.

Cappella, E., & Weinstein, R.S. (2001). Turning around reading achievement: Predictors of high school students' academic resilience. *Journal of Educational Psychology, 93,* 758–771.

Catterall, J.S. (1998). Risk and resilience in student transitions to high school. *American Journal of Education, 106,* 302–333.

Connell, J.P., Spencer, M.B., & Aber, J.L. (1994). Educational risk and resilience in African-American youth: Context, self, action, and outcomes in school. *Child Development, 65,* 493–506.

Dillon, S. (2003, February 16). Thousands of schools may run afoul on new law. *The New York Times,* A33.

Finn, J.D., & Rock, D.A. (1997). Academic success among students at risk for school failure. *Journal of Applied Psychology, 82*, 221–234.

Franklin, W. (2000). Students at promise and resilient: A historical look at risk. In M.G. Sanders (Ed.), *Schooling students placed at risk. Research, policy, and practice in the education of poor and minority adolescents*, (pp. 3–16). Mahwah: NJ: Erlbaum.

García Coll, C., Lamberty, G., Jenkins, R., McAdoo, H.P., Crnic, K., Waski, B.H., & Vázquez García, H. (1996). An integrative model for the study of developmental competencies in minority children. *Child Development, 67*, 1891–1914.

Howard, S., & Johnson, B. (2002). What makes a difference? Children and teachers talk about resilient outcomes for children 'at risk.' *Educational Studies, 26*, 321–337.

Jimerson, S., Egeland, B., & Teo, A. (1999). A longitudinal study of achievement trajectories: Factors associated with change. *Journal of Educational Psychology, 91*, 116–126.

Kenny, M.E., Gallagher, L.A., Alvarez-Salvat, R., & Silsby, J. (2002). Sources of support and psychological distress among academically successful inner-city youth. *Adolescence, 37*, 161–182.

Luthar, S.S., Cicchetti, D., & Becker, B. (2000a). The construct of resilience: A critical evaluation and guidelines for future work. *Child Development, 71*, 543–562.

Luthar, S.S., Cicchetti, D., & Becker, B. (2000b). Research on resilience: Response to commentaries. *Child Development, 71*, 573–575.

Masten, A.S. (2001). Ordinary magic: Resilience processes in development. *American Psychologist, 56*, 227–238.

Masten, A.S., & Coatsworth, J.D. (1998). The development of competence if favorable and unfavorable environments. *American Psychologist, 53*, 205–220.

Masten, A.S., Coatsworth, J.D., Neemann, J., Gest, S.D., Tellegen, A., & Garmezy, N. (1995). The structure and coherence of competence from childhood through adolescence. *Child Development, 66*, 1635–1659.

McClendon, C., Nettles, S.M., & Wigfield, A. (2000). Fostering resilience in high school classrooms: A study of the PASS program (Promoting Achievement in School through Sport). In M.G. Sanders (Ed.), *Schooling students placed at risk. Research, policy, and practice in the education of poor and minority adolescents*, (pp. 289–307). Mahwah: NJ: Erlbaum.

Miller, M. (2002). Resilience elements in students with learning disabilities. *Journal of Clinical Psychology, 58*, 291–298.

Montgomery, D., Miville, M.L, Winterowd, C., Jeffries, B., & Baysden, M.F. (2000). American Indian college students: An exploration into resiliency factors revealed through personal stories. *Cultural Diversity and Ethnic Minority Psychology, 6*, 387–398.

Morrison, G.M., Robertson, L., Laurie, B., & Kelly, J. (2002). Protective factors related to antisocial behavior trajectories. *Journal of Clinical Psychology, 58*, 277–290.

Noam, G.G., & Hermann, C.A. (2002). Where education and mental health meet: Developmental prevention and early intervention in schools. *Development and Psychopathology, 14*, 861–875.

O'Connor, C. (1998). Resilience despite reproductive notions of risk: A case of Black inner-city youth. In L.K. Wong (Ed.), *Advances in Educational Policy Vol. 4, Perspectives on the social functions of schools* (pp. 51–86). Stamford, CT: JAI Press.

Richardson, G.E. (2002). The metatheory of resilience and resiliency. *Journal of Clinical Psychology, 58*, 307–321.

Turner, J.E., Husman, J., & Schallert, D.L. (2002). The importance of students' goals in their emotional experience of academic failure: Investigating the precursors and consequences of shame. *Educational Psychologist, 37*, 79–89.

Turner, J.E., & Schallert, D.L. (2001). Expectancy-value relationships of shame reactions and shame resiliency. *Journal of Educational Psychology, 93*, 320–329.

Waller, M.A., Okamoto, S.K., Hankerson, A. a. Hibbeler, T. Hibbeler, P.s, McIntyre, P., & McAllen-Walker, R. (2002). The hoop of learning: A holistic, multisystemic model for facilitating educational resilience among indigenous students. *Journal of Sociology and Social Welfare, 29,* 97–116.

Weinstein, R.S. (2002). *Reaching higher. The power of expectations in schooling.* Cambridge, MA: Harvard University Press.

Winerip, M. (2003, February 19). Defining success in narrow terms. *The New York Times,* B7.

Chapter 18

Enhancing Child and Adolescent Resilience through Faith-Community Connections

Celeste C. Owens, Tanya N. Bryant, Sylvia S. Huntley,
Elizabeth Moore, Tom Sloane, Alvin Hathaway,
and Mark D. Weist

INTRODUCTION

There has been a resurgence of interest in the unique ability of the faith community to support youth and promote their healthy development. Faith-based organizations (FBOs) according to White (1998) are "organizations or programs which claim to be affiliated with a religious congregation, or those organizations that are independent from a religious congregation or order, but who express a religious motivation for working with at-risk youth." Recently, the U.S. federal government has expressed clear support for the role of FBOs in community efforts to improve health and life functioning for children and adults. In 2001, President George W. Bush submitted an executive order that created the White House Office of Faith-Based and Community Initiatives. According to Jim Towey, director, this proposal was designed to make federal funds available to FBOs instrumental in providing a variety of community services that the federal and state governments have been unsuccessful in implementing (Abernethy, 2003). The Bush administration is adamant that funds will not be used to fund "clearly religious" programs but to fund those aspects or parts of programs that instead support programs that address human needs. Furthermore, organizations are forbidden from using federally supported programs as a means of proselytizing to recipients and/or promoting the organization's religious beliefs.

The Faith Based Initiative of the Bush administration is not without controversy, with those opposed to the initiative expressing concerns that it is blurring the line of separation between church and state. Others are concerned that the government's sudden interest in FBOs is self-serving and a quick answer to recent reductions to funding in state and federal assistance programs. Still others worry that the church does not have adequate resources to effectively deal with the social problems facing our communities (e.g., Winston, 1992).

Nonetheless, the need for effective programming is great and the demand for services far outweighs the resources currently available to youth. For example, African Americans and Latinos are 4 to 5 more times likely to live in poverty than Whites (Bureau of the Census, 1998; Cook, 2000) and the percentages are suspected to be higher in urban areas. A disparity in unemployment rates for youth is also evident with White youth ages 16–19 at 15% and African American youth ages 16–19 at 37% (Bureau of Labor Statistics, 2003).

The U.S. government recognizes that no single group or organization can sufficiently reduce the social distresses facing our youth; therefore funding is first available to FBOs that collaborate on a common project with other agencies. Likewise, the federal government has a long history of contracting with FBOs (e.g., The Salvation Army, Catholic Charities and Lutheran Family Services) to provide childcare, foster care and other services (Shirk, 2000). Therefore, it is vital that the faith, mental health, education, and other child serving communities (e.g., juvenile justice, child welfare) explore ways of collaborating on a shared agenda to promote holistic and synergistic approaches to improving child and adolescent functioning and enhancing resilience. The present chapter will highlight the contributions of the faith community in fostering positive mental health for children, particularly within the context of research on the beneficial effects of religiosity in promoting resiliency in youth. Secondly, the chapter will emphasize the importance of collaboration, as well as outline the steps necessary to forge successful collaborations with the faith community.

RESILIENCY: THE POWER FROM WITHIN AND WITHOUT

It is well known that youth exposed to chronic and serious problems and risks, such as youth in poverty, and/or exposed to high levels of crime and violence are at increased risk to show a range of emotional and behavioral problems, and problems in life, including drop out, criminality, and increased morbidity and early mortality (Werner, 1995). However, despite the overwhelming odds against youth in these conditions, substantial proportions go on to become healthy, well-adjusted adults (Werner, 1995). In fact, at least half of children at risk for later emotional/psychological problems do not repeat the cycle and improve their conditions considerably (Benard, 1996). As found throughout this book, this ability of children to endure extreme stress, to overcome adversity despite overwhelming risk factors, and to go on to be productive adults is called resilience.

Three important factors work together to promote resilient behavior in youth, these include the individual characteristics of the child, family characteristics, and community supports (e.g., school and faith). Although resilience was once thought to be an innate trait that only some children possessed (Cook, 2000), it is now apparent that resilience is reinforced by external support systems such as the family network, school and faith communities (Garmezy & Masten, 1991; Larson & Johnson, 1998). In fact, it is now believed that these external factors are just as, if not more, important for strengthening resiliency in children and adolescents than the individual internal factors. As individual and school/community characteristics are discussed at length in other chapters in this book, the following will focus on the ways in which religious faith can be a protective factor.

Religious Faith as a Protective Factor

Religious faith or spirituality is a strong protective factor against high-risk behavior for adolescents who endorse an affiliation with religious institutions (Resnick, Harris, & Blum, 1993). Importantly, religious faith and involvement involves many of the individual, family, and school/community resilience factors reviewed in this volume. For example, youth involved in religious organizations learn social skills (such as respectful, behavior during services), experience a sense of meaning in life, experience positive family routines and rituals, and connect with positive adults. In fact, studies have found that the promotion of spirituality by parents and the religious community for youth can serve to promote positive peer and adult relationships (Cook, 2000), altruistic/prosocial behavior (Benson, Donahue, & Erickson,1989; Donahue & Benson, 1995), and decrease the commitment to problematic behaviors including substance use (Booth & Martin, 1998; Jang & Jonhson, 2001), violent behavior (Cook, 2000; Jagers, 1996), and sexual behavior (Donahue & Benson, 1995; Benson et al., 1989; Whitehead, Rostosky, Randall, & Wright, 2001; Moore, Hair, Bridges, & Garrett, 2002). Additional findings supporting the benefit of religious faith include decreased stress (Cook, 2000), decreased likelihood of psychological problems including depression (Koenig, George, & Peterson, 1998; Brown, Ndubuisi, & Gary, 1990), decreased rates of suicide (Donahue & Benson, 1995) and higher levels of self-esteem (Payne, Bergin, Biellema, & Jenkins, 1991). Likewise, the literature reports several ways in which the faith community can help to foster resiliency in youth, including the development of structured community programming (e.g., youth groups, gang prevention, mentoring, and tutoring), fostering identity development, and opportunities for positive relationships with supportive adults. These areas are reviewed in the following.

Structured Community Programming

Providing youth with structured community programming is crucial to their healthy development. The faith community has continued to provide these services through various activities and programming including after school tutoring and safe houses. A critical mass of FBOs in Washington D.C. provides a wealth of services to inner-city youth for this very reason. An intensive survey of these FBOs (not including schools) indicated that programming fell into five major categories: tutoring programs (56%), youth groups (21%), evangelization (5%), gang violence prevention (3%) and mentoring (5%) (White, 1998). The staff consists of a variety of paid and unpaid workers from 129 programs with a majority of the staff volunteering (56%). Most of these programs endeavor to provide services that supply meals to children, motivate them to achieve, and keep them off the streets.

Another form of structured community programming is regular church attendance, which has also been reported to have negative effects on delinquency and criminal behavior. Larson and Johnson (1998) examined the National Bureau of Economic Research survey of children that was implemented in Boston, Chicago and Philadelphia. The survey was designed to examine joblessness in Black youth in the U.S. by examining three factors that typically put youth at risk for criminal behavior: delinquency, drug use, and alcohol use. The surveyors also collected information on family composition, family size, welfare status and the youth's involvement with other community entities including the church. Findings indicated that church attendance was a strong protective factor against delinquency, drug use, and alcohol use even when controlling for other variables such as age, family structure, family size, and opportunities for illegal behavior. This is a significant finding considering that most research studies have focused on school and family as agents of social control on criminal behavior, with relatively few focusing on the role of religious institutions. In urban areas where schools and families are at times chaotic, utilizing churches, synagogues, mosques and other religious institutions to influence positive development in youth may bolster these weakened social control agents by providing youth with opportunities to develop strong social bonds and increase their involvement in constructive social activities.

Identity Development

Erikson (1968), in his study of the stages of human development, describes adolescence as a time of identity versus diffusion. During this psychosocial crisis, youth seek to answer the question of purpose, "Who am I?" Most adolescents participate in some minor delinquency, but if successful role identity is formed the adolescent will adopt a constructive identity as opposed to a negative/delinquent identity.

A sense of identity and belonging is a normative part of development in adolescents. Therefore, when the primary family structure is dysfunctional or unavailable youth often turn to gangs or other deviant groups for support, identity and guidance. In his study of gang members, Goldstein (1991) reported that former members identified the church as being instrumental in providing a new/restructured identity that allowed them to find a sense of purpose in their lives. Furthermore, some would argue that those youth who allow the church to provide a "frame for identity" (Cook, 2000) would have a better chance of avoiding prison, school dropout, drugs and other negative outcomes (McLaughlin & Heath, 1993).

Walker and Pitts (1998), in their study of religious/spiritual practices of adolescents, reported that religiosity was correlated with healthy identity development in adolescents. High school students from Los Angeles were asked to report on the sense of purpose and meaning in their lives as well as prosocial beliefs and attitudes, as measured by the Life Regard Index. Results indicated that religious identity was correlated with one's sense of purpose and meaning in life and a sense of purpose and meaning was correlated with empathy.

Opportunities for Relationships with Supportive Adults

The presence of supportive adults who provide caring relationships to children experiencing adversity is identified in the literature as one of the primary protective factors that fosters resilience (Benard, 1996; Werner, 1995; Resnick et al., 1993). In fact, Henderson and Milstein (2003) assert that it is virtually impossible for youth to overcome adversity without caring and supportive adults. The faith community can assist youth by fostering a sense of belonging and connectedness to a significant other, which can facilitate positive peer and adult relationships and influence social decision-making (Resnick et al., 1993). They can also act as a resource to provide youth with opportunities to interface with positive, supportive adults via mentoring programs, supportive after school programming and other activities.

INTERPERSONAL CONNECTION: FAITH FACILITATING PARTNERSHIPS

Since the 1990s policymakers and researchers have begun to examine the potential of the faith community as an agent for change and improvement in social problems (White, 1998). However, the importance of religious faith and spirituality in the protection of youth from delinquency, drug use, pregnancy and other problematic behaviors has often been overlooked by policy makers and system leaders at local, state and national levels (Bridges & Moore, 2002) despite strong evidence of the potential religious faith and FBOs to contribute to life success for troubled and non-troubled youth (see Cook, 2000; Donahue & Benson, 1995; Freeman, 1986; Koenig, George, & Peterson, 1998; Payne et al., 1991).

The role of FBOs in the facilitation of interagency communication has been well documented in the sociology and social work literature (e.g., Frazier, 1974; Lincoln & Mamiya, 1990). This literature emphasizes the primary role of faith institutions in addressing difficult issues such as civic and political concerns, educational pursuits and economic and community development by encouraging interpersonal communication between organizations for the purpose of collaboration. Furthermore, the literature has listed several instances where the faith community, in an effort to support families and children has become involved and partnered with education, mental health and other agencies within the local community (Shirley, 2001).

In one such example, the University of Maryland School Mental Health Program partnered with the Pennsylvania Avenue Zion AME Church in order to conduct a series of focus groups, which served to inquire about the economical, educational and mental health needs of the community in West Baltimore. The Pennsylvania Avenue Zion AME Church, a well-respected congregation in the community, was instrumental in rallying neighborhood mental health stakeholders including school personnel, district representatives, the Police Athletic League (P.A.L.), parents, and other concerned community members. Focus group participants were asked to comment on the social ills of youth, challenges to youth success in the community, ways to promote resilience, and the promotion and delivery of mental health services in the community. Participants identified the main stressors and risk factors for youth as drugs, violence, and poverty. They also reported that funds would be best used to provide affordable, safe housing, more effective drug treatment programs, and additional mentoring programs (Axelrod, Bryant, Lever, Lewis, Mullett, Rosner, Wiest, Sorrell, & Hathaway, 2002). The faith organization's ability to interface with members of various groups and to facilitate open dialogue around difficult subject matter is supported by the success of these focus groups. In fact, we would argue that the faith community often brings two ingredients to multi-agency efforts: interpersonal connections and passion to address social problems affecting community members.

Given the research (as we have reviewed) supporting the power of religious faith and FBOs to promote positive outcomes and life success for youth and families, why are faith and FBOs often not represented in youth-focused community efforts? What hinders the development of successful partnerships and what may be possible solutions to these hindrances?

BARRIERS TO AND SOLUTIONS FOR EFFECTIVE COLLABORATION

Historically, collaboration between religious organizations, education, mental health and other child serving professionals have been rare, due in part to a lack of understanding and insight about the ways in which each entity has the potential to offer substantial benefits to youth. Unfortunately, most clinical training programs for both medicine and mental health do not offer seminars in client spiritual or religious issues (Lannert, 1991). Further, a surprising 50% of psychologists report no religious preference (Shafranske, 1996).

On the other hand, Americans continue to be a religious people with the 1997 CNN/USA TODAY Gallup Poll reporting that 97% of adults surveyed admitted believing in God or a universal spirit. On average 65% of adults reported being a member in a church, temple, mosque or similar place of worship. Likewise, the number of Americans believing that religion is vital to solving social problems is substantial (60% of all Americans, 80% of African Americans). In another poll, 76% of adolescents in the United States reported believing in a personal God, 74% reported praying at least occasionally, 48% reported attending a church or temple weekly, and 27% reported a higher interest in religion than their parents (Gallup & Bezilla, 1992).

Lack of Understanding of the Role of Clergy as it Relates to Mental Health

Barriers

Mental health professionals often do not have an accurate understanding of the prominent role that clergy have within their communities. Not only are they the spiritual leaders of the community but also instrumental in providing a wealth of other services including mental health counseling. In the U.S., more than 400,000 clergy and religious workers allocate a significant portion of their time (up to 20%) for these services (Weaver, 1995; Weaver, 1998) and counsel on a wide range of personal issues including depression, alcohol/substance abuse, marital and family conflict and unemployment (Taylor, Ellison, Chatters, Levin, & Lincoln, 2000). Clergy and religious leaders within FBOs are obvious first choices for mental health services for many reasons. Sherman (2003) reports that FBOs are usually in walking distance of those in need, which make it easier for people in the community to get help and there services are typically free. They are able to provide help that tends to be structured to fit individual lifestyles instead of the rigor of other secular-based programs. Lastly, clients find hope in working with people who are steeped in faith.

Solutions

Clergy frequently act as a gatekeeper to the delivery of mental health services either by facilitating such services in house or as a mechanism for referral to outside agencies. Additionally, clergy are among the most trusted professionals in society (Gallup, 1990) and FBOs usually have a long-standing relationship within the community allowing parents and children to trust that they have the community's best interest in mind. Mental health professionals desiring to increase their presence within communities and to improve service delivery would benefit from a collaborative relationship with the faith community. A solution would be for mental health providers to network with key persons within the faith community and become actively involved with meetings sponsored by the faith organization in order to assess the needs and identify ways to provide effective assistance. Also, mental health professionals can provide informational packets on culturally sensitive information (e.g., parenting workshops, depression) with outside referral information.

Separation of Church and State

Barriers

The American ideal of limited religious involvement in governmental agencies is very much entrenched (Prodente, Snader, Hathaway, Sloane, & Weist, 2000) and fueled by myths and misconceptions surrounding the First Amendment of the U.S. Constitution, or the law mandating the separation of church and state. Many agencies, including public schools, fear legal repercussions should they attempt to partner with FBOs.

Solutions

However, the true meaning of the First Amendment is to protect religious freedom for all by discouraging the development of a state or national church. Thus, in community efforts, as long as FBOs are not attempting to indoctrinate participants and are providing secular services (e.g., mentoring, childcare, foster care) the First Amendment should not be an impediment to their strong participation in youth-focused community efforts. In these community collaborations, FBOs are to adhere to the same government rules and professional guidelines for the provision of services including peer review, licensure, and liability (Prodente et al., 2000).

The U.S. Department of Education (2000) provides guidelines for school officials, volunteers and mentors participating in public school community partnerships that are relevant to connections with FBOs. These guidelines require participants to: 1) maintain secular purpose, 2) remain neutral when selecting partners, 3) select students without regard to their religious affiliation, 4) make sure that jointly sponsored programming is completely secular, 5) make sure space used for children is safe and secure, 6) make sure that spaces used within public schools is free of religious symbols, and 7) put the partnership agreement in writing.

The federal government has also made guidelines for the faith community when partnering with groups. They assert that 1) FBOs do not have to change their places of worship into secular havens, 2) FBOs do not have to alter or conceal religious language or symbols on the buildings, and 3) the volunteers are not to proselytize to the youth, participate in prayer, or encourage attendance at religious services (White House, 2003).

Limited Awareness of Children's and Adult's Mental Health Issues

Barriers

As emphasized in this chapter, the role of FBOs, specifically clergy (e.g., pastors, rabbis, ministers, priests) in addressing the mental health needs of participants is long standing however there is little empirical evidence supporting the efficacy of these services. While clergy typically encounter clients that are similar to those encountered by mental health professionals with respect to both type and severity of psychiatric symptoms (Larson et al., 1988) they may be unfamiliar with various forms of psychopathology and symptoms associated with severe mental illness (Gottlieb & Olfson, 1987). This matter is further complicated by the spiritual community's interpretation of mental health problems, with a tendency to view these problems as manifestations of spiritual issues. This philosophy lends itself to the underestimation of the severity of mental health problems by faith leaders (e.g., interpreting hallucinatory behaviors as evidence of religious conflict; Larson, 1968) as compared to other mental health service practitioners (e.g., psychologists, social workers, physicians).

Solutions

As an example of clergy's limited preparedness to deal with mental health problems and their associated stress conditions, Bruns et al. (2003) conducted a focus group with 11 clergy members of multiple religious affiliations (e.g., Baptist, Catholic, Muslim, Presbyterian, Universal Life) on the needs of sexual assault victims and their preparedness to address those needs. Overall, these clergy emphasized that they are grossly under prepared to assist these victims, and acknowledge a strong need for increased training in this area, and more broadly in mental health.

Clinicians' Perceptions of Partnering with the Faith Community

A study was conducted at the University of Maryland Baltimore (UMB) that sought to gauge clinicians' views on partnering with the faith community as well as to gather information about clinicians' perceptions of the religious and spiritual practices of their clients. The survey was developed in conjunction with the Faith-Education Partnership for West Baltimore Youth, which includes participants from various religious backgrounds and beliefs and professional disciplines (e.g., clergy, mental health, education, family advocates). The mission of the group is to provide services to children that foster their growth academically, psychologically, and spiritually via the combined efforts of the faith-based, mental health and education communities. The information from this survey was used to inform the members of the partnership of clinicians' perspectives on collaborating on a shared project with the faith community.

The participants in the study consisted of 31 school-based mental health therapists who worked in the Baltimore City Public Schools. The majority were hired through the University of Maryland Baltimore and housed in the school or schools they serve, but four therapists were school-hired professionals. The participants were male and female, African American and White, and they had various degrees, which ranged from the Bachelors to Doctoral level. Fifteen percent of the clinicians' revealed that they initiated discussion about faith in therapy and 77% revealed that the student is usually the first to initiate discussion of faith. Nearly 20% of the clinicians surveyed were uncomfortable incorporating faith into mental health treatment. Clinician concerns included whether all religions would be represented and whether FBOs would force their views and doctrines on the youth taking part in the programs sponsored by FBOs. The clinicians' hopes included wanting collaboration with FBOs to assist in making more supportive resources available to youth and families, and to help families feel more comfortable about seeking mental health services (see Larson & Johnson, 1998).

COLLABORATIVE ENDEAVORS

Faith-Mental Health Partnership

The P.R.A.I.S.E. Project (Providing Resource Alternatives in Spiritual Education) formerly called Project H.O.P.E. began in 1999. The P.R.A.I.S.E. Project's goal is to diffuse the stigma, educate youth about mental health and integrate the powerful relationship between spirituality and mental health care. This unique partnering is designed to serve populations who are less likely to seek mental health care because of misperceptions, and diverse cultural beliefs. This project links faith organizations and the mental health community. In an effort to educate, research and build bridges between the faith community and mental health, P.R.A.I.S.E. is affiliated with many agencies such as: Johns Hopkins Medical Institution, Core Service Agency of Hartford County, First Southern District of Maryland, and the University of Maryland.

The P.R.A.I.S.E. has also partnered with the Institute for Mental Health Ministry, Inc. Their philosophy is referred to as the "Biopsychospiritual Model." This model assumes that each individual is comprised of three dimensions: spirit, mind and body. The Institutes' mission is to promote a greater awareness of mental health issues within the faith community, to promote a greater awareness of the spiritual dimension among mental health providers and to provide mental health services that meet the needs of individuals seeking spiritually sensitive and inclusive treatment. Their ultimate goal is the improvement of the well being and quality of life of individuals, families and communities.

Faith-Education Partnerships

The Industrial Areas Foundation (IAF), a political organization, is working collaboratively with the faith community to improve academic achievement in underserved, low-income communities in Texas (Shirley, 2001). Morningside Middle School in Fort Worth, Texas was a recipient of such efforts. Via the partnership, which included several churches from the local community, the school went from a state of crisis to a thriving "community" school. The leaders of the school emphasized the importance of education, as well as the role of parents and the community in the students' success. Members of congregations participating in the partnership joined school personnel in visiting the homes of the students and hosting parent/family assemblies. Preliminary evaluation data from the project suggested improved standardized test scores and a reduction in failed subjects for participating students.

Academic Achievement Award Foundation, Inc.

The Academic Achievement Award Foundation, Inc. (AAAF) was founded in Baltimore in 1988 as a collaborative endeavor between education and the faith communities to provide incentives to students that achieve academically. The students recognized are those who consistently score at the top of their grade level. Over its twenty-five-year history, the AAAF has provided incentives to over 4,000 elementary school students via its Annual Awards Ceremony in Baltimore, Maryland. The initiative is also seeking to enhance supportive resources in participating elementary schools, including mental health resources.

CONCLUSION

The problems of today's youth may seem insurmountable in the environment of extremely limited resources for them found in most communities. It is clear that traditional child serving systems such as education and mental health cannot even approach meeting the needs of youth when working in isolation. While there are increasing efforts to integrate these systems (see Lever et al., 2003), the integration of faith perspectives, faith leaders, members of congregations and faith-based organizations (FBOs) into such systems, improvement remains at a primitive level.

Our literature review confirmed that both religious faith and FBOs can and do serve to promote resilience and life success for youth and families. This literature underscores the untapped resource of partnerships with FBOs to enhance the integration of community systems (e.g., through the interpersonal connections of religious communities), but also points to barriers that mitigate against such integration. These barriers (e.g., poor knowledge of faith resources by mental health staff and vice versa; limiting ideas regarding the separation of church and state) along with ideas for overcoming them need to be brought to the fore in discussions of community systems improvement for youth. As examples of successful FBO-child serving systems collaboration advance, mechanisms are needed to describe lessons learned and to broadly share information on the ingredients of successful collaborations. Clearly, an interconnected agenda of awareness training, research, program/initiative development, and policy enhancement in this area is needed. We hope that this chapter provides helpful ideas in advancing this critically important agenda for our youth and families.

REFERENCES

Abernethy, B. (2003). Jim Towey: Faith Based Initiative. *Religion and Ethics News Weekly*, http://www. pbs.org/wnet/religionandethics/week635/perspectives.html.

Axelrod, J., Bryant, T., Lever, N., Lewis, C., Mullett, E., Rosner, L., Weist, M., Sorrell, J., & Hathaway, A. (2002). Reaching out to school and community stakeholders to improve mental health services for youth in an urban US community. *The International Journal of Mental Health Promotion*, 4(4), 49–54.

Benard, B. (1996). Resilience research: A foundation for youth development. *New Designs Newsletter*, Summer 1996.

Benson, P.L., Donahue, M.J., & Erickson, J.A. (1989). Adolescence and religion: A review of the literature from 1970 to 1986. *Research in the Social Scientific Study of Religion, 1*, 153–181.

Booth, J., & Martin, J.E. (1998). Spiritual and religious factors in substance use, dependence, and recovery. In H.G. Koenig (Ed.), *Handbook of religion and mental health* (pp. 175–200). San Diego: Academic Press.

Bridges, L.J., & Moore, K.A. (2002). Religious Involvement and children's well-being: What research tells us (and what it doesn't). *Child Trends Research Brief.* Washington, DC: Child Trends, Inc.

Brown, D.R., Ndubuisi, S.C., & Gary, L.E. (1990). Religiosity and psychological distress among Blacks. *Journal of Religion and Health, 29*, 55–68.

Bruns, E.J., Lewis, C., Kinney, L.M., Rosner, L., Weist, M.D., & Dantzler, J. (2003). Clergy members as responders to victims of sexual abuse and assault. Manuscript submitted for publication.

Bureau of the Census (1998). *Statistical abstract of the United States: 1998* (118th ed.). Washington, DC: U.S. Government Printing Office.

Bureau of Labor Statistics (February, 2003). *Labor for statistics for the current population survey* [On-line data]. Washington, DC: Bureau of Labor Statistics. Available: http://stats.bls.gov:80/webapps/legacy/cpsatab2.htm.

Cook, K.V. (2000). "You have to have somebody watching your back, and if that's God, then that's mighty big": The church's role in the resilience of inner-city youth. *Journal of Substance Abuse Treatment, 19*, 347–354.

Donahue, M.J., & Benson, P.J. (1995). Religion and well-being in adolescents. *Journal of the Scientific Study of Religion, 15*, 29–45.

Erikson, E.H. (1968). *Identity: Youth and crisis.* New York: Norton.

Frazier, E.F. (1974). *The Negro church in America.* New York: Schocken.

Freeman, R.B. (1986). Who escapes? The relation of church-going and other background factors to the socioeconomic performance of black make youths from inner-city poverty tracts. In R.B. Freeman (Ed.), *The black youth employment crisis (pp. 353–376).* Chicago: Chicago University Press.

Gallup, G.H. (1990). *Religion in America: 1990.* Princeton, NJ: Gallup Organization.

Gallup, G.H., & Bezilla, R. (1992). *The religious life of young Americans.* Princeton, NJ: George Gallup International Institute.

Garmezy, N., & Masten, A.S. (1991). The protective role of competence indicators in children at risk. In E.M. Cummings, A.L. Greene, & K.H. Karraker (Eds.), *Life span development psychology: Perspectives on stress and coping* (pp. 151–174). New Jersey: Lawrence Erlbaum Associates.

Goldstein, A.P. (1991). *Delinquent gangs: A psychological perspective.* Champaign, IL: Research Press.

Gottlieb, N.H., & Olfson, M. (1987). Current referral practices of mental health care providers. *Hospital and Community Psychiatry, 38*, 1171–1181.

Henderson, N., & Milstein, M.M. (2003). *Resiliency in schools: Making in happen for students and educators.* California: Corwin Press, Inc.

Jagers, R.J. (1996). Culture and problem behaviors among inner-city African-American youth: Further explorations. *Journal of Adolescence, 19*, 371–381.

Jang, S.J., & Johnson, B.R. (2001). Neighborhood disorder, individual religiosity, and adolescent use of illicit drugs: A test of multilevel hypotheses. *Criminology, 39*, 109–143.

Koenig, H.G., George, L.K., & Peterson, B.L. (1998). Religious importance and remission of depression in medically ill older patients. *American Journal of Psychiatry, 155*, 536–542.

Lannert, J.L. (1991). Resistance and countertransference issues with religious and spiritual clients. *Journal of Humanistic Psychology, 31*, 68–76.

Larson, D.B., & Johnson, B.R. (1998). Religion: The forgotten factor in cutting youth crime and saving at-risk urban youth. *The Jeremiah project, An initiative of the center for civic innovation, report 98–2*, www.manhattan-institute.org.

Larson, D.B., Hahmann, A., Kessler, L., Meadon, K., Boyd, J., & McSherry, E. (1988). The couch and the cloth: The need for linkage. *Hospital and Community Psychiatry, 39*, 1064–1069.

Lever, N.A., Adelsheim, S., Prodente, C., Christodulu, K.V., Ambrose, M.G., Schlitt, J., & Weist, M.D. (2003). System, agency and stakeholder collaboration to advance mental health programs in schools. In M.D. Weist, S.W. Evans, & N.A. Lever (Eds.), *Handbook of school mental health:*

Advancing practice and research (pp. 149–162). New York, NY: Kluwer Academic/Plenum Publishers.

Lincoln, C.E., & Mamiya, L.H. (1990). *The Black church in the African American experience.* Durham, NC: Duke University Press.

McLaughlin, M.W., & Heath, S. (1993). Casting the self: Frames for identity and dilemmas for policy. In S.B. Heath & M.W. McLaughlin (Eds.), *Identity and inner-city youth: Beyond ethnicity and gender* (pp. 210–239). New York: Teachers College Press.

Moore, K., Hair, E., Bridges, L., & Garrett, S. (2002). Parent religious beliefs and adolescent outcomes. *Poster presentation at a meeting of the Population Association of America,* Atlanta, May.

Payne, I.R., Bergin, A.E., Biellema, K.A., & Jenkins, P.H. (1991). Review of religion and mental health: Prevention and the enhancement of psychological functioning. *Prevention in Human Services, 9,* 11–40.

Prodente, C.A., Sander, M.A., Hathaway, A.C., Sloane, T., & Weist, M.D. (2002). Children's mental health: Partnering with the faith community. In H.S. Ghuman, M.D. Weist, & R.S. Sarles (Eds.), *Providing mental health services to youth where they are* (pp. 209–224). New York: Brunner-Routledge.

Resnick, M., Harris, L., & Blum, R. (1993). The impact of caring and connectedness on adolescent health and well-being. *Journal of Pediatrics and Child Health, 29,* 53–59.

Shafranske, E.P. (1996). *Religion and the clinical practice of psychology.* Washington, DC: American Psychological Association.

Sherman, A.L. (2003). Faith in communities: A solid investment. *Society, 40*(2), 19–26.

Shirk, M. (2000). Faith-based youth work wins more converts. *Youth today: The newspaper on youth work, December/January, 9*(1).

Shirley, D.L. (2001). Faith-based organizations, community development, and the reform of public schools. *Peabody Journal of Education, 76*(2), 222–240.

Taylor, R.J., Ellison, C.G., Chatters, L.M., Levin, J.S., & Lincoln, K.D. (2000). Mental health services in faith communities: The role of clergy in black churches. *Social Work, 45*(1), 73–87.

U.S. Department of Education, (2000). *Guidelines for school officials, volunteers and mentors participating in public school community partnerships.* (Available from the Federal Department of Education, http://www.ed.gov/inits/religionandschools/v-guide.html)

U.S. Department of Education (1999). *How faith communities support children's learning in public schools.* www.ed.gov/inits/religionandschools/faith-support.pdf.

Walker, L.J., & Pitts, R.C. (1998). Naturalistic conceptions of moral maturity. *Developmental Psychology, 34,* 403–419.

Weaver, A.J. (1995). Has there been a failure to prepare and support parish-based clergy in their roles as front-line community mental health workers?: A review. *Journal of Pastoral Care, 49,* 129–149.

Weaver, A.J. (1998). Mental health professionals working with religious leaders. In H. Koenig (Ed.), *Handbook of religion and mental health.* San Diego, CA: Academic Press.

Werner, E.E. (1995). Resilience in development. *Current Directions in Psychological Science, 4,* 81–85.

White, J. (1998). Faith-based outreach to at-risk youth in Washington, D.C. *The Jeremiah project: An initiative of the center for civic innovation, report 98-1,* www.mahattan-institute.org.

White House, (2003). *Guidance to faith-based and community organizations on partnering with the federal government.* www.whitehouse.gov/government/fbci/guidance_document.pdf.

Whitehead, B.D., Wilcox, B.L., Rostosky, S.S., Randall, B., & Wright, M.L.C. (2001). *Keeping the faith: The role of religion and faith communities in preventing teen pregnancy.* Washington, DC: National Campaign to Prevent Teen Pregnancy.

Winston, D. (1992). Churches endure as havens of hope. *Progressions: The Black Church in America, 4,* 1–4.

Chapter 19

A Whole-School Approach
to Mental Health Promotion
The Australian *MindMatters* Program

ELIZABETH MULLETT, STEVEN W. EVANS, AND MARK D. WEIST

Across the United States, there is growing recognition of the need to promote the mental well-being of children and adolescents (New Freedom Commission on Mental Health, 2003). Approximately one-third of children and adolescents will experience a diagnosable mental health disorder in their lifetime; however, 75–80% of these children do not receive appropriate interventions (Department of Health and Human Services, 1999, 2000; Pelosi, 1996). Time trend analysis reveals that the prevalence of mental health disorders among youth is not improving (Fombonee, 1994; Australian Bureau of Statistics, 1991; Rutter, 1994), causing researchers to examine the contributing factors to these mental health problems and how to prevent them.

Of further concern is the detrimental impact that mental health problems can have on adolescents' academic achievement. "Children cannot reach their academic potential if they have social, emotional, and physical problems that interfere with their learning" (National Commission on the Role of the School and Community in Improving Adolescent Health, 1990). Students who are experiencing serious emotional difficulties are at a decreased capacity to concentrate on their school work, complete tasks, or even attend school. Furthermore, recent federal initiatives and educational trends in the United States such as the No Child Left Behind Act place increasing pressure on schools to be accountable for their students' academic performance.

The growing mental health needs of youth and the impact of mental health problems on student's academic performance result in a natural union between schools and mental health programs and staff. There are many examples of mental health providers and educators taking advantage of this mutually beneficial coll-aboration resulting in the development, implementation, and evaluation of ex-panded school mental health programs (ESMH; Weist, Evans, & Lever, 2003). Ideally, ESMH programs provide a broad array of services to youth in both gen-eral and special education ranging from school-wide efforts to promote the mental health and school success of all students (e.g., Molina, Smith, & Pelham, 2003) to intensive services for youth with serious emotional and behavioral problems (e.g., Nyre, Vernberg, & Roberts, 2003). Expanded school mental health is gain-ing momentum in the U.S. related to data supporting advantages such as improv-ing access to care and outreach to underserved youth (Diala et al., 2002; Evans, 1999; Weist, Myers, Hastings, Ghuman, & Han, 1999), enhancing productivity of program staff (Flaherty, & Weist, 1999; Jennings, Pearson, & Harris, 2000), promoting the generalization of behavioral change (Evans, Langberg, & Williams, 2003) and leading to improved emotional, behavioral, and academic outcomes in students (Armbruster & Lichtman, 1999; Evans, Axelrod, & Langberg, in press; Illback, Kalafat, & Sanders, 1997; Jennings et al., 2000; Nabors & Reynolds, 2000).

A very promising development was the recent report of the President's New Freedom Commission on Mental Health, which included as one of their recom-mendations, "Improve and expand school mental health programs" (New Freedom Commission on Mental Health, 2003; p. 62). In the U.S., federal support is also reflected in the funding of two national centers for mental health in schools at the University of Maryland, and the University of California Los Angeles (UCLA), and the Safe Schools/Healthy Students initiative to provide school mental health and violence prevention in over 150 communities.

However, in spite of this progress, the school mental health field remains young, and there is much progress to be made in all areas, with a particular need to advance whole-school mental health promotion approaches. While there are excel-lent school-based prevention programs reviewed in the literature (e.g., Cowen et al., 1996), frequently these programs function as a series of well-meaning, short-term initiatives that are not sufficiently linked to the mission of the school (Greenberg et al., 2003). Based on the results of their meta-analysis of 130 universal, selected or indicated prevention programs for school-aged children, Greenberg, Domitrovich, and Bumbarger (2001) made the following conclusions about effective programs: a) multi-year programs are more likely to have long-term effects than short-term programs, b) prevention programs should focus on the multiple domains that a child is involved in, such as school, family and community, c) a central focus of the prevention program should be on the school environment, and d) emphasis should be made on enhancing child, family and teacher behavior, while building home-school-community relationships.

Although broad whole-school mental health promotion programs are lacking in the U.S., a number of countries outside of the United States have already begun developing full-continuum programs and services that emphasize environmental change, focus on early intervention, utilize a strength-based model and are based on empirical evidence (Weist, Johnson, Lowie, Lever & Rowling, 2002). International dialogue and collaboration regarding mental health and schools, with a particular emphasis on whole-school mental health promotion is being facilitated by the newly developed International Alliance for Child and Adolescent Mental Health in Schools (Intercamhs; Weist et al., 2002). Intercamhs currently has over 200 members from over 40 countries with an advisory panel of international leaders from 15 nations (see www.intercamhs.org). Within Intercamhs, one whole school mental health promotion program—*MindMatters* has received the most attention. *MindMatters* was developed in Australia, and is now being implemented throughout this country and a number of European nations including Ireland, Germany and Switzerland. Whole-school mental health promotion offers much promise as a strategy to promote resilience in youth. The purpose of this chapter is to review the *MindMatters* program, discuss ideas related to its implementation in the U.S., and to review findings from a qualitative research project that assessed school stakeholder perspectives from four U.S. communities on the feasibility and potential value of the program.

THE AUSTRALIAN "*MINDMATTERS*" PROGRAM

MindMatters is a national mental health promotion program, based on the concept of the "Health Promoting School." A "Health Promoting School" is one that takes action and places priority on creating an environment that will have the best possible impact on the health of students, teachers and other school community members, and which recognizes the interaction and connections among its curriculum, policies, practices and partnerships with families (World Health Organization [WHO], 1997). Health Promoting Schools utilize a comprehensive approach to strengthen life skills and resilience and foster a school environment and culture that promote school-community partnerships (WHO, 1997).

The goal of *MindMatters* is to provide the framework and resources for the school to develop a comprehensive approach to mental health promotion. Using the health promoting schools' framework, *MindMatters* audits, plans and implements mental health promotion structures, policies and activities. The audit focuses on the three "spheres" of practice that interact to create a health promoting school: 1) curriculum, 2) teaching and learning; school organization, ethos and environment; and 3) partnerships and services (Wyn, Cahill, Holdsworth, Rowling & Carson, 2000). The results of the audit aid the school in developing a comprehensive, multi-year strategy to enhance the mental health and well-being of its students, and to promote the mental health of families and school staff.

MindMatters provides two levels of resources to the school to aid in the school-wide promotion of mental health and well-being. The first level of resources includes comprehensive information to aid in the whole-school audit of current mental health promotion policies and practices and assists with the identification of areas in need of additional support. There are four major whole-school resources which schools can use based on their needs:

1) *SchoolMatters: Mapping and Managing Mental Health in Schools* involves a comprehensive document and framework for a "core team" to audit existing programs, and develop partnerships in the school and community to broadly promote mental health for all members of the school community.

2) *CommunityMatters* provides a resource for school leaders to use with the school and community to support *MindMatters* and provides education about diverse groups of students in the school and suggests strategies for managing their well-being needs. In addition, information is given on how to create family and community partnerships with the school.

3) *Educating for Life: A Guide for School-Based Responses to Preventing Self-Harm and Suicide* provides an overview of the policies and practices involved in suicide prevention, including managing crises, preventing self-harm and recognizing signs of possible suicidal behavior by students.

4) *A Whole-School Approach to Dealing with Bullying and Harassment* includes a booklet to guide schools in comprehensively addressing bullying and harassment, and a checklist to guide policy and practice.

The second level of resources aid teachers in the effective implementation of curricula that promote the mental health and well-being of their students. The decision to implement a specific curriculum is based on the result of the audit conducted by the school.

The five curriculum modules to be implemented by teachers in classrooms are:

1) *Enhancing Resilience 1: Communication, Changes and Challenges* focuses on enhancing resilience via enhancing communication skills, promoting team building, and exploring personal, social and cultural identity issues.

2) *Enhancing Resilience 2: Stress and Coping* provides training on stress, stress management, coping, help seeking, peer support and goal setting.

3) *A Whole-School Approach to Dealing with Bullying and Harassment* includes focused curriculum units for use in Health, English and Drama

classes which teach students how to cope with bullying and harassment.

4) **Understanding Mental Illnesses** aims to increase students' understanding of mental illnesses and mental health problems, reduce the stigma of having mental health problems, and increase help-seeking behavior among those who may present emotional/behavioral problems.

5) **Loss and Grief** focuses on increasing awareness of the connection between loss and depression, assists in identifying students who may be "at risk," and promotes an open environment for discussion of grief and loss issues.

The Development of the *MindMatters* Program

A consortium of Australian health and education experts, working closely with school and community staff, stakeholders and government officials, conducted a comprehensive review of relevant literatures, and developed the *MindMatters* program. The program has been improved and refined since its inception in 1997, including an extensive pilot evaluation, and is well supported by the government of Australia and leadership in diverse sectors and systems from across the country. All 24 education systems in each state and territory of Australia are either implementing *MindMatters* in their secondary schools or have agreed to/are planning to implement it. *MindMatters* recognizes that the success of an initiative is based on teachers' professional development and comfort level in implementing a curriculum. Therefore, a country-wide infrastructure has been established to support the initiative including a National *MindMatters* Team, professional development and training mechanisms in every state and territory, a comprehensive evaluation strategy and resources to assist schools/communities in conducting evaluations, a website (www.curriculum.edu.au/*MindMatters*), and a range of communication mechanisms. Please note that through the just mentioned websites, all of the *MindMatters* resource and training materials can be downloaded free of charge. At present, there are various levels of evaluation of the *MindMatters* program, including descriptive, qualitative, and preliminary outcome data. Major findings include:

1) The program's structure and curricula have been well received by participating schools (*MindMatters* Evaluation Consortium, 2000);

2) Qualitative evaluation of the program by stakeholders within schools has been positive (Wyn et al., 2000);

3) Teachers who are trained to use the program gain confidence in the procedures, and are inclined to use the curriculum resources (Wyn et al., 2000);

4) Increased school-community partnerships are being documented (Hazel, Vincent, Waring, & Lewin, 2002);

5) Following participation in the program, students in some schools have expressed increased willingness to seek help for mental health issues (*MindMatters* Evaluation Consortium, 2000);

6) Many schools reported positive changes (e.g., improved student learning, staff attitudes, school policies) from participating in the program (*MindMatters* Evaluation Consortium, 2000); and

7) Circumstances for optimal implementation of the program have been identified (Wyn et al., 2000).

Levels of Whole-School Change

MindMatters is influenced by the World Health Organization's whole-school approach to school change (WHO, 1997). This model is represented by a triangle that describes the four levels at work in the whole-school approach to mental health promotion: 1) the school environment, 2) curricula, 3) providing additional support, and 4) assessment and referral (*MindMatters* Consortium, 1999).

School Environment

The top and broadest level of the triangle represents the school environment. According to the World Health Organization, school environment is the first and most important aspect of promoting the mental health of students (WHO, 1997). Mental health promotion involves the entire school community and addresses the quality of life for students and staff. The *MindMatters* program emphasizes this level of intervention as the school environment and culture can directly affect the mental health and well-being of its staff and students (*MindMatters* Consortium, 1999). The program encourages teachers to teach "for mental health promotion," meaning that they should help foster an environment where children feel safe and secure, implement curricula that encourage student participation and challenge students to excel, and create a classroom climate that promotes mental health and learning. In addition, *teaching for mental health* uses mental health strategies to aid in learning (e.g., systematic problem solving), and elaborates on important mental health themes through study in other areas (e.g., characters that show resilience, overcome depression in literature). The program also suggests that a supportive school environment may be fostered through school-wide activities such as community forums, mental health days, multicultural events, art shows, peer support groups, mentoring programs, and effective critical incident management plans (*MindMatters* Consortium, 1999). These activities are intended to help students and faculty feel safe and valued in their school.

Curricula

The second level of the triangle represents the school curriculum. *Mind-Matters* suggests that the curriculum should be designed to "promote mental health via the development of communication, help-seeking and problem-solving skills" (MindMatters Consortium, 1999). The *MindMatters* curriculum modules as reviewed previously (two units on resilience, one on bullying, one on understanding mental illness, and one on dealing with loss and grief) model ways to teach both for and about mental health. Interactive lessons are often used to promote excitement about the material, enhance learning and skill acquisition, and foster group interactions and interconnectedness. Guided discussions are used to help students reflect about the topics of interest and aid students and teachers in talking about common changes and challenges that adolescents face (MindMatters Consortium, 1999). The lessons are meant to be integrated into the curriculum so activities that promote mental health education and foster a supportive environment happen as part of daily lessons and are not an "add-on." Obviously, to implement such training through curricula taught by educators, requires considerable training, ongoing support, and resources for classroom teachers (see Greenberg, Domitrovich, & Bumbarger, 2001).

Providing Additional Support

A positive school environment and effective curriculum programs can benefit all students, including those at risk or encountering specific learning or life challenges; however, some students may require additional support. The third layer of the triangle therefore concentrates on the mechanisms designed to identify, and provide support for, those students who are contending with learning, social, emotional and/or mental health problems (MindMatters Consortium, 1999). It is important for schools to review the process by which students are identified and referred for further services so that students do not "fall through the cracks" and fail due to unrecognized or unmet mental health needs. Teachers may need additional training to identify students who are at risk for major psychological or emotional problems. Targeted programs aimed at providing individual counseling or consultation with parents may need to be developed or enhanced. Referrals to and partnerships with outside agencies can also be a powerful way to enhance mental health services to students or provide additional supports during challenging life situations (MindMatters Consortium, 1999).

Assessment and Referral (and Treatment)

The fourth and smallest layer of the triangle pertains to the small percentage of students who require referral for professional assessment or treatment of mental health problems (MindMatters Consortium, 1999). In Australia, these referrals are often to mental health staff in other community settings. As mentioned, in the U.S., when the school has a full expanded school mental health program, referrals are often to staff working within the school, again suggesting a complementary relationship between whole-school mental health promotion and ESMH (Weist, Evans, & Lever, 2003), which should be explored and researched (e.g., are approaches such as *MindMatters* facilitated in schools already taking an ESMH approach?).

In schools in the U.S. without ESMH, educators and school mental health professionals sometimes struggle with the issue of which community provider(s) to refer to, since such referrals implicitly convey endorsement of that provider's services. An additional dimension when students are referred to outside community providers is ensuring adequate school-provider communication to enhance assessment, treatment, and follow-up. Frankly, this communication is often related to practical difficulties, such as arranging phone calls between teachers (who have difficulty accessing a phone) and community providers (who are often in session). A recent report describes an internet-based system of coordinating care and communicating progress (Evans, Serpell, Schultz, & Williams, in press) that may help facilitate these efforts.

IMPLEMENTING THE *MINDMATTERS* PROGRAM

Schools have unique backgrounds with regard to curriculum innovation and the implementation of policies designed to address health and mental health issues. Hence, *MindMatters* was designed to build upon existing programs and structures already in place to promote the mental well-being of students and staff. For example, one school may have well developed policies defining mental health and well-being that are reflected in their school's mission statement. Other schools may have policies that are less well developed, but have developed an environment that promotes mental health and the well-being of all school members. Given the differences among schools and their individual needs, plans to promote mental health promotion need to be tailored to each school.

MindMatters provides education about various aspects of mental health promotion in schools and a framework by which schools can evaluate their school's environment, practices and policies. Resources are given to aid schools in the development and/or revision of policies, programs and practices in the school. Lesson plans are provided to facilitate the implementation of the *MindMatters* curriculum units; however, schools can decide which lessons would be the most beneficial for their students.

With this in mind, the implementation of the *MindMatters* program begins with an assessment of the school by a core team, or group of diverse stakeholders including administrators, teachers, students, parents, community members and others who have an investment in the school. The purpose of the core team is to identify the school's current strengths and areas in need of development. The team is guided in their assessment by the materials presented in the *SchoolMatters* document (one of text in the *MindMatters* curriculum). The core team can utilize this framework to audit, plan and implement mental health promotion structures, policies and activities based on the needs of their individual school.

Once the core team has assessed the school's strengths and areas in need of development, they develop a plan to implement the *MindMatters* whole school approach and curriculum modules that address their specific needs. For example, if a school decides that more work is needed to address a school environment issue such as bullying, they can utilize *The Whole School Approach to Bullying and Harassment* audit, address issues related to diversity in the school community via the *CommunityMatters* resources, and implement one of the three curriculum units provided in the module that addresses bullying and harassment.

ADAPTING *MINDMATTERS* FOR USE IN THE UNITED STATES

In the 2002–2003 academic year, we conducted four discussion groups with school stakeholders (administrators, teachers, parents and students) from large and small urban, suburban and rural school districts in the U.S. The goal of these meetings was to begin to assess the feasibility of implementing the *MindMatters* program in American secondary schools. In each of the four communities, participants attended a meeting where the materials were presented and explained. Before the meeting, each participant received materials including a comprehensive review of the *MindMatters* program, and full curriculum materials for assigned segments (e.g., some were assigned the Resilience 1 segment, others were assigned the Bullying segment). This plan ensured that each curriculum unit was reviewed by at least three people before each of the meetings. After carefully discussing the materials, the participants provided feedback about the potential obstacles and benefits of implementing this program in U.S. schools.

Overall, preliminary data suggest that participants were enthusiastic about the program and indicated that adapting the program for use in their schools seemed feasible. Several aspects of the program made it particularly appealing for use in the U.S. For example, participants valued the fact that the *MindMatters* is a whole-school approach and addresses more than just curriculum issues. In that regard, they reported that the program appears to be much more comprehensive than existing school-based mental health programs. They also appreciated that the program provides an overarching framework for evaluating existing programs in the school and that action plans can be tailored to the needs of the individual school. The teacher training materials were well-received and filled a need area, as teachers reported that they generally were not trained to deal with student mental health issues. Students reported that the topics covered in the curriculum materials addressed important developmental issues. The overall consensus at each discussion group was enthusiasm and a request to be involved in continued efforts to bring *MindMatters* to secondary schools in the U.S.

While the majority of the feedback was positive, there were areas of concern. Participants pointed out that the information on cultural issues needed to be revised to reflect the cultural diversity of the United States instead of Australia. Information regarding lesbian, gay, bisexual, transgendered, and questioning students (LGBTQ) also needed to reflect the particular experience that students have in the U.S. rather than Australia. Research shows, for instance, that gay and lesbian youth are two to three times more likely to attempt suicide than their heterosexual peers and may comprise as much as 30% of suicides among youth in the United States each year (Gibson, 1989). There are also safety issues for LGBTQ youth that need to be considered in the context of the U.S. educational system. Garofalo, Wolf, Kessel, Palfrey, & DuRant (1998), for instance, conducted a study at a Massachusetts high school and found that nearly one-third of gay teens had been threatened with a weapon in the past month in comparison to 7% of heterosexual students. *CommunityMatters* (a handbook for helping teachers manage the well-being of students who are often marginalized), offers education to teachers on how students who are attracted to the same-sex may be bullied, issues related to their resiliency, and loss and grief issues these students may face.

The area of greatest concern in each of the discussion groups was the demand on time and resources involved in using *MindMatters*. A great deal is expected of teachers and the recent focus on standardized test scores has added considerable stress to all school staff. Members of the discussion groups described the prioritization of scores on standardized tests as overwhelming and indicated that this has led to the elimination of many aspects of schools that focused on anything that did not directly teach an answer to questions on these tests. Efforts to attend to students' health and mental health were described as frequent casualties of this trend. Therefore, while there was a great deal of enthusiasm about bringing *MindMatters* to schools in the U.S. because it is sorely needed, this enthusiasm was coupled with concerns about both who would be able to implement it and how it would be implemented.

Interestingly, for each barrier that participants identified, they also made suggestions for overcoming this barrier. Due to the mounting pressures on teachers to increase test scores, a number of participants at each site noted that the manner in which *MindMatters* is presented to the school staff may be crucial to the acceptance of the program. Numerous participants suggested that *MindMatters* be described to staff as a "resource for teachers" instead of as a "program" in order to avoid the perception that *MindMatters* would either create more work for teachers or detract from teaching students what they need to know for testing purposes.

Participants also suggested that *MindMatters* first be implemented to fit within the existing structures of the school. For example, teachers should be trained to use *MindMatters* during a few of the continuing education days that school districts set aside each year. Since many teachers are not comfortable implementing material related to mental health issues, several discussion group participants suggested that *MindMatters* first be implemented by the counselor in conjunction with the classroom teacher. Other groups suggested that teachers notify counselors when they are implementing a potentially sensitive unit, such as Grief and Loss, so that counselors can help students who may need to talk more in depth about an issue.

The *MindMatters* program has gained widespread acceptance in Australia and a modified version is now being implemented in Ireland, Germany and Switzerland. Important steps are necessary before widespread implementation in the U.S. is recommended. First, as mentioned, the materials need to be modified to make them relevant to diversity in the U.S. Second, there should be some evaluation of the modified version to ensure that it is indeed leading to positive outcomes for U.S. schools and students. This is particularly important, because evaluation data on the program thus far do not support that it could be viewed as "evidence based" according to U.S. standards. Notwithstanding these cautions, we hope that this chapter will provide the impetus for school communities here to begin exploration of whole-school mental health promotion approaches as in *MindMatters*. These approaches hold considerable promise to enhance global collaboration in improving schools and promoting child and family resilience, mental health and school success.

ACKNOWLEDGEMENT

Logistical support for the four stakeholder meetings referred to herein was provided by the Center for Mental Health Services (CMHS), Substance Abuse and Mental Health Services Administration (SAMHSA), and the United States Department of Health and Human Services (DHHS). However, the content of the paper does not necessarily reflect the views of DHHS/SAMHSA/CMHS, nor should any endorsement by those organizations be implied. We thank Dr. Louise Rowling of the University of Sydney for her valuable guidance in conducting this project.

REFERENCES

Armbruster, P., & Lichtman, J. (1999). Are school based mental health services effective? Evidence from 36 inner-city schools. *Community Mental Health Journal, 35*, 493–504.
Australian Bureau of Statitics (1991). *Mortality Statistics for Australia:1991*. Canberra: Commonwealth of Australia.

Commonwealth Department of Health and Family Services (1996). *Promoting mental health and emotional well-being within a health promoting schools framework, draft guidelines*. Canberra: Australian Government Printing Services.

Cowen, E.L., Hightower, A.D., Pedro-Carroll, J.L., Work, W.C., Wyman, P.A., & Haffey, W.G. (1996). *School-Based prevention for children at risk: The primary mental health project*. Washington DC: American Psychological Association.

Department of Health and Human Services. (1999). *Mental health: A report of the Surgeon General*. Rockville, MD: Substance Abuse and Mental Health Services Administration, Center for Mental Health Services, National Institutes of Health, National Institute of Mental Health.

Department of Health and Human Services. (2000). *Healthy People 2010: Conference editions Volume I and II*. Washington, DC.

Diala, C.C., Muntaner, C., Walrath, C., Nickerson, K., LaVeist, T., & Leaf, P. (2002). Racial/ethnic differences in attitudes toward seeking professional mental health services. *American Journal of Public Health, 91*(5), 805–807.

Evans, S.W. (1999). Mental health services in schools: Utilization, effectiveness, and consent. *Clinical Psychology Review, 19*, 165–178.

Evans, S.W., Axelrod, J.L., & Langberg, J. (in press). Efficacy of a school-based treatment program for middle school youth with ADHD: Pilot data. *Behavior Modification*.

Evans, S.W., Langberg, J., & Williams, J. (2003). Treatment generalization in school based mental health. In M.D. Weist, S.W. Evans, & N.A. Lever (Eds.), *Handbook of School Mental Health*. New York: Kluwer Academic/Plenum Publishers.

Evans, S.W., Serpell, Z., Schultz, B., & Williams, A. (2003). Developing and transitioning school-based treatment: The Challenging Horizons Program example. *Report on Emotional & Behavioral Disorders in Youth*.

Fombonne, E. (1994). Increased rates of depression: Update of epidemiological findings and analytical problems. *Acta Psychiatrica Scandinavica, 90*, 145–156.

Garofalo, R., Wolf, C., Kessel, S., Palfrey, J., & DuRant, R.H. (1998). The Association between health risk behaviors and sexual orientation among a school-based sample of adolescents, *Pediatrics, 101*, 895–902

Gibson, P. (January, 1989). *Gay male and lesbian youth suicide: report of the secretary's task force on youth suicide* (pp. 110–142). Washington, DC: United States Department of Health and Human Services.

Greenberg, M.T., Domitrovich, C.E., & Bumbarger, B. (2001). The prevention of mental disorders in school-aged children: Current state of the field. *Prevention and Treatment, 4*, Article 1. Retrieved August 22, 2003, from http://journals.apa.org/prevention/volume4/pre0040001a.html.

Greenberg, M.T., Weissberg, R.P., O'Brien, M.U., Zins, J.E., Fredericks, L., Resnik, H., & Elias, M.J. (2003). Enhancing school-based prevention and youth development through coordinated social, emotional and academic learning. *American Psychologist, 58*, 466–474.

Hazell, T., Vincent, K., Waring, T., & Lewin, T. (2002). The challenges of evaluating national mental health promotion programs in schools: A case study using the evaluation of MindMatters. *International Journal of Mental Health Promotion, 4*, 21–27.

Illback, R.J., Kalafat, J., & Sanders, D. (1997). Evaluating integrated service programs. In R.J. Illback, C.T. Cobb, & H.M. Joseph (Eds.), *Integrated services for children and families: Opportunities for psychological practice* (pp. 323–346). Washington, DC: American Psychological Association.

Jennings, J., Pearson, G., & Harris, M. (2000). Implementing and maintaining school-based mental health services in a large urban school district. *Journal of School Health, 70*(5), 201–296.

MindMatters Consortium (1999). *Mindmatters: A whole-school approach promoting mental health and well-being*. Melbourne: Youth Research Centre.

MindMatters Evaluation Consortium (2000). *Report of the MindMatters (National Mental Health in Schools Project) Evaluation Project, vols 1–4*. Newcastle, Australia: Hunter Institute of Mental Health, 2000.

Molina, B.S.G., Smith, B.H., & Pelham, W.E. (2003). *A school-wide program to improve behavior and achievement in a public middle school: Implementation, satisfaction, and effectiveness.* Manuscript submitted for publication.

Nabors, L.A., & Reynolds, M.W. (2000). Program evaluation activities: Outcomes related to treatment for adolescents receiving school-based mental health services. *Children's Services: Social Policy, Research, and Practice, 3*(3), 175–189.

National Coodinating Technical Assistance Center for Drug Prevention and School Safety Program Coordinators. (2003). Frequently asked questions. Retrieved August 22, 2003, from http://www.k12coordinator.org/faqs.asp.

New Freedom Commission on Mental Health (2003). *Achieving the Promise: Transforming mental health care in America. Final report.* Rockville, MD: DHHS Pub. No. SMA-03-3832.

Nyre, J.E., Vernberg, E.M., & Roberts, M.C. (2003). Serving the most severe emotionally disturbed students in school settings. In M. Weist, S. Evans, & N. Lever (Eds.), *Handbook of School Mental Health: Advancing Practice and Research.* New York: Kluwer Academic/Plenum Publishers.

Pelosi, N. (1996). Reducing risks of mental disorders. *American Psychologist, 51,* 1128–1129.

Rutter, M. (1994). Beyond longitudinal data: Causes, consequence, changes and continuity. *Journal of Consulting and Clinical Psychology, 62,* 928–940.

Weist, M.D., Evans, S.W., & Lever, N.A. (2003). Advancing mental health practice and research in schools. In M.D. Weist, S.W. Evans, & N.A. Lever (Eds.), *Handbook of school mental health: Advancing practice and research* (pp. 1–8). New York, NY: Kluwer Academic/Plenum Publishers.

Weist, M.D., Johnson, A., Lowie, J.A., Lever, N.A., & Rowling, L. (2002). Building an international network for mental health in schools. *International Journal of Mental Health Promotion, 4,* 34–39.

Weist, M.D., Myers, C.P., Hastings, E., Ghuman, H., & Han, Y. (1999). Psychosocial functioning of youth receiving mental health services in the schools vs. community mental health centers. *Community Mental Health Journal, 35*(5), 69–81.

World Health Organization (1997). The Jakarta Declaration on leading health promotion into the 21st century, Presented at the Fourth International Conference on Health Promotion, *Jakarta, 21–25,* July 1997.

World Health Organization: What is a health promoting school? Retreived from: http://www.who.int/school_youth_health/gshi/hps/en/ on October 30, 2003.

Wyn, J., Cahill, H., Holdsworth, R., Rowling, L., & Carson, S. (2000). MindMatters, a whole-school approach promoting mental health and wellbeing. *Australian and New Zealand Journal of Psychiatry, 34,* 594–601.

Chapter 20

Home, School, and Community
Catalysts to Resilience

MICKEY C. MELENDEZ AND SAUNDRA TOMLINSON-CLARKE

RISK AND RESILIENCE IN STUDENTS

As the demographic profile of the United States continues to change, so do the challenges associated with the health and well-being of our youth in United States society. Differences in racial/ethnic background, region, socio-economics, language, values, and ability are among the issues of cultural diversity that are represented by children and their families. As a result, each year an increasing number of students are entering schools with life circumstances that teachers and school personnel are not prepared to address (Costello, 1996). These multiple and interlocking aspects of cultural diversity have been associated with the ability of children to succeed in school and in life. Consequently, a major focus in the education and psychological literature is the overall health and well-being of children and youth in a changing society. Research in this area has focused on two critical aspects affecting overall health and development. First, researchers have identified at-risk factors that interfere with healthy development in children and adolescents (Thompson, 2002). Secondly, protective factors that increase the likelihood that children and youth will succeed in school and in life have been studied (Barr & Parrett, 2001). Following this line of research, this chapter highlights stressors in schools, families, and communities that threaten the health and well-being of youth in today's society. Protective factors or characteristics of resilience that help in overcoming potential stressors are reviewed. Finally, building support networks at home and in schools, and mentoring relationships that promote healthy academic, social and emotional well-being are discussed.

Stressors among Children and Youth

Frymier and Gansneder (1989) compiled a comprehensive list of 45 at-risk factors that today's youth might experience. These factors cover a wide range of parameters, which are ranked from most serious to least serious. Factors that place youth at risk include: attempted suicide, drugs and alcohol use and abuse, risky sexual activity, school violence and safety issues, tobacco use, and poor nutrition. Other researchers have categorized at-risk factors as academic or non-academic, identifying at-risk behaviors that are school related, and others that are related to family and community. Academic factors associated with at-risk students include low achievement, retention in grade level, behavior problems, poor attendance in school, and attending school with a large number of poor students (Slavin & Madden, 1989). Non-academic factors associated with the health and well being of children and youth include poverty, welfare dependence, the absence of both parents in the home, unmarried mothers, and undereducated parents (Barr & Parrett, 2001; Lambie, Leone, & Martin, 2002; McPartland & Slavin, 1990; McWhirter, McWhirter, McWhirter, & McWhirter, 1998; Rak & Patterson, 1996). These factors are interrelated and affect the quality of an individual's life. For example, some children may experience supportive family networks and early educational and social preparation, resulting in the ability to meet the demands of school and to succeed in other areas of life. Other children may experience a lack of family supportive networks and an absence of early and on-going educational and social interventions, resulting in the inability to adjust and succeed in school. Consequently, factors affecting the ability to achieve in school set the foundation for the ability to succeed in life. Therefore, schools have been shown to have a critical impact on students identified as at-risk (The U.S. Department of Education, 1998). Effective schools have been shown to provide all students with opportunities to learn, promoting healthy psychological development and assisting with enhanced academic achievement (Barr & Parrett, 2001).

However, in examining the overall plight of youth within the context of school and community, Thompson (2002) stated that... "the self-defeating, self-destructive potential of youth is a growing threat to the welfare of the nation. The growing concern over suicide rates, substance abuse, violence, alienation, victimization and abuse, family dysfunction, truancy, and dropout rates continues to demonstrate that relationships between youth and adults and among youth peers are significantly strained" (p. 37). The combined and cumulative effects of at-risk factors to which many children encounter on a daily basis puts our nation's youth in dire circumstances regarding their future life. From a systems perspective, one must be mindful that children and youth in our society may mirror the dysfunction and turmoil that currently exists in society as a whole. McWhirter et al. (1998) cautioned that the United States is an at-risk society, as evidenced by the epidemic proportions of unhealthy behaviors affecting a large segment of the population.

Consequently, behaviors that members of society engage in will continue to have a significant impact on overall health and psychological well-being.

Existing Limitations of the Research

Definitional variance exists in the use of the term "at-risk", which has served to confound research outcomes. In order to avoid making stereotypical generalizations about an individual based solely on life circumstances, it is critical to understand how and from what perspective the term "at-risk" is used in the research.

Research on children and youth that is intended to be proactive and preventative, uses the term "at-risk" to identify factors that have the potential to disrupt the social, emotional, academic, and health-related development of children and youth. Intervention strategies based on a preventative approach are designed to buffer the negative effects of problematic areas that are identified as at-risk. To this end, the term is used only as a description of circumstances and events associated with the potential to interfere with health and well-being. In other research studies, however, the term "at-risk" has been used as a prediction for a child's outcome in school (McPartland & Slavin, 1990; Slavin & Madden, 1989), level of educational achievement and attainment, and productivity as a citizen in society (Liontos, 1991). In addition, the term "at-risk" has been used as a catchall label for a variety of negative behaviors, inclusive of emotional and adjustment problems, health concerns, and absence of appropriate learning skills (McWhirter et al., 1998).

Many of the studies examining at-risk children and youth focus on the life circumstances of racial/ethnic minority groups, specifically, African Americans and Latinos. Pallas, Natriello, and McDill (1989) suggested the interrelation of risk factors, identifying five key characteristics that place a child at risk: (a) minority, racial, or ethnic group identity; (b) living in poverty; (c) living in a single-parent family; (d) having a poorly educated mother; and (e) having a non-English language background. Too often, researchers studying racial-ethnic minority youth have used at-risk as a connotation for deficiency. Deficit models were quite prevalent in education when describing and labeling racial/ethnic minority youth, leading to biased assumptions about culture and ability. From this perspective, associating the term "at-risk" in describing a child may negatively bias the expectations of teachers and other significant adults in the child's life, leading to negative outcomes.

It is important to consider that the common factor that shapes the lives' of many racial-ethnic minority youth is class or socio-economic status. A disproportionate number of African American and Latino youth live in poverty, increasing the potential for exposure to and participation in behaviors that are stressors. However, higher socio-economic status is not a protective shield against dysfunction. Any child may experience stress regardless of economics, gender, race/ethnicity, or family structure (McWhirter et al., 1998; Sinclair & Ghory, 1987).

Proactive Intervention Model for Youth Who Face Stress

McWhirter et al. (1998) offer a continuum approach to help in identifying and examining at-risk factors. This model examines at-risk behaviors within a cultural context, and is consistent with a proactive, preventative framework. Steps along the continuum range from minimal risk to at-risk. The descriptors for each category on the continuum are as follows:

1. Minimal risk characterized by favorable demographics and limited stressors,
2. Remote risk characterized by less favorable demographics, less positive family, school, and social interactions, with some stressors,
3. High risk characterized by negative family, school and social interactions, numerous stressors and development of personal at-risk behaviors,
4. Imminent risk characterized by a progression of negative personal behaviors,
5. At-risk characterized as participation in behaviors associated with an at-risk category. Behaviors at this stage of the continuum are no longer at-risk, but are considered to be maladaptive. Youth exhibiting maladaptive behavior in one category are at-risk for maladaptive behavior in other categories (p. 7–9).

The steps along the continuum are not meant to be diagnostic or to be used to label individuals. The steps are useful in assessing potentially problematic behaviors from a proactive stance, and developing effective strategies for intervention based on the amount of stressors in the child's life.

Interventions targeted for home, school, and community provide supports that aid children and youth in developing characteristics that are associated with the likelihood that they will engage in positive behaviors rather than at-risk behaviors. The Developmental Assets Survey (Benson, Galbraith, & Espeland, 1998) measures forty assets directly related to behaviors experienced by youth. The dimensions of the Survey include Supportive Assets, Empowerment Assets, Boundaries and Expectations Assets, and Constructive Use of Time. Also, twenty personal internal assets inclusive of commitment to learning, positive values, social competence and positive identity that influence behavior are identified. The goal of this assessment is to increase opportunities that foster positive characteristics in children and youth.

TOWARDS POSITIVE MODELS OF HEALTH: RESILIENCE IN CHILDREN AND YOUTH

Resilience is simply defined as "beating the odds" (Haggerty, Sherrod, Garmezy & Rutter, 1994; Wang & Haertel, 1995). However, similar to studies using the term "at-risk" there is no agreed upon definition for resilience (Clauss-Ehlers, this volume). Although much of the resilience research has focused on African American and Latino youth in inner city communities (Clauss-Ehlers & Lopez Levi, 2002a, 2002b; Wang, Haertel, & Walberg, 1995) these studies have focused on the positive strengths that an individual utilizes to cope with difficult life circumstances, thus eliminating the use of deficit and disease models in examining minority youth. Furthermore, resilience as a health promotion model to understanding health and well-being is consistent with counseling psychology and other preventative approaches.

Developing Resiliency

Consistent with identifying developmental assets associated with the increased likelihood that children and youth will engage in positive behaviors (Benson et al., 1998), many researchers have identified characteristics associated with resiliency (Bernard, 1991; Rak & Patterson, 1996; Werner, 1984). Characteristics of resiliency are considered to be protective factors that help in overcoming negative life events, enabling youth to succeed in life. In developing a list of resilient characteristics, researchers have typically examined children who succeed despite the presence of at-risk factors in school, in the family and within the community (Thompson, 2002). Among the attributes that youth develop in coping with adversity are:

1. Social competency, good interpersonal skills, a responsive style, empathy and humor;
2. Problem-solving skills, critical thinking abilities, and a proactive perspective;
3. A strong self-esteem, a sense of personal power, independence and autonomy;
4. A sense of purpose, goal directed behavior, and optimism regarding the future;
5. A positive vision of a meaningful life, and
6. An ability to seek out novel experiences.

Protective Mechanisms

McWhirter et al. (1998) isolated five overlapping competencies that discriminate high-risk youth from low-risk youth. They refer to these characteristics as the "five C's of competency," stating that, "These characteristics discriminate between youngsters who move through life with a high potential for success and those who are not doing well" (p. 83). These competencies are: (a) critical school competencies, (b) concept of self and self-esteem, (c) communication with others, (d) coping ability and, (e) control.

While poverty and racism are factors that many children contend with, other salient psychosocial factors may also be at work during the process of resiliency development. For example, Rak and Patterson (1996) identified salient personal, family, and environmental protective factors involved in fostering resiliency in children. Some of the factors highlighted by the authors included:

1. An active, evocative, approach to problem solving (personal);
2. An optimistic view of negative experiences (personal);
3. An ability to maintain a positive vision of a meaningful life (personal);
4. An ability to gain others positive attention (personal);
5. Age of the opposite sex parent (males benefited from younger mothers, females benefited from older fathers) (family);
6. Not more than four children in the family, spaced two or more years apart (family);
7. Little prolonged separation from the primary caregiver and focused nurturing during the first year of life (family);
8. Alternate caregivers (e.g.: grandparents, siblings, neighbors) who stepped in when the parents were not consistently available (family);
9. Identified role models outside of the family (environmental).

Rak and Patterson also recommend adopting a strength, as opposed to illness, perspective when considering the plight of children under stress. Taken together, these factors speak to the complexity of resilience as a construct, and to the different influences that shape its development.

A Sociocultural Perspective

Recent research has questioned the notion of resilient characteristics. Clauss-Ehlers (this volume) suggested a sociocultural perspective in addressing the dynamic nature of the construct of resilience, proposing a *Culturally-focused Resilient Adaptation* (CRA) model of resilience. She views resilience as a process of interaction between the individual and the larger sociocultural context, which is reflective of the relevant resources and stressors of the child's experience. This model differs dramatically from trait-based models, in that the focus is not placed solely on the individual child in developing resilient characteristics, but on culturally responsive individual, family, and community interventions. However, current interventions designed to foster protective factors through "resilience building experiences" and life skills training are based on previous research and remain focused primarily on the individual. Also, due to the influence of schools in the lives of children, resilience-building experiences are often taught to students through school-based interventions, with a goal of helping students to develop those characteristics associated with resiliency.

McWhirter et al. (1998) identified three areas in a child's life that are related to developing resiliency. These areas are identified as (a) the social environment inclusive of school, work and church; (b) the family or significant relationships with adults that build trust at an early age, and (c) personal characteristics. Although parent involvement has been directly associated with increasing school achievement (Carlson & Lewis, 2002), parents are not considered to be the only resource for developing resiliency in children and youth. Parents do provide direct and indirect influences related to resilience, however, McWhirter et al. (1998) noted that parents are not the only adults that can help to build trusting relationships which foster resiliency in children. Research suggests that resilient children often develop a supportive, trusting, mentoring relationship outside of the family (Wolin & Wolin, 1993). Mentoring, therefore, provides a fruitful avenue for having an impact on the interaction between the child and the sociocultural environment. Mentoring relationships can build upon resources and help the child to learn strategies for reducing a variety of stressors in one's life. A lack of research, however, has focused on resilience building experiences taught through mentoring, specifically mentoring through group involvement, such as sport participation, or other extracurricular activities.

PRACTICAL CONSIDERATIONS OF RESILIENCY DEVELOPMENT: BUILDING SUPPORT NETWORKS

Understanding and fostering resilience in at-risk children has become a focus of academics, teachers, parents, clinicians, clergy, and any individuals or groups concerned with the plight of children in our society. To that end, Hirayama and Hirayama (2001) recommend that individuals working to foster resiliency in children adopt a systems approach, reasoning that resiliency may only be enhanced through numerous interactions between the individual, the family, the school, and the community. More specifically, parents, teachers, coaches, community leaders, and other mentors play an imperative role in helping construct protective mechanisms to children living under stress.

Fostering resiliency in children requires the construction of resilience networks. Incorporating family, school, and community resources, resilience networking allows for the collaboration of parents, teachers, community leaders, and other mentors, for the purposes of building social, emotional, and psychological supports for children who face substantial stressors.

Building Support at Home: Parents and Family

The role of parents and family in the development of resilience in children is an important area of consideration for individuals working with children under stress.

A number of key familial factors have recently been identified in the literature. Gordon Rouse Longo, & Trickett (1999a) generated a list of recommendations for fostering competence and resilience in children based on familial and environmental factors. These recommendations included:

1. Establishing a strong care taking bond between child and primary caregiver soon after birth;
2. Fostering positive healthy relationships with extended kin;
3. Establishment of daily and weekly routines;
4. Promoting two way communication between parents (caregivers) and children;
5. Establishing discipline and structure with rational limits in the home;
6. Involving children in chores and hobbies;
7. Establishing external supports;
8. Fostering a strong work ethic through role modeling;
9. Involving children with spirituality and religion;
10. Participating in family activities;
11. Promoting egalitarian values;
12. Valuing education.

Although not an exhaustive list, these recommendations were intended to focus attention on the familial environment, as opposed to individual characteristics, as a pathway to resilience for any child.

Other researchers offered more specific strategies for developing familial support for children. Brooks and Goldstein (2001), based on their "resilient mindset" model, offer five strategies for helping children become more resilient. They are: (a) teaching empathy and practicing empathy through role-modeling, (b) teaching responsibility and encouraging contributions in areas of competence (islands of competence), (c) teaching decision-making and problem-solving skills while also reinforcing self-discipline, (d) offering encouragement and positive feedback, and (e) helping children deal with mistakes. According to the authors, these strategies are intended to help develop an increased sense of self-worth and competence in children, while also promoting a sense of optimism, ownership, and self-control.

Rak and Patterson (1996) discussed how counselors might assist families in fostering resilience in children. They suggested that school and agency based counselors offer individual and group consultation to parents, focused on communication, empathy, support, and other parenting skills. In addition, the authors recommend that parents consider seeking professional help with their own individual, marital, and family based concerns. Issues such as family and marital discord, anxiety, depression, alcoholism, and emotional instability can often hinder parents' abilities to create safe and accepting environments for their children.

School Factors Effecting Resiliency

Schools and school systems can play an important role in the development of resiliency in at-risk children as well. School related factors can help foster resiliency by protecting students from negative consequences and outcomes such as problems with social skills and academic performance. For example, school size, academic standards, and levels of support are all related to resilience in the literature (Gordon Rouse, Longo & Trickett (1999b). In addition, other studies point to the importance of teacher support, effective teacher feedback, and teacher communication as important factors in the enhancement of resilience in children (Werner, 1984; Werner, 1990).

Social skill development and background characteristics are also influencing factors for resilience. The ability of all children to transition from grade to grade is influenced, in part, by the mastery of certain school-related social behaviors. For elementary school children, the development of social competence and help seeking skills are imperative. For middle school aged children, school norms and relationships with peers are thought to have more influence on resiliency (Winfield, 1994).

Race/ethnicity can also play a role in the development of resiliency in schools. For instance, greater numbers of African Americans, Latinos, and Native Americans live in poverty, which puts them at greater risk due to limited resources and limited access to health (Fraser & Galinsky, 1997). Documented differences in behavior patterns between African American and White children, along with teacher's belief systems regarding differences in intelligence across race can influence what is expected, and observed, from racial/ethnic minority children (Winfield, 1994).

Other, more internally focused, indices of success can influence resilience as well. Research has indicated that children who experience success in an area of competence such as cognitive, spiritual, behavioral, social, emotional, or physical competence, tend to be more resilient than those who do not (Kumpfer, 1999; Resiliency in Children, 2002). School resources play a key role in the development of many of these competencies. However, family and community resources are equally important in the overall development of resiliency.

Building Support in Schools: Teachers and Counselors

Schools occupy a central role in the development of resiliency. Research has revealed that family and school occupy more of children's and adolescent's time than any other factors, followed by television and sports (Danish, Nellen, & Owens, 1996). Building school-based supports from a systems perspective, in turn, should incorporate aspects of all of these important influences in children's lives. Within any given community, schools, along with churches, often serve to connect the community with the family. Therefore, the influence of the family and the community must also be considered when building school-based supports.

A number of recommendations for building support for the development of resiliency in schools have been offered in the literature. For example, Gordon Rouse et al. (1999b) suggested the following practical considerations for fostering resiliency in schools:

1. Smaller school sizes, or in larger schools, smaller classes and greater access to guidance counselors;
2. Setting higher academic standards and providing the support needed to achieve them;
3. Increase support to students and families by providing assistance programs and setting up additional services;
4. Provide opportunities for positive peer interactions;
5. Create a supportive general atmosphere in the school;
6. Provide opportunities for accomplishment and success, both through academics and extracurricular activities;
7. Employment of specific feedback in describing how student contributions resulted in successful outcomes;
8. Application of fair and even discipline standards for all students.

Teachers play an imperative role in addressing these considerations, and in the subsequent development of resiliency, according to the authors. Teachers are often the only consistent and supportive adult role models in the lives of many children, and must therefore assume a variety of proactive and supportive roles.

Certain school systems have begun to employ system-wide policies to promote resilience. For example, the Minneapolis Public School system has adopted resilience-building strategies (North Central Regional Educational Laboratory, 1994) to "help kids build social skills, reduce stress, and increase their sense of skill mastery" (p. 3). The strategies included (a) offering opportunities to develop attachment relationships with caring adults, (b) increasing student's sense of mastery in their lives by providing opportunities for success, (c) building social competencies as well as academic skills, (d) reducing unnecessary stressors from children's lives, and (e) generating school and community resources to support the needs of children. The authors also revealed that teachers were trying to "reorient toward positive values, rather than focus on problems" (p. 4). Additional resilience strategies suggested by the authors included: the development of peer support programs, the development of learning approaches that build on prior cultural knowledge, the pursuit of topics of personal interest for each child, and the integration of social services into the schools.

In sum, school based support programs are currently being employed in school districts across in the US. In addition, several authors have recommended both family and community participation with the schools in the development of resiliency (Brooks & Goldstein, 2001; Gordon Rouse, 1999a; NCREL, 1994).

Building Support in the Community: Leaders and Mentors

Community support is, in part, related to the type of the external supports available to children and their families. According to Hirayama and Hirayama (2001) the presence of persons and networks that provide financial, physical, emotional, social, and spiritual supports is important. Friends, relatives, community groups, and community agencies can supplement the support networks available in the home. Government can also play a role by adopting, and funding, comprehensive, integrated, long-term, research based policies that support child development from birth to adulthood (Steinhauer, 1996).

In addition, a community needs to help create opportunities for at-risk children to develop resilience. Teachers, church leaders, volunteers, and other community mentors can play an important role in this capacity. After school programs that create opportunities for children to develop their interests and competencies are also needed. Organizations such as Big Brothers, Big Sisters, and Boy/Girl Scouts of America were created to directly supplement the mentoring provided by parents (Rak & Patterson, 1996). One previously underutilized area of opportunity for mentoring and fostering resilience in children exists within local youth sport programs.

Sport Participation and Resilience

Although, athletic participation has been researched as a potential factor in childhood and adolescent development (Smith & Smoll, 1996), less is known about sport as a building block for resiliency in children. Playing a sport may act as a buffer or protective mechanism for children, especially boys, allowing for increased self-esteem, resilience, and adolescent identity (Braddock, Royster, Winfield, & Hawkins, 1991; Melendez, 2001; Taylor, 1995).

Braddock et al. (1991) determined that persistence developed through athletic participation in students was closely related to academic resilience. Their findings revealed that sport participation was positively related to aspirations to enroll in academic programs, complete high school, and foster positive peer relations among schoolmates. In addition, participants (eighth grade African American boys) reported looking forward to attending classes more, and were judged by their teachers as working harder.

Lending support to Braddock et al. (1991), Winfield (1994) highlighted specific benefits of athletic participation to resiliency development in children. Accordingly, athletic involvement may play an effective buffering role and may facilitate academic resilience and attachment for African-American boys in several ways. First, sport involvement is typically contingent upon students' meeting minimal academic requirements. Second, certain behaviors acquired through sport participation are generalizable to classroom behaviors, such as: (a) conditioning [oneself for optimal performance]; (b) self-discipline; (c) adherence to rules; (d) a propensity for hard work; (e) an ability to persist even when one loses (fails); and (f) an ability to analyze why one lost (failed) and compensate for it. According to the author, "these are many of the critical skills and strategies for students to learn if they are to be successful" (p. 5).

Other authors have built on a theorized link between athletic participation and self-esteem. Athletic participation has been theorized to positively influence self-esteem and college adjustment in student athletes (Melendez, 2001). In addition, Taylor (1995) determined that athletic participation was one of several factors that lead to increased levels of self-esteem for college students. Finally, Parham (1993) stated that "involvement in athletics seems to satisfy several basic human needs, including those having to do with success, approval, validation from others, recognition, and feeling a part of someone or something" (p. 417).

Coaches and Mentors

Coaching youth sport can provide other opportunities for adults to foster resilience in children. The importance of "alternate caregivers" who were available to step in when parents were not consistently available, and "mentors outside of the family" who served as potential buffers for vulnerable children, has been addressed in the literature (Rak & Patterson, 1996). Also, research on sport participation shows that that it can have an important role in the development of children's self-concept and self-esteem (Smith & Smoll, 1996). Therefore, coaches have a unique opportunity to nurture children and help them increase their self-esteem, thus fostering resilience.

Coaches can serve as mentors by providing ongoing supportive relationships that children can depend on. In addition, coaches can help teach and role model other important life skills, such as: discipline, determination, focus, leadership, and cooperation. Hedge (1998) offered several recommendations to help coaches become better mentors. These included:

1. Praise each child often, and not just for successes;
2. Be patient when teaching skills, let children know how important their understanding is to you;
3. Keep sport participation child focused, and keep it fun;
4. Treat every player equally, and with respect, regardless of ability;
5. Foster a sense of teamwork by encouraging every player to try every position;

6. Foster a sense of responsibility by allowing each child to help evaluate their own performance;
7. Offer support to children who are struggling and allow them to recommend changes;
8. Be sincere, and remember that winning is not the primary reason for playing a sport.

In sum, coaches can be an integral part of the community resilience network. Along with parents, teachers, extended family members, and friends, coaches can help establish and maintain the types of secure and supportive relationships needed to foster resilience in all our children. In addition, coaches can also be mentors for children, helping them to gain confidence and self-worth through participation in organized sport.

REFERENCES

Barr, R.D., & Parrett, W.H. (2001). *Hope fulfilled for at-risk and violent youth: K-12 programs that work* (2nd ed.). Boston, MA: Allyn and Bacon.

Benson, P.L., Galbraith, J., & Espeland. (1998). *What kids need to succeed.* Minneapolis, MN: Free Spirit Publications.

Braddock, J.H., Royster, D.A., Winfield, L.F., & Hawkins, R. (1991). Bouncing back: Sports and academic resilience among African-American males. *Education and Urban Society*, 24, 113–131.

Brooks, R., & Goldstein, S. (2001). *Risk, resilience and futurists: Changing the lives of our children.* Retrieved January 7, 2003 from the Center for Development and Learning. Web site: http://www.cdl.org/resources/reading_room/print/risk_resilience.html

Clauss-Ehlers, C.S. (2004). Re-inventing resilience: A model of culturally-focused resilience adaptation. In C.S. Clauss-Ehlers & M.D. Weist (Eds.), *Community planning to foster resilience in children* (pp. 27–41). New York: Kluwer Academic/Plenum Publishers

Clauss-Ehlers, C.S., & Lopez Levi, L. (2002a). Violence and community, terms in conflict: An ecological approach to resilience. *Journal of Social Distress and the Homeless*, 11, 265–278.

Clauss-Ehlers, C.S., & Lopez Levi, L. (2002b). Working to promote resilience with Latino youth in schools: Perspectives from the United States and Mexico. *International Journal of Mental Health Promotion*, 4, 14–20.

Costello, M.A. (1996). *Critical issue: Providing effective schooling for students at risk, pp. 1–9.* Retrieved 12/10/00 from: http://www.ncrel.org/sdrs/areas/issues/ students/atrisk/at600.html

Danish, S.J., Nellen, V.C., & Owens, S.S. (1996). Teaching life skills through sport: Community based programs for adolescents. In Van Raalte, J.L., & Brewer, B.W. (Eds.), *Exploring sport and exercise psychology.* (pp. 205–225). Washington, DC: American Psychological Association.

Fraser, M.W., & Galinsky, M.J. (1997). Toward a resiliency based model of practice. In M.W. Fraser (Ed.) *Risk and resilience* (pp. 265–275). Washington, DC: NASW Press.

Frymier, J., & Gansneder, B. (1989). *The Phi Delta Kappa study of students at-risk.* Delta Kappan, 71, 142–146.

Gordon Rouse, K.A., Longo, M., & Trickett, M. (1999a). *Fostering resiliency in children: Familial environmental factors.* The Ohio State University: Bulletin 875–99. Retrieved on January 7, 2003 from http://ohioline.osu.edu.b875/b875_3.html

Gordon Rouse, K.A., Longo, M., & Trickett, M. (1999b). *Fostering resiliency in children: Academic environmental factors.* The Ohio State University: Bulletin 875-99. Retrieved on January 23, 2003 from http://ohioline.osu.edu.b875/ b875_4.html

Haggerty, R.J., Sherrod, L.R., Garmezy, N., & Rutter, M. (1994). *Stress, risk, and resilience in children and adolescents: Processes, mechanisms, and interventions.* Cambridge, UK: Cambridge University.

Hedges, D.D.L. (1998). *Coaches need to mentor, too.* Retrieved February 18, 2003, from Montana State University, Communication Services Web Site: http://www.montana.edu/wwwpb/home/coach.html

Hirayama, H., & Hirayama, K. (2001). Fostering resiliency in children through group work: Instilling hope, courage and life skills. In T.B. Kelly, T. Berman-Rossi, & S. Palombo, (Eds.) *Group work: Strategies for strengthening resiliency.* (pp. 71–83). New York: Hawthorne Press.

Kumpfer, K. (1999). Factors and processes contributing to resilience: The resilience framework. In M.D. Glanzt, & J.L. Jonson, (Eds.), *Resilience and development: Positive life adaptations.* (pp. 179–224). New York: Plenum Publishers.

Lambie, R.A., Leone, S.D., & Martin, C.K. (2002). Fostering resilience in children and youth. In J. Carlson & J. Lewis (Eds.), *Counseling the adolescent: Individual, family and school interventions.* (4th edition, pp. 87–119). Denver, CO: Love Publishing.

Liontos, L.B. (1991). *Involving the families of at-risk youth in the educational process.* (ERIC Document Reproduction Service No. ED 328 946).

McPartland, J.M., & Slavin, R.E. (1990). *Policy perspectives: Increasing achievement of at-risk students at each grade level.* Washington, DC: U.S. Department of Education.

McWhirter, J.J., McWhirter, B.T., McWhirter, A.M., & McWhirter, E.H. (1998). *At risk youth: A comprehensive response* (2nd ed.). Pacific Grove, CA: Brooks/Cole.

Melendez, M.C. (1991). *The social experiences of African American football players on an Eastern university campus: A qualitative approach.* Unpublished manuscript, Boston University.

Melendez, M.C. (2001/2002). *Contributions of gender, ethnic status, athletic participation, and athletic identity to college adjustment.* (Doctoral dissertation, Michigan State University, 2001). Dissertation Abstracts International, 62 (12-B), 5973.

North Central Regional Educational Laboratory (NCREL)(1994). *Resilience research: How can it help city schools?* Retrieved on January 23, 2003 from http://www.ncrel.org/sdrs/cityschl/city1_1b/htm

Pallas, A.M., Natriello, G., & McDill, E.L. (1989). The changing nature of a disadvantaged population: Current dimensions and future trends. *Educational Researcher*, 18, 16–22.

Parham, W.D. (1993). The intercollegiate athlete: A 1990's profile. *The Counseling Psychologist*, 21, 411–429.

Rak, C., & Patterson, L.E. (1996). Resiliency in children. *Journal of Counseling and Development*, 74, 368–373.

Rutter, M. (1985). Resilience in the face of adversity: Protective factors and resistance to psychiatric disorders. *British Journal of Psychiatry*, 147, 598–611.

Resiliency in children (2002). Retrieved January 30, 2003, from http://www.stolaf.edu/depts/cis/wp/millersa/resiliencyinchildren.html

Sinclair, R.L., & Ghory, W.J. (1987). *Marginal students: A primary concern for school renewel.* Berkeley, CA: McCutchan.

Slavin, R., & Madden, N. (1989). What works for students at risk: A research synthesis. *Educational Leadership*, 48, 71–82.

Smith, R.E., & Smoll, F.L. (1996). Psychosocial interventions in youth sport. In J.L. Van Raalte, & B.W. Brewer (Eds.), *Exploring sport and exercise psychology* (pp. 205–225). Washington, DC: American Psychological Association.

Steinhauer, P.D. (1996). *Methods for developing resiliency in children from disadvantaged populations.* Retrieved January 30, 2003, from http://www.sparrowlake.org/docs/resil.htm

Taylor, D.L. (1995). A comparison of college athletic participants and non-participants on self-esteem. *Journal of College Student Development*, 35, 444–451.

Thompson, R.A. (2002). *School counseling: Best practices for working in the schools* (2nd ed.). New York: Brunner-Routledge.

U.S. Department of Education. (1998). *Turning around low-performing schools. A guide for state and local leaders*. Washington: DC: Author.

Wang, M.C., & Haertel, G.D. (1995). Educational resilience. In M.C. Wang, M.C. Reynolds, & H.J. Walberg (Eds.), *Handbook of special education and remedial education: Research and practice* (2nd ed., pp. 159–200).

Wang, M.C., Heartel, G.D., & Walberg, H.J. (1994). Educational resilience inner cities. In M.C. Wang & E.W. Gordon (Eds.), *Educational resilience in inner city America: Challenges and prospects* (pp. 45–72). Hillsdale, NJ: Lawrence Erlbaum.

Werner, E.E. (1984). Resilient children. *Young Children*, 40, 68–72.

Werner, E.E. (1990). Protective factors and individual resilience. In S.J. Miesels & J.P. Shonkoff (Eds.), *Handbook of Early Childhood Intervention*, (pp. 97–116). Cambridge: Cambridge University Press.

Wolin, S., & Wolin, S. (1993). *The resilient self: How survivors of troubled families rise above adversity*. New York: Villard.

Winfield, L.F. (1994). *Developing resilience in urban youth*. Retrieved January 13, 2003 from http://ericeece.org/pubs/books/resguide/winfield2.html

Chapter 21

Enhancing Student Resilience through Innovative Partnerships

JENNIFER AXELROD, ROBERT BURKE, JOANNE CASHMAN,
STEVEN EVANS, JAMES KOLLER, EDWIN MORRIS, CARL
PATERNITE, KAY RIETZ, AND MARK WEIST

The urgent need for reforms in the provision of child and adolescent mental health services was recently highlighted in the president's New Freedom Commission on Mental Health Report, released in 2003. This report delineates the fragmented, frequently stigmatized, and under-resourced nature of mental health service provision in the United States; in addition, it lays the foundation for innovative models of prevention and intervention to promote healthy outcomes for youth. Like the Surgeon General's document that preceded this commission's report, the roles of school-based personnel as major sources of support for students were emphasized; further, the need to create innovative models and to improve the translation of science into practice was clearly articulated. The report illuminates the impact of mental health on children's academic, health, and life success: "While schools are primarily concerned with education, mental health is essential to learning as well as to social and emotional development. Because of this important interplay between emotional health and school success, schools must be partners in the mental health care of our children" (President's New Freedom Commission on Mental Health, 2003, p. 58).

Furthermore, research has highlighted the protective role that schools may play in the lives of children. As nurturing, caring learning communities, schools play a critical role as a source of support for youth and frequently have been cited in the resiliency literature as a critical element (Henderson, Benard, Sharp-Light, 2000). Healthy schools have the ability to provide for at-risk youth the majority of the factors that have been linked to resiliency: 1) caring, supportive relationships with adults, 2) challenging environments with high expectations, and 3) opportunities for active involvement in learning and in impacting the environment that surrounds them. The question then becomes one of how to translate this ambitious agenda of creating healthy, positive schools into a pragmatic reality in the lives of all children. The importance of school-based mental health programs (Adelman & Taylor, 2000) has been bolstered by three recent trends; first, the widening gap between children's mental health needs and the availability of relevant services; second, the heightened national emphasis on the twin aims of promoting mental wellness and preventing mental illness; and third, the growing recognition that emotional and behavioral problems often act as significant barriers to learning.

In an effort to enhance educational success while simultaneously promoting the health and well-being of students, schools and the people who work in them have been the focus of considerable attention by researchers, program developers, and policymakers. Teachers and other school personnel are increasingly viewed as essential partners in school-based mental health services. Due to their daily roles in the lives of students, teachers are uniquely positioned to influence their mental health and school success. However, their potential contributions are often undermined because teachers are undervalued as collaborators, appear unaware of their invaluable roles, and lack relevant training and skills related to children's social and emotional health (Paternite & Johnston, in press). Additionally, there are the well-documented difficulties of collaborating with school and school staff including limited resources and time, competing agendas, and a failure on the part of those who seek to work with schools to be grounded in the ecology of the school environment (Elias, Zins, Graczyk, & Weissberg, 2003).

In addition, the research literature documents that although numerous prevention and treatment programs related to children's mental health demonstrate efficacy in clinical settings, they are rarely implemented effectively in the schools. Specifically, the disconnect between science and practice occurs when research-based projects fail to be adequately translated into the school setting, resulting in diminished outcomes. This "science-practice gap" has garnered considerable attention and prompted controversy in recent years. Although sustained attention and effort have been directed at transporting evidence-based practices to provider settings, numerous problems have been reported in this process including the drift away from manualized procedures (Henggeler, Schoenwald, Liao, Letourneau & Edwards, 2002), and systemic issues in schools that create barriers to effective implementation and integration of the practice (Elias, Zins, Gracyk & Weissberg, 2003). In addition, schools are highly fluid human and political environments often characterized by changes in students, staff and initiatives; this fluidity and the accompanying general lack of hospitable infrastructures for school mental health create daunting barriers to the transport of effective practices into schools.

School-based mental health initiatives that aspire to include teachers, counselors, and administrators face similar challenges. Educators have limited time and resources. Also, local communities and their surrounding public schools have historically prioritized teaching and learning of the mandated academic curriculum over the social and emotional dimensions of schooling. Nevertheless, teachers are frequently asked to try a new program or intervention that taxes their time, demonstrates minimal or no impact, and within two to three years is never mentioned again. The complexity of working within a school system is often further strained by the attitudes and opinions of those individuals and organizations that attempt to improve the health and well-being of students, but do so without adequately understanding the school climate or assessing the existing resources. One typical scenario that transpires when "outside experts" enter a school system is that they tend to approach school staff with the agenda that they will "teach" the teachers how to do a better job with certain children. This approach frequently appears arrogant and naïve to teachers, and there is some validity to this perception. First, teachers spend more time with children (including problematic children), which provides educators with valuable information and judgment that should not be minimized. Second, one of the main tenets of evidence-based treatment [the careful assessment of presenting problems prior to implementing treatment] is frequently ignored. Instead, spending time in schools working with teachers as well as learning the culture, obstacles, language, social norms, and strengths and weaknesses are important prerequisites to both claiming expertise and establishing collaborative relationships.

TOWARDS EFFECTIVE COLLABORATION

Increasingly, researchers, policymakers, educators, human service personnel and families recognize that both academic and non-academic barriers threaten students' school achievement and fulfilling community participation. For these reasons, policies in education, and in health and human services have encouraged cooperation, collaboration, cost sharing and, in some cases, consolidation of services (Cashman, 2003a; 2003b). However, in reality, efforts to assist youth are often characterized by multiple staff from different agencies working in an uncoordinated and/or duplicative fashion (Annie E. Casey Foundation, 2003). Though child agency staff often serve the same consumer, the efficacy of their efforts is typically reduced due to ill- defined agency roles and responsibilities as well as sketchy cross-agency integration. This issue is particularly salient in public schools, where "no agency or system is clearly responsible or accountable for young people with serious emotional disturbances. They are invariably involved with more than one specialized service system, including mental health, special education, child welfare, juvenile justice, substance abuse, and health" (President's New Freedom Commission on Mental Health, 2003, p. 58).

With greater frequency, common goals and shared work are being recognized as pathways to achieving positive outcomes for children, youth and families. In the following sections, descriptions of illustrative local and state initiatives reflecting the complexity of developing partnerships to enhance resiliency and positive outcomes for youth are provided.

Community of Practice as a Mechanism for Change

While dialogue and sharing of information between individuals and organizations are essential elements in crafting new approaches to collaboration, they are insufficient for stimulating the kinds of new models necessary for educational reform geared towards promoting a shared agenda for youth and schools. To achieve such innovative partnerships, agencies and organizations are looking to external domains for effective models of engaged learning and collaboration. A "community of practice" is an example of a business model being translated into the educational/mental health communities. Within communities of practice, groups of people who share a concern, a set of problems, or a passion about a topic recognize that they can deepen their understanding by interacting on a regular basis (Wenger, McDermott, & Snyder, 2002). More precisely, communities of practice are formed around a common set of perplexing issues which, through analytical dialogue and critical reflection, are transformed via novel solutions. These communities are composed of diverse individuals who are united by an intense desire to generate change (Wesley & Buysse, 2001). While the concept of communities of practice is not new (i.e., all individuals participate in groups that have meaning) utilization of the model to support, for example, resilient schools and communities, is a novel approach to systems change within the education and mental health fields.

In an environment where needs exceed resources; where issues are complex and interrelated; and where important work is distributed across personnel in many fields, communities of practice hold real promise. Wenger, Mc Dermott and Snyder (2002) suggest that cultivating communities of practice is a practical way to manage knowledge as an asset, in parallel fashion to the way that other assets are managed. Furthermore, through engagement with communities of practice, individuals become "co-constructors of knowledge and [create] a mechanism for shared inquiry, and learning as a means of improving practice" (Wesley & Buysse, 2001, p. 120). In this model, the distinction between novice and expert (or researcher and practitioner) is broken down, with the knowledge translation process viewed as bi-directional (Buysee, Sparkman, & Wesley, 2003). Some communities are transactional in nature. They focus on sharing to improve practice among individuals in like roles or engaging in like work. Other communities are more transformational and are expressly formed for the purpose of transforming systems that provide services (Cashman, 2003a; Cashman 2003b). Both kinds of communities can and should be encouraged at local, state, and/or national levels for the purpose of promoting innovative thinking and generating new partnerships. Examples of communities of practice, including initial outcomes of efforts to promote children's education, health and well-being, are given in the following sections.

A Local Model of Collaboration as an Example of a Community of Practice

The Challenging Horizons Program (CHP) is a school-based treatment program for middle school youth with attention-deficit/hyperactivity disorder (AD/HD). Initial attempts to implement the CHP relied upon university graduate and undergraduate students to staff an after-school model of the program. However, after-school programs are labor intensive and relatively expensive; thus, they may be beyond the reach for many middle schools. Therefore, the initial strategy was to develop, refine, and evaluate the interventions, using an after-school model only until the data suggested that the program was effective and user-friendly.

To promote the use of the program in public middle school settings, a process involving the use of Community Development Teams was established (Evans et al., 2003). The team membership included local educators, administrators, parents, mental health counselors, and physicians. Their purpose was to work with the investigators in revising the CHP after-school treatment manual for use in an integrated model, in which teachers, school counselors, and administrators implemented the CHP interventions during the school day.

The Community Development Team met monthly with CHP leaders over a one-year period of time. They reviewed the treatment manual and listened to presentations describing AD/HD and the specific interventions in CHP. A website established for members of the Community Development Team included a discussion board and places to post documents. During the year, project leaders worked with the team to revise the manual, incorporating their suggestions regarding practical and feasible use by educators. Project leaders wrote drafts and modified procedures, subsequently posting them on the web page for review. Feedback from the team came via messages on the discussion board and during the meetings. An attempt was made to balance the feedback regarding feasibility with the need to keep the salient characteristics of the treatment procedures intact. The result was a manual that a team of educators and other community stakeholders believed was effective and practical.

Members of the Community Development Team were asked to provide written feedback and videotaped testimonials about the process and resulting product. This information was incorporated into the training sessions and training materials used with the participating schools. While the initial training occurred in workshops shortly before the start of a new school year, the majority of the training support occurred on a continuous basis through a school consultant. The school consultant was a research funded position filled by a school psychologist with experience working in the after-school model of the CHP. This person spent between 75 and 90 percent of his time at the schools implementing the program. His role was not to directly provide the interventions, but to work with teachers to help them implement the procedures. Providing this type of support was seen as essential by the Community Development Team to increase the likelihood of adherence to treatment procedures.

Bringing evidence-based treatments to schools and evaluating their effectiveness and feasibility is critical, but this process is very labor intensive and involves many risks. Project leaders or research staff must be willing to relinquish some control over their procedures. Allowing people only token input is likely to be readily apparent and will rapidly compromise collaboration. Further, public schools have numerous other agendas. These agendas can compromise procedures and projects; nevertheless, developing and evaluating prevention and treatment procedures under real-world school conditions is essential since these are the settings in which they are intended to operate. This principle has been central to achieving generalization of treatment gains, but its adoption for the generalization or dissemination of prevention and treatment procedures has been slow.

Promoting Communities of Practice: State Level Initiatives

In an effort to address the fragmentation in the field at the state and national level and to promote a common framework for meeting the social, emotional, and academic needs of youth, the National Association of Mental Health Program Directors (NASMHPD) and the National Association of State Directors of Special Education (NASDSE), spearheaded a national discussion of shared work through the development of a concept paper, *Mental Health, Schools and Families Working Together: Toward a Shared Agenda.* This document was developed through the sustained interaction of researchers, policymakers, administrators, direct service providers and families in both the education and mental health fields with the goal of targeting state level policymakers and implementers, and national organizations encouraging state level dialogue and the development of state-specific strategies. The concept paper expressed ideas that were promoted by the organizations representing those individuals in positions of influence and authority over services in state child serving systems, bringing high level visibility to the report and its recommendations.

Translating Ideas into Action Initiatives

Realizing the need for concrete examples, NASMHPD and NASDSE offered small 'seed grants' to states to work on cross-agency and cross-stakeholder issues and act on the system recommendations articulated in the shared agenda (See Table 1). These grants were funded through the Policymaker Partnership, an investment by the Office of Special Education Programs (OSEP) dedicated to finding cross-stakeholder solutions to persistent problems in implementing The Individuals with Disabilities Education Act (IDEA). The Policymaker Partnership was one of four collaborations created under the IDEA Partnerships. The NASDSE/ NASMHPD initiative is an example of the innovative collaborations envisioned by OSEP in funding the Partnerships. OSEP recognized that implementers and consumers are more open to influence if the messages come from groups with which they are voluntarily affiliated. The Partnerships were born to explore that premise and apply the learnings to common issues and shared interests. In many ways, this investment was the foundation for discovering the power of 'communities of practice' as a technical assistance strategy that should be supported with public investments.

For NASDE and NASMHPD, the decision to shape their initiative around small grants was also a strategic consideration. The two organizations tested their assumption that states and stakeholders would come together because of the 'value added' for each, rather than because of funding provided. With this understanding, NASMHPD and NASDSE awarded grants to six states, Missouri, Ohio, Oregon, South Carolina, Texas, and Vermont. In 2002, these six states were awarded small grants to join education, mental health and family organizations in advancing mental health in the schools. System leaders within state agencies and family leaders were united in a shared effort to create new knowledge by sharing the work and creating new communication mechanisms that would build the infrastructure for sustained efforts.

Within states, the creation of networks and action teams was an essential first step. The realities of implementation had to be meaningfully addressed if the lessons learned were to transfer across sites, issues and groups. In these states, implementers and consumers honored the expertise that each brought to the effort, while forging opportunities for building new, shared knowledge. Agencies, organizations and consumers within the state moved beyond their personal and organizational agenda to shared interests. Interviews with participants across states consistently showed that stakeholders discovered their commonalities; and in that discovery, they forged powerful linkages (McLaughlin & Schuyler, 2003; Cashman, 2003a; 2003b). Networks and workgroups were transformed into 'communities' with the potential to transform practice. Policymakers, implementers and consumers recognized their new ability to work together to garner attention, stimulate dialogue, impact decisions and create new resources (Cashman, 2003a; 2003b).

The Policymaker Partnership promoted both within-state and cross-state learning communities of practice through the shared agenda with mental health and family organizations. The Partnership hypothesized that by bringing the stakeholders in the six states together routinely; they would discover commonalities across states and stakeholder groups. Furthermore, they posited that by inviting the national technical assistance providers and federal agency staff to interact with the states and follow their progress, they could leverage cross-system support for the communities approach to shared work. The Partnerships believed that through interaction, agencies, states and stakeholders would find meaning and develop outcome-oriented affilations that could be supported in cost effective ways.

The results over one year provided some important first insights into processes of community building within and across states. In routine communication among all states and stakeholders, federal officials and national technical assistance providers celebrated and reinforced the evolving work of the six states. Monthly, key leaders from education, mental health and family organizations from each of the states shared their progress. Gradually, they began to advise each other as they moved from technical assistance providers in both education and mental health joined the monthly calls and began to connect the work in the six states to other efforts conducted by federal investments with aligned purposes. In a short time, the community developed a 'high profile' and representatives were asked to present at national meetings. Back in the state, this national attention fueled interest in the state effort. The state leaders and stakeholders were consistently reinforced for dispositions and skills that undergird successful collaborations.

In evaluative interviews, participants articulated four factors associated with the success of the within-state and cross-state communities that included: 1) The attention of national professional organizations and federal agencies, 2) small seed grants to focus the effort, 3) committed participation of state leaders, implementers and consumers, and 4) community sponsorship by the Policymaker Partnership (Mc Laughlin & Schuyler, 2003; Cashman, 2003a; Cashman 2003b). At the conclusion of the first year, two states crafted legislative initiatives to better align their education and mental health systems, and three states stimulated state/community collaboration to address persistent challenges. One state engaged higher education institutions in developing the competencies required of early care workers and educators in meeting the needs of children with emotional disturbances. While these achievements are impressive, it is even more impressive to note that state teams report that the efforts are sustainable. By pursuing shared work that was largely accomplished through leveraging of existing resources and by adopting a community-building strategy that united stakeholders, states have created the visibility and support required to ensure that issues remain on the public agenda.

Missouri's Experience

Recognizing the unmet needs of youth in the State of Missouri, former Governor Carnahan identified children's health and school success as a top priority for his administration. In response, the strategic plan developed by the Missouri Department of Mental Health (DMH) identified two objectives related to improving a school-linked mental health agenda: (1) to formalize a System of Care (Stroul & Friedman, 1986) structure across the State, and (2) to address school-based

Table 1. The Logic and Design for Promoting a Shared Agenda

Tool	Rationale	Strategy
Develop a concept paper that outlines a shared agenda for schools agencies and families	Articulate shared goals, garner cross sector support; ground the work in the laws and regulation of each system; bridge policy research and practice	Engage policymakers, researchers, administrators, service providers, and family groups in education and mental health
National distribution and cross-stakeholder presentation at high profile meetings	Stimulate national dialogue; create national interest, invite likeminded organizations and technical assistance providers	Create links to existing networks that have allied purposes; build a critical mass of groups that share the understandings and voluntarily affiliate with one another
Develop small 'seed grants' to states that want to pursue a shared agenda	Provide concrete examples of the action rooted in the beliefs, ideas and recommendations articulated in the concept paper	Provide small allocations so that states and organizations would leverage existing resources; create a cross-stakeholder team that includes decision makers, practitioners and families that learn by doing; put a 'national spotlight' on the groundbreaking work
Grow communities of practice among individuals doing shared work	Build on the collective expertise of the stakeholders; demonstrate the 'value added' in cross stakeholder work; sustain cross-stakeholder efforts	Monthly conference calls; designated participation in meetings with report back to the community; invitations to present at high profile national meetings; sharing the lessons learned across states, national organizations and federal agencies; communicating with the broader network of allied groups

prevention efforts. Similarly, the Missouri Department of Elementary and Secondary Education (DESE) identified several objectives to increase student success, including (1) to increase the percentage of students achieving the Show-Me Standards at targeted performance levels in the Missouri Assessment Program, and (2) to decrease the state's annual dropout rate. From a national perspective, both the DMH and DESE objectives complement the concepts and approaches articulated in the document entitled *Mental Health, Schools and Families Working Together for All Children and Youth: A Shared Agenda* (2001).

As mentioned, during 2002–2003, Missouri became one of six states in the nation to receive a Shared Agenda seed grant from the Policy Maker Partnership (PMP). This funding provided the opportunity to engage interested stakeholders in a process of conducting multi-dimensional focus groups across different geographic regions statewide in order to better understand the needs and perspectives of families, school-based personnel and professionals across agencies, including general and special education, rehabilitation, social services and mental health. Under the direction of the Center for the Advancement of Mental Health Practices in the Schools, three sites were selected to "pilot" the focus group approach in order to ensure participation that reflected the diverse geography, demography, and school districts of Missouri. Stakeholders that participated in each "grass roots" local focus group included teachers, school administrators, local mental health agency staff, families and advocacy representatives.

The pilot focus group process led to the identification of local and state needs, barriers and specific recommendations for implementing the *Shared Agenda*. Regardless of participant affiliation, six common themes emerged as "barriers": (1) Communication and Collaboration, (2) Mental Health Stigma, (3) Lack of Training, (4) Family Respect and Support, (5) Support for Children, and (6) Support for Schools.

From these common themes, participants were explicitly asked for their recommendations to create a true shared agenda in the State of Missouri at both the state and local level. Five major recommendations were developed:

1. **Make mental health training a priority.** Although it is important to understand mental *illness*, the primary focus of training should be the promotion of mental *health* in *all* children and youth, focusing on prevention and wellness. Examples include: a) Provide pre-service and in-service competency-based training for teachers and others who work in schools (Mental health training must become a requirement for teacher certification at all levels); b) Provide crisis intervention training in all schools; c) Integrate mental health awareness training into the classroom curriculum; d) Provide parent training to "empower" parents whose children are affected by mental health problems; e) Provide mental health training to all new state legislators; f) Provide mental health training to all new school board members; g) Provide training on school structure and

practice to mental health personnel; and h) Provide training focused on the establishment of effective state agency collaborations across systems.

2. **Make the prevention of mental illness a priority by:** a) Including mental health promotion in the K-12 health curriculum for all children and youth; b) Increasing resources for early identification of at-risk children; and c) Providing mental health information and support for early childhood educators.

3. **Empower and support families at all levels by:** a) Promoting increased family involvement in policy groups and decision making at the state level; b) Providing additional funding for parents to attend conferences, workshops, and policy meetings; c) Emphasizing parent and family respect in schools and mental health agencies; and d) Ensuring that all schools have information on parent advocacy and support groups (e.g., National Alliance for the Mentally Ill, Missouri Statewide Parent Advisory Network, Missouri Parents Act) to disseminate to families in need.

4. **Create a statewide system of care network for the implementation of a shared agenda process by:** a) Utilizing state and regional System of Care teams as coordinating bodies; b) Creating School-based System of Care teams within each district; c) Establishing mental health information and support funnels from the state level through regional levels, down to local levels; d) Creating a "blueprint" for a shared agenda at the state level (with regional and local input) and disseminate to all School-based System of Care teams; e) Using the System of Care network to create a statewide protocol for services with the goal of improving accessibility to and consistency of mental health services across Missouri; and f) Create a database of mental health services available in each region that can be accessed by any school or child-serving agency.

5. **Develop a statewide campaign to promote mental health awareness and reduce the stigma of mental illness by:** a) Creating public service ads for television and radio; and b) Creating collaborative panels composed of family members, mental health professionals and school professionals to make presentations on mental health issues at a variety of venues across the state.

As Missouri's effort becomes systemic across all fronts, it is clear that teacher and other school-based state accrediting agencies, as well as national organizations (e.g., National Council for Accreditation of Teacher Education [NCATE] and Interstate New Teacher Assessment and Support Consortium [INTASC]) must provide the leadership in requiring competency-based training in the areas of mental health prevention for all school personnel. As a result, public schools that mandate professional training in mental health and that work proactively to reduce the stigma of mental illness will have opportunities to create safe and stimulating environments, thereby fostering the acquisition of resiliency skills in youth.

Ohio's Experience

Ohio has been nationally recognized for leadership in working to build and expand collaboration across education, mental health and family serving organizations in developing a shared agenda for children's mental health and school success. Similar to Missouri, Ohio was awarded a grant in October, 2002 from the Policymaker Partnership. In Ohio the policymaking leadership of education, mental health and family serving organizations is engaging with state and local partners to generate a commitment to address non-cognitive barriers to learning to support successful academic achievement for all children and youth.

In 2001 the Ohio Department of Mental Health, in partnership with the Ohio State University Center for Learning Excellence (CLEX), and with participation of the governor's office and the Ohio Department of Education (ODE), convened a hearing that served as a "call to action" for Ohioans to improve mental health and school success for all children. The resulting hearing summary and resource guide, and a more recent follow-up publication, have been disseminated widely throughout the state (Ohio Department of Mental Health [ODMH], 2001, 2003). Concurrent with the 2001 hearing, the Ohio Mental Health Network for School Success was formed, consisting of action networks spearheaded by affiliate organizations in six regions of the state. Currently, the Network is funded jointly by ODMH and ODE, and is co-lead by CLEX and the Center for School-Based Mental Health Programs at Miami University. The mission of the Network is to help Ohio's school districts, community-based agencies, and families work together to achieve improved educational and mental health outcomes for all children. The current Network action agenda is available for review at http://www.units.muohio.edu/csbmhp/network.html and http://altedmh.osu.edu/omhn/omhn.htm.

Ohio's shared agenda initiative, funded in part by the NASMHPD/PMP grant, is being implemented within the collaborative infrastructure of the Network. The three phases of the grant implementation thus far have included: 1) a statewide forum (March 3rd, 2003) for leaders of mental health, education, and family policymaking organizations and entities; 2) six regional forums (April-May, 2003) for policy implementers and consumer stakeholders; and 3) a legislative forum (October 9th, 2003) involving key leadership of relevant house and senate committees. The Appreciative Inquiry model for promotion of systems-level change and transformation informed the process for the forums (Cooperrider & Whitney, 1999).

Phase I was completed with a Policymakers' Forum in the State capital (Columbus) on March 3, 2003. One hundred and twenty five policymakers attended the forum, including representatives from education, families, mental health and other child-serving systems and advocacy organizations. National experts in school-based mental health offered national policy perspectives in keynote speeches. In addition, promising work in Ohio was showcased. Facilitated discussion during the forum was structured to create a collective vision among all stakeholders, build a sense of mutual responsibility for reaching the vision, and instill hope that systemic change is possible.

In Phase II, following the state-wide forum, six regional forums highlighted a variety of themes related to advancing a shared agenda. Across the six regional forums various features included cross-stakeholder panel discussions, youth and parent testimony, showcasing of promising work in Ohio, and facilitated discussion structured to promote collaboration and problem-solving regarding implementation issues. Approximately 725 stakeholders participated in the Phase 1 and Phase II forums. The evaluation data were quite positive, reflecting a strong sense that processes of the initiative assist with the development of more effective collaboration. Several recommendations were derived from the facilitated discussion of the forums, which provided the framework for the fall, 2003 Legislative Forum. These recommendations included the following:

1. **A statewide effort should be undertaken in Ohio to disseminate knowledge about links between mental health and school success and the importance of School-Based Mental Health (SBMH) services by:** a) Reducing stigma for children in Ohio who need mental health services; b) Promoting a better understanding of children's mental health needs, the risks of suicide, and mental health barriers to learning; c) Educating school personnel in Ohio (board members, administrators, teachers, and other staff) about the impact of children's mental health concerns on academic performance and school success; and d) Educating the public in Ohio about the need for SBMH services.

2. **The educational and mental health systems in Ohio must challenge existing ideas and practices of "traditional" education and mental health services by:** a) Identifying and serving children in Ohio with mental health needs early, not late, and considering school-based screening for behavioral disorders; b) Providing better training for educators, mental health providers, and families, emphasizing mental health and school success; c) Improving availability of and access to SBMH services for all children in Ohio who need care; d) Improving quality and community-relevance of mental health efforts in Ohio's schools; e) Encouraging schools to incorporate awareness of mental health in the local health education curriculum for all children (K-12th grade); f) Identifying funding and policy barriers that interfere with children's mental health service delivery and with mental health—education collaboration; and g) Increasing collaboration between education, mental health, and alcohol and drug prevention/treatment at the state and local levels.

3. **Educators, mental health professionals and families in Ohio should work together to shape and implement policies and practices that comprehensively address children's well-being by:** a) Increasing family involvement in school mental health and educational programs in Ohio, including policy making on the state and regional levels; b) Empowering and supporting parents to be involved, in partnership with the schools and mental health providers, in promoting the mental health and school success of their children; c) Actively encouraging parent involvement in advocacy and support groups; d) Actively soliciting and appreciating student input in program planning; and e) Improving collaboration between SBMH services and community-based services in Ohio.

Following the regional meetings, Phase III of the initiative was a Legislative Forum in which a panel of 16 key legislators in Ohio was convened. Presentations to the forum were made by national, state and local leaders as well as students and families. The recommendations reviewed above were presented to the legislators. At the time of this writing, findings and recommendations derived from the Legislative Forum were being developed into an action plan. An important immediate goal has been to raise public awareness and build advocacy for fiscal and policy support and practices in order to better align education and mental health in the next biennial budget process.

CONCLUSION

Communities of practice that bring together local, state, and national agendas to improve the health and well-being of children and youth have the potential to create long-term systematic change. This change process focuses on collaboration and partnership in meaningful ways and goes beyond the traditional literatures on collaboration to illustrate the impact of new models of partnering of systems of care. Through these partnerships, supportive structures needed to promote resiliency in youth via empowering individuals to work together in meaningful ways have been created. Traditionally, schools have not been very attentive to promoting resiliency or being resilient; however the concepts of resiliency have been argued as being the core of schooling. This chapter argues that schools can become more resilience-engendering communities through the use of communities of practice models for professional development and knowledge enhancement. The implications of communities of practice for school-community partnerships and other systematic change processes are illustrated in the three examples provided in the chapter.

- At the local community level, the Challenging Horizons Program and the corollary Community Development Team were created in order to build classroom, school, family, and community support for middle school students with Attention-Deficit/Hyperactivity Disorder [AD/HD]; in addition, the CHP incorporated a research component examining the effectiveness and feasibility of the treatment approach.

- At the national level, the Policymaker Partnership [PMP] led a collaborative effort that resulted in a document entitled *Mental Health, Schools and Families Working Together: Toward a Shared Agenda*. This document provided the conceptual foundation for a series of collaborative conversations and actions simultaneously occurring at state and national levels. An important theme that emerged from these initiatives was consensus that the "Community of Practice" model holds great promise for future work in this area.

- As recipients of grants from the PMP, the states of Missouri and Ohio designed and implemented integrative activities and programs whose outcomes would best meet their unique needs and circumstances. While informative details of their state-level plans are provided, the differences between them highlight the importance of creating programs responsive to the issues and needs present in the local communities which collectively constitute each state.

In light of the well-documented contemporary crisis in child and adolescent mental health explained here the need for innovative, cross-disciplinary approaches to addressing and ameliorating these concerns is now recognized by steadily increasing numbers of individuals and stakeholder groups at the local, state, and national levels. However, the field has moved beyond mere recognition and surface attempts at collaboration to a deeper understanding of the intensive work and long-term commitment that promoting resiliency and healthy outcomes for children and youth entails. Furthermore, communities of practice ensure that the needs of the targeted community are being addressed rather than a one-size-fits-all approach to programmatic change. Too often, mandates or extant practice are the critical determents of the programming; however, embedding these collaborative efforts in the communities responsible for long-term sustainability greatly enhances both the feasibility of the design as well as the buy-in (both financially and emotionally) to persevere with the initiatives. Presented here are exemplars of promising, innovative policy and programmatic initiatives that have demonstrated potential to affect positive change in the lives of our children and youth as well as the people who care for them.

REFERENCES

Adelman, H.S., & Taylor, L. (2000). Promoting mental health in schools in the midst of school reform. *Journal of School Health, 70*, 171–178.

Annie E. Casey Foundation, (2003). The unsolved challenge of system reform: The condition of the frontline human service workforce. Available online: www.aecf.org

Buysee, V., Sparkman, K., & Wesley, P. (2003). Communities of practice: Connecting what we know with what we do. *Council for Exception Children, 69(3),* 263–277.

Cashman, J. (2003a, Spring). Special education and school-based mental health: Bringing shared meaning to implementation. *On the Move, The Newsletter of The Center for School Mental Health Assistance, 7.*

Cashman, J. (2003b, July). *Communities of practice: The human side of implementation.* Presentation at the Office of Special Education Programs, National Monitoring Academies Baltimore, Maryland and Salt Lake City, Utah.

Cooperrider, D.L. & Whitney, D. (1999). *Appreciative inquiry.* San Francisco: Berrett-Koehler.

Elias, M., Zins., J., Graczyk, P., & Weissberg, R. (2003). Implementation, sustainability, and scaling up of social-emotional and academic innovations in public schools. *School Psychology Review, 32,* 303–319.

Evans, S.W., Serpell, Z., Williams, A., Gearing, F., Swensson, K., & Ingram, R. (2003, June). *Using community development teams to transport science to practice.* Poster presented at ISRCAP: 11th Scientific Meeting, Sydney, Australia.

Henderson, N., Bernard, B., & Sharp-Light, N. (2000). *Mentoring for resiliency.* Rio Rancho, NM: Resiliency in Action.

Henggeler, S.W., Schoenwald, S.K., Liao, J.G., Letourneau, E.J., & Edwards, D.L. (2002). Transporting efficacious treatments to field settings: The link between supervisory practices and therapist fidelity in MST programs. *Journal of Clinical Child and Adolescent Psychology, 31,* 155–167.

Mc Laughlin, J., & Schuyler, J. (2003). *An evaluation of Communities of Practice funded by The Policymaker Partnership.* Unpublished Document.

Ohio Department of Mental Health (2001). *Mental health & school success: Hearing summary & resource guide.* Columbus, OH: Author.

Ohio Department of Mental Health (2003). *Mental health & school success: What we are learning.* Columbus, OH: Author.

President's New Freedom Commission on Mental Health (2003). *Achieving the promise: Transforming mental health care in America.* Final Report for the President's New Freedom Commission on Mental Health (SMA Publication No. 03-3832). Rockville, MD: Author.

Stroul, B.A., & Friedman, R.M. (1986). *A system of care for severely emotionally disturbed children and youth.* Washington, D.C.: Georgetown University, Child Development Center.

Wenger, E., McDermott, R., & Snyder, W. (2002). Cultivating communities of practice: A guide to managing knowledge. Boston, MA: Harvard Business School Press.

Wesley, P., & Buysse, V. (2001). Communities of practice: Expanding professional roles to promote reflection and shared inquiry. *Topics in Early Childhood Special Education, 21,* 114–123.

Chapter 22

Resilience-Building Prevention Programs that Work
A Federal Perspective

CHARLES G. CURIE, PAUL J. BROUNSTEIN, AND NANCY J. DAVIS

Attempts to promote mental health, to foster resilience, and to prevent mental, behavioral, and substance use disorders probably have been made throughout human history. In the last few decades, these attempts have become more formalized into specific programs, with an increasing emphasis on the need for these programs to be based on sound scientific principles and rigorously evaluated. Noted Dutch researcher, Dr. Clemens Hosman, describes the early days of the current activities, which are generally referred to as "promotion and prevention," as follows:

> During the optimistic 1970s, . . . we invented program after program with a minimal scientific opinion and unhindered by a knowledge of epidemiology because that knowledge was not available. . . . No one asked us for evidence on the outcomes of our investments; at that time, there was no realistic understanding of all the investments in personnel and money and all the research effort that is needed to establish significant and evidence-based reductions in mental health problems in local communities (Hosman, 2002, p. 33).

Times clearly have changed. In the 1980s, the field known as prevention science, an interdisciplinary science that includes epidemiology, developmental psychology, sociology, and clinical and community psychology, began to emerge, and with it, considerable scientific rigor was introduced. Scientific rigor has come about, in part, because researchers have developed better techniques for measuring the effects of their programs and because government and private funding agencies have begun to require that grantees use programs and approaches that have passed stringent efficacy and effectiveness trials. These factors have dramatically increased community awareness of such evidence-based interventions and interest in implementing them. Many reports have documented the efficacy of prevention programs for both preventing mental and substance use disorders and promoting positive functioning and resilience (Mrazek & Haggerty, 1994).

Although many other Federal agencies and departments are actively involved in promotion and prevention, the Substance Abuse and Mental Health Services Administration (SAMHSA) has primary responsibility for promoting mental health and preventing mental, behavioral, and substance use disorders. Within SAMHSA, promotion and prevention programs are housed primarily in the Center for Mental Health Services (CMHS) and in the Center for Substance Abuse Prevention (CSAP). The third component of SAMHSA, the Center for Substance Abuse Treatment (CSAT), is actively involved in preventing comorbidity of mental and substance use disorders through both the treatment of substance abuse problems and the prevention of relapse into substance use disorders. SAMHSA's framework for preventing mental and behavioral disorders and for increasing resilience in children, families, and communities is based on the public health model. This framework puts a strong emphasis on promoting resilience by reducing risk factors and increasing protective factors (Curie, 2003).

THE PUBLIC HEALTH APPROACH AND THE ISSUE OF RISK AND PROTECTION

Successful promotion and prevention programs take a public health approach. This approach consists of at least four core elements:

1. *Conducting surveillance* by determining the major problems to be targeted, the risk and protective factors associated with those problems, and the readiness of the community to implement an evidence-based program;
2. *Selecting and implementing the appropriate evidence-based program*;
3. *Monitoring and evaluating* both the process and outcomes of the program to ensure its proper implementation and to determine its effectiveness in the given community; and
4. *Educating professionals and the general public* about the importance of prevention and ways to implement it effectively.

At this point in the development of prevention science, decreasing risk factors and increasing protective factors are at the heart of promotion and prevention interventions based on the public health model. In the words of Olds and his colleagues (1999), the "most useful investigations have focused on risk and protective factors that, *at a group level*, can be traced developmentally to predict adaptive and maladaptive functioning" (p. 4). One cannot assume, however, that decreasing risk factors or increasing protective factors, or both, will *inevitably* lead to improved mental health *for a given individual*. The myriad factors involved in the development of any single human being, and the resources available to him or her at any given time, are too great to predict outcomes with any degree of certainty, especially when the individual is young.

SPANNING THE GREAT DIVIDE

A number of highly influential publications—for example, *Reducing Risks for Mental Disorders* (Mrazek & Haggerty, 1994), the *Global Burden of Diseases* (Murray & Lopez, 1996), and the *Diagnostic and Statistical Manual of Mental Disorders—Fourth Edition* (American Psychiatric Association, 1994)—include substance use disorders under the broader category of mental illnesses. But, beginning in the 1930s, for a multitude of reasons beyond the scope of this chapter, training programs and treatment facilities were developed for people with such mental illnesses as depressive disorders, anxiety disorders, and schizophrenia separately from those for people with alcohol and other substance use disorders. The attempt to dichotomize the understanding and treatment of these disorders has been truly devastating. Only in the last decade have significant steps been taken to develop programs for people with co-occurring disorders, to train substance abuse counselors about broader aspects of mental health, and to train mental health professionals about the interaction between alcohol and other drugs and psychiatric symptoms (Substance Abuse and Mental Health Services Administration [SAMHSA], 2002b).

Unfortunately, the great divide has been perpetuated in the prevention field. Beginning in the 1980s, the Federal Government and other funding agencies targeted substance abuse as the priority problem for prevention, rather than conditions such as depression or anxiety. In response, prevention researchers developed substance abuse prevention programs and evaluated and reported outcomes primarily for substance abuse. Because *early* substance abuse prevention programs were directed primarily at adolescents (ages 14–18), researchers tended to target risk factors that occur in that developmental stage. Similarly, policymakers focused on this age group. The 1992 Congressional language instructing SAMHSA/CSAP to develop substance abuse programs for high-risk youth lists 10 risk factors. A person at high risk, it said, is one who

1. is identified as a child of a substance abuser;
2. is a victim of physical, sexual, or psychological abuse;
3. is economically disadvantaged;
4. has dropped out of school;

5. has become pregnant;
6. has committed a violent or delinquent act;
7. has experienced mental health problems;
8. has attempted suicide;
9. has experienced long-term physical pain due to injury; and
10. has experienced chronic failure in school (United States Statutes at Large, 1992).

Although the first three factors may be present from birth, the other seven usually occur during late childhood or adolescence. Researchers who have focused mainly on mental health promotion and disorder prevention have argued that interventions need to target the earlier risk factors (Greenberg, Domitrovich, & Bumbarger,1999; Webster-Stratton & Taylor, 2001). Doing so, they say, will build resilience, will reduce risks, and will increase protective factors for both mental and substance use disorders because

• Conduct problems predict the initiation of alcohol use as well as greater escalations of alcohol use over time (Costello, Erklani, & Federman, 1999; Hussong, Curran, & Chassin, 1998).
• First-graders with the combination of hyperactivity and social problem-solving deficits have been found to have a greatly increased rate of drug and alcohol use when they are between 11 and 12 years old (Kaplow, Curran, Dodge, & The Conduct Problems Prevention Group, 2002).
• First-grade children with conduct problems, anxiety or depression, or Attention Deficit Hyperactivity Disorder (ADHD) have approximately twice the risk of first tobacco use during grades 4–7 of children without these early emotional disorders (McMahon, Collins, Doyle, & The Conduct Problems Prevention Group, 2002).
• Social impairment in childhood is a critical predictor for later substance use disorders (Greene et al., 1999).
• Children who lack prosocial behavior skills are likely to be rejected by their peers and to gravitate toward other rejected children. These deviant peer groups, in turn, promote substance abuse and involvement in antisocial activities (Keenan, Loeber, Zhang, Stouthamer-Loeber, & Van Kammen, 1995).

It should be noted that some risk factors are unique to substance abuse, such as misinformation on the normative rate of use of alcohol and other drugs. To address this concern, many adolescent substance abuse prevention programs provide information on normative behavior; that is, for example, most teens don't binge drink. This information, combined with effective cognitive, social, and emotional skills training, greatly strengthens the programs.

WHAT IS A "*RESILIENCE*-BUILDING PREVENTION PROGRAM"?

The title of this chapter raises the definitional dilemma that plagues the constructs of mental health promotion, substance abuse and mental illness prevention, and resilience. Not only is each construct multifaceted, the overlap among them is substantial. For the 1994 IOM report, *Reducing Risks for Mental Disorders,* the IOM Committee decided not to include *mental health promotion* because

> health promotion is not driven by an emphasis on illness, but rather by a focus on the enhancement of well-being. It is provided to individuals, groups, or large populations to enhance competence, self-esteem, and a sense of well-being rather than to intervene to prevent psychological or social problems or mental disorders (Mrazek & Haggerty, 1994, p. 27).

In marked contrast, the Australian Mental Health Initiative actually includes prevention in its definition of mental health promotion:

> Mental health promotion needs to be seen in two contexts: promoting positive mental health and preventing the development of mental health problems and disorders. These two contexts are inextricably linked... to the extent that initiatives aiming to promote positive mental health will also impact upon the prevention of mental health problems and disorders. Similarly, initiatives aiming to prevent mental health problems and disorders will also impact upon promoting positive mental health (Scanlon, Williams, & Raphael, 1997, p. 7).

Historically, the term *primary prevention* has referred to prevention before the onset of a disorder; *secondary prevention* has referred to early identification and treatment of a disorder; and *tertiary prevention* has referred to the prevention of disability from or relapse of a disorder. More recently, the IOM Committee recommended using "prevention" to refer only to those interventions that occur *before the initial onset* of a disorder (Mrazek & Haggerty, 1994, p. v), and many researchers follow this definition. The National Institute of Mental Health Ad Hoc Committee on Prevention endorsed a broader definition: "Prevention refers not only to interventions that occur before the initial onset of a disorder, but also to interventions that prevent comorbidity, relapse, disability, and the consequences of severe mental illness [or substance abuse] for families" (National Institute of Mental Health, 1998). In short, considerable controversy continues to surround the definition of this term. Interestingly, while the term *substance abuse prevention* refers to prevention of *initial onset* of substance use, a study of more than 10,000 youth (ages 10–17) in 48 programs found that the greatest impact of prevention activities was with youth who had already initiated use. The programs were extremely effective in preventing these young people from proceeding to problem use or dependence (Sambrano, Springer, Sale, Kasim, & Hermann, 2002).

The operating definition of resilience for this chapter is that it is the *interaction between individual traits and environmental resources* that promotes resilience and healthy development. Most developers of prevention programs do not describe their programs as "programs to foster resilience." One who does, however, is Dr. Karol Kumpfer, the developer of the *Family Strengthening Program* (Kumpfer, Alvarado, Smith, & Bellamy, 2002). Kumpfer clarifies the resilience and prevention issue as follows:

> Luckily, although not specifically designed to increase resilience, most prevention programs *logically or intuitively focus on increasing protective mechanisms*. Many of these protective mechanisms are synonymous with resilience mechanisms. Hence, increasing research findings about resilience building processes should better inform prevention program design and increase program effectiveness (Kumpfer, 1999).

Scientific inquiry aims to establish linkages between cause and effect. A major strength of the scientific method is that it uses strictly defined, standardized procedures to determine how events are causally related to one another. This approach may be seen most clearly in experiments in the "hard sciences" such as physics, chemistry, and biology. Cause and effect relationships in the "soft sciences"— psychology, sociology, and economics, for example—are more complex and often harder to discern because each involves human interactions and because many practical factors affect the rigor of the research design and the degree of confidence in the findings.

Despite these difficulties, prevention science can and does use methods appropriate for inferring causal relationships in mental health and substance abuse programs with a satisfactory degree of certainty. For example, researchers are able to use relatively homogeneous samples such as third-graders in an economically disadvantaged neighborhood. Certain research designs, if implemented well, are more likely to produce definitive results than others. "Experimental" designs or randomized controlled trials (RCTs) are considered the gold standard, and random assignment often is possible at the individual or group level (e.g., classrooms in a school or elementary schools in a unified school district). Even when it is impossible to control all the factors that may moderate the outcome of the study, sufficient comparison designs and/or measurement and statistical control of these factors may be quite feasible. That is, "quasi-experimental" designs including multiple time-series analyses, repeated cross-sectional surveys, cohort or case-control analytic studies, and meta-analytic methods can demonstrate the effectiveness of interventions for individuals, peer groups, families, schools, or a whole community.

The Importance of Evidence-Based Programs

Beginning in the early 1990s, Federal agencies and other organizations that provide funds for community-based prevention programs decided the taxpayer would get more for his money if they funded only evidence-based programs, that is, programs that had been shown through rigorous testing to be efficacious under ideal circumstances and effective in the "real world." Various organizations, most of which are government agencies, then crafted a set of criteria for use in identifying what they considered to be effective programs, usually for the prevention of violence or substance abuse, or both. These organizations, and contact information for their programs, are presented in the Resources Appendix.

Although lists of "promising," "model," "effective," or "exemplary" programs differ in some respects, what is striking is how much agreement exists among reviewers. In 2002, Taylor, Metzler, and Eddy reviewed 11 of these lists and identified the "Top 21 Evidence-Based Family-Focused Programs," presented in the Resources Appendix. Not surprisingly, several well-known programs appear on multiple lists. For example, Nurse Family Partnerships appears on 7 of the 8 lists for which it is eligible, The Incredible Years on 8 of the 11 lists for which it is eligible, and Preparing for the Drug Free Years (now known as Guiding Good Choices) on 7 of the 10 lists for which it is eligible.

Lists of programs are useful, but many are static, one-time-only projects. Once a program gets on a list, it is likely to stay, even if it encounters problems. Moreover, a list cannot include programs created after it was developed, and most lists focus on only one concern even though the risk and protective factors for that concern may apply to a variety of problems. In 1998, in an attempt to avoid the problems inherent in lists, SAMHSA/CSAP developed National Registry of Effective Programs (NREP). NREP's evaluation and appropriateness criteria are reviewed annually and revised as necessary to reflect progress in prevention science. The criteria assess several factors in order to draw conclusions about two primary dimensions: (1) scientific credibility—the extent to which the design, implementation, and evaluation of the research provide a reasonable means of assessing change over time attributable only to the program, and (2) utility of findings—the magnitude, valence, and consistency of findings across measurement domains and/or across replications and adaptations. Together, these two overall criteria convey the level of confidence that a program will accomplish its aims. (The current NREP review criteria may be found at www.modelprograms.samhsa.gov.) As of this writing, NREP evaluates programs for substance abuse prevention and treatment, co-occurring disorders, mental health treatment, and promotion and prevention in mental health. Program developers may submit their programs for review through a "prevention portal" at www.modelprograms.samhsa.gov. All programs are provided feedback on each review criterion. Table 1 presents NREP programs that address both mental and substance use disorders.

Contemporary promotion and prevention programs for both mental health and substance abuse generally focus on *promoting healthy family relationships or developing social and emotional skills (especially in children), or both.* One extremely influential program listed above that focuses on family relationships

Table 1. Prevention Programs for Both Mental and Substance Use Disorders

Depression	Anxiety	Conduct	Substance
Child Development Program	Child Development Program	Child Development Program	Child Development Program
Dare To Be You	*Dare To Be You*	*Dare to Be You*	*Dare To Be You*
Family Effectiveness Training	*Family Effectiveness Training*	*Family Effectiveness Training*	*Family Effectiveness Training*
Families & Schools Together	*Families & Schools Together*	*Family & Schools Together*	*Families & Schools Together*
Guiding Good Choices	*Guiding Good Choices*	*Guiding Good Choices*	*Guiding Good Choices*
The Incredible Years	*The Incredible Years*	*The Incredible Years*	*The Incredible Years*
Nurse Family Partnership	*Nurse Family Partnership*	*Nurse Family Partnership*	*Nurse Family Partnership*
Parenting Wisely	*Parenting Wisely*	*Parenting Wisely*	*Parenting Wisely*
Promoting Alternative Thinking Strategies (PATHS)	Promoting Alternative Thinking Strategies (PATHS)	Promoting Alternative Thinking Strategies (PATHS)	Promoting Alternative Thinking Strategies (PATHS)
Positive Action		*Positive Action*	*Positive Action*
Reconnecting Youth	Reconnecting Youth	Reconnecting Youth	Reconnecting Youth
Strengthening Families Program	*Strengthening Families Program*	*Strengthening Families Program*	*Strengthening Families Program*
		Across Ages	Across Ages
		All Stars	All Stars
		Early Risers	Early Risers
		High/Scope Perry Preschool Program	High/Scope Perry Preschool Program
		Life Skills Training	Life Skills Training
		Project Achieve	Project Achieve
		Responding in Peaceful Positive Ways	Responding in Peaceful Positive Ways
		Second Step	Second Step
		Olweus Bullying Prevention Program	Olweus Bullying Prevention Program
		Students Managing Anger & Resolution Together (SMAST)	Students Managing Anger & Resolution Together (SMART)

Note: Italics indicate a program that involves family members.

and that shows positive results in mental health and substance use is the *Nurse-Family Partnerships* that started in Elmira, New York, in 1977. This program focuses on prenatal care, early attachment processes, and maternal life course. When compared to control groups, its many positive outcomes are striking:

- An 80% decrease in child abuse and neglect;
- A decrease in maternal depression;
- Lower rates of conduct problems and delinquency in adolescence;
- Significantly fewer reported arrests, convictions, and violations of probation in adolescence; and
- Lower consumption of alcohol and less cigarette smoking in adolescence (Olds et al., 1998).

Promotion and prevention programs that focus on *social and emotional skills* help people develop the ability to understand, manage, and express one's social and emotional life to successfully manage life tasks (Elias, 1997). A comprehensive perspective on social and emotional skills is provided by the Collaborative for Academic, Social, and Emotional Learning (CASEL) (www.casel.org). An excellent example of a program developed to prevent substance abuse that combines social and emotional skills training with education about how to resist social and media influences to use alcohol, tobacco, and other drugs is *Life Skills Training* (LST). Numerous evaluations have shown that LST prevents or reduces use of these substances, and recent research indicates that social and emotional skills are an important mediator of the effectiveness of LST (Botvin, Baker, Dusenberry, Botvin, & Diaz, 1995).

Common Elements of Successful Programs

In 1990, Dryfoos summarized the following common findings regarding successful prevention programs for young people:

- No single program component can prevent multiple high-risk behaviors. Each community requires a package of coordinated, collaborative programs.
- Short-term preventive interventions produce time-limited benefits, at best, with at-risk groups, whereas multiyear programs are more likely to foster enduring benefits.
- Preventive interventions should be directed at risk and protective factors rather than at categorical problem behaviors. With this perspective, it is both feasible and cost-effective to target multiple negative outcomes in the context of a coordinated set of programs.
- Interventions should be aimed at changing institutions, environments, and individuals.

A 2002 SAMHSA study found five science-based program components to strengthen programs significantly and to produce consistent and lasting reductions in substance use:

- Promotion of protective factors including attitudinal and behavioral life skills;
- Emphasis on building connectedness to positive peers and adults through team and interpersonal activities;
- Coherent program design, training, and implementation within a clearly articulated and coherent prevention theory;
- Introspective orientation that encourages youth to use self-reflection in examining their behaviors and in determining the impact of their behaviors on others or themselves; and
- Intensive contact of 4 hours or more per week with youth. Programs that delivered fewer than 20 hours total did not achieve meaningful effects, regardless of other characteristics.

This study further found that programs delivered in after-school settings tended to be more effective than those delivered in school, probably because they incorporated more of the effective characteristics listed above, and because the frequency and duration of the sessions tended to be greater. Schools apparently found it hard to devote the time necessary to implement the program correctly (SAMHSA, 2002c).

Few researchers and community implementers would question the value of any of the above-mentioned components. However, *building connectedness to positive peers and adults* is a critical component of a very large number of promotion and prevention programs. Of the 22 programs in Table 1, shown previously, 9 involve family members. This is a real plus for these programs because experts maintain that involving parents in their children's lives throughout adolescence is critically important in enabling teens to avoid high-risk behaviors.

MAKING RESILIENCE-BUILDING PREVENTON PROGRAMS WORK

Community stakeholders often ask why they cannot create their own programs. After all, they know their local community better than any outside program developer does. The answer is that they *can* create their own programs, and many do. The drawback of this approach, which was the case with early researchers, is that people who have never developed a program before rarely have a "realistic understanding of all the investments in personnel and money and all the research effort that is needed to establish significant and evidence-based reductions in mental health problems in local communities" (Hosman, 2002, p. 33).

The process of making resilience-building prevention programs work in community settings often is referred to as a *Science to Service Cycle.* This complex process involves translating scientifically validated efficacy studies into tools for communities to provide effective services. It also involves supporting the development of an evidence base among community implementers so that practice can help inform the nation's scientific agenda.

The Fidelity/Adaptation Dilemma

The critical issue in resilience-building prevention programs today is not so much finding programs or knowing how to assess whether or not they work. The field has become fairly sophisticated at these tasks. However, good programs sometimes do not work in all settings. Relatively little scientific information exists about just why that is, but researchers and implementers suspect that the problems most likely lie in the fidelity/adaptation dilemma. Fidelity of implementation is essentially the degree to which a program is conducted as it was originally designed and tested. Problems with fidelity may occur for many reasons. Sometimes, a community chooses a program that simply won't work with its population. For example, "talking" interventions rarely work with people possessing only limited verbal skills. Similarly, it is extremely difficult to conduct programs that require parents to participate fully if those parents are preoccupied by crises, a common situation for many families targeted by promotion and prevention programs. In addition, it is critical to match program capabilities and requirements with clients' and implementers' needs and resources.

Fidelity is compromised further when inadequately trained staff alter the content of a program or decrease the number, frequency, and/or duration of the sessions. Unenthusiastic leaders of the implementing agency sometimes do not allow needed scheduling flexibility, or the agency may be so disorganized that it can provide no support for staff trying to implement the program. Funding may not be available to strengthen the organization's infrastructure so that an evidence-based program can be successfully implemented.

Greenberg and his colleagues note "prevention practice will reach its full maturity only when effective programs are *implemented with integrity* in the various contexts of children's lives. This goal will require an unprecedented focus on the science and practice of implementation" (Greenberg, Domitrovich, Graczyk, & Zins, in press). Fortunately, many researchers now focus on these areas and have developed ways to evaluate implementation fidelity. These evaluations include *measures of the program delivery itself,* for example, adherence to curricula, frequency, duration, and number of sessions delivered, and *measures of the support system for training and consultation.* In addition, fidelity evaluations look at the *influences external to the actual program* that may greatly impact the quality of program implementation. (For a discussion of contextual factors that may affect the intervention process or program quality, see Greenberg et al., in press.)

Adapting Programs for Cultural, Gender, Age, and Situational Appropriateness

Adaptation is the degree to which a program implementer modifies the program, for whatever reason (Emshoff, Blakely, Gray, Jakes, Brounstein, Coulter, in press). Altering a program by decreasing the number, frequency, or duration of sessions is widely seen as a threat to fidelity. Perhaps the most controversial adaptations are those that alter the program so that it will better match certain community characteristics. For example, if a program was designed for and tested on an African American population, an American Indian tribe might alter the program in some way to make it more acceptable to—and possibly more effective with—the American Indian population. Strong arguments for adaptations to achieve cultural competence are that the community will feel more of a sense of ownership and that participants will be more engaged.

The problem with any type of adaptations is that people sometimes intentionally or unintentionally alter the core components of the program and then wonder why the program does not work in their community. An even greater problem, and one that generates tremendous controversy among researchers, is that very little research exists that identifies the "core elements" that cannot be modified without sacrificing fidelity (Greenberg et al., in press). Researchers who are skeptical of adaptations—often because they have seen adaptations with disastrous consequences—point out that the only way we can know for sure what the core components of any program are is through scientific research.

Community implementers, especially psychologists and other social scientists, may find that they debate the fidelity/adaptation dilemma within themselves. They value adapting programs because they know the importance of ecology and context in understanding phenomena and because program adaptation empowers local communities. Yet, as social scientists, they value empirical data that link specific interventions with specific outcomes. They also recognize that programs often are diluted when implemented at sites other than the original test site (Emshoff et al., in press). It seems prudent to reframe the fidelity/adaptation debate as a *need for fidelity/adaptation balance* (Backer, 2001a; Backer 2001b). Researchers certainly must continue to identify the core components of various programs and to determine whether and how a given program might be adapted to serve a population other than that for which it was originally designed and tested.

A key component of the successful *implementation* of an evidence-based program is that connections must be built among the program developer, implementers, and other community stakeholders. This step often is complicated because these individuals not only have different roles, but they also speak the "languages" associated with these roles (Emshoff et al., in press). Even if they have the interest, busy community stakeholders rarely have the time to learn the esoteric language of prevention science, so it is incumbent upon the scientists to "sell the stakeholders on the idea that fidelity is absolutely essential if the program is going to be successful in their agency" (Greenberg et al., in press).

Another critical activity that increases fidelity is training and ongoing consultation and supervision by the developer. The developer absolutely must be involved in any adaptations the community implementers wish to make. The evaluators of a major SAMHSA study concluded that "while the written manuals were fairly detailed, there appears no substitute for the value of human interaction between the original program developer and the adopting site" (Emshoff et al., in press, p. 26). These evaluators further found, to no one's surprise, that the closer the implementation was to the original program, even when targeting somewhat different populations than the original program, the better the program outcomes.

THE COMMUNITY CONTEXT

A critical element in getting resilience-building prevention programs to work in a given community is to get adults to talk to each other. Evidence-based programs often are only one of many important components of a broader community initiative to foster resilience, to promote mental health, and to prevent substance abuse, violence, teen pregnancy, and other maladaptive behaviors among young people. Early intervention, ongoing treatment, jail diversion, and other services often are provided in well-functioning communities through coalitions of caring adults. Creating a community coalition and keeping it functioning well over time can be an arduous task. Research on community coalitions has identified eight characteristics associated with success:

- A comprehensive vision that covers all segments of the community and aspects of community life;
- A widely held vision agreed on by groups and individuals across the community;
- A strong core of committed partners from the outset;
- An inclusive and broad-based membership, welcoming all segments of the community;
- Avoidance or resolution of severe conflicts that might reflect misunderstandings about a partnership's basic purpose;
- Decentralized units that encourage participation and action at small-area or neighborhood levels;
- Reasonable, non-disruptive staff turnover; and
- Extensive prevention activities and support for local prevention policies, reaching a large number of people for as many extended contact hours as possible (SAMHSA, 2002c).

PROMOTION AND PREVENTION PROGRAMS ARE COST EFFECTIVE

Cost-benefit analyses are extremely difficult and expensive to conduct, but they are often worth the effort. Several analyses have found that many promotion and prevention programs more than pay for themselves. Researchers in Washington State reviewed programs for children and adolescents and found significant economic benefits from *reductions in the costs of crime alone.* For example, the benefits per dollar spent on the Nurse Family Partnership Program was $3.06; on the Seattle Social Development Project, $4.25; and on the Big Brothers/Big Sisters program, $5.29 (Aos, Phipps, Barnuski, & Lieb, 2001). Specific programs for juvenile offenders such as Multisystemic Therapy, Functional Family Therapy, Aggression Replacement Training, and coordinated services have been found to produce benefit-to-cost ratios that *exceed 20 to 1.* That is, a dollar spent on these programs today can be expected to return to taxpayers and crime victims *twenty or more dollars* in the years ahead (Aos et al., 2001).

FUNDING PROGRAMS THAT WORK

If prevention science has progressed to the point that significant savings are possible in both human suffering and health care dollars, one might wonder why all communities are not clamoring for programs. The short answer is that a great many are. In 2003, a youth violence prevention grant announcement issued by SAMHSA/CMHS generated 580 applications. Funds were available to award 25 grants.

The more complete and complex answer is that funding and infrastructure for promotion and prevention in the United States are sorely lacking. Not only is the nation's mental health *treatment* system "fragmented and in disarray" (New Freedom Commission on Mental Health, 2003, p. 3), but funding for promotion and prevention is even more limited and fragmented. Services are not well coordinated, and local communities usually must deal with multiple funding sources that cannot always provide a consistent stream of money. Because many early prevention programs were neither well evaluated nor held accountable for failures, and because program developers and community implementers have not been good marketers of their successes, the awareness of and respect for promotion and prevention are seriously limited.

Despite these problems, many positive activities are under way. As noted earlier, SAMHSA is the primary federal agency charged with promoting mental health and preventing mental and substance use disorders. Both SAMHSA/CMHS and SAMHSA/CSAP provide substantial funding for promotion and prevention grant programs administered solely by the Centers. However, understanding the power of coalitions, the Centers also partner with each other, with other Federal agencies, and with national organizations to develop technical assistance and promote evidence-based promotion and prevention services. Furthermore, noting that, all too often, the agencies within HHS "have remained cocooned within our agency-specific knowledge," SAMHSA Administrator Charles Curie has called for "a common framework from which all of us [DHHS agencies] can address the range of risk-taking behaviors, protective factors, and positive choices to achieve healthy outcomes and well-being for our youth" (Curie, 2003). Consistent with the goal of greater inter-agency collaboration, SAMHSA has partnered with both the National Institutes of Health (NIH) and the Agency for Healthcare Research and Quality (AHRQ) in leading a Science to Services Initiative that systematically attempts to strengthen and accelerate the widespread adoption of effective and evidence-based interventions for the prevention and treatment of mental and addictive disorders.

CONCLUSION

We conclude on an optimistic note. Not only do many evidence-based resilience-building prevention programs exist, but researchers and implementers also are increasingly working together to ensure fidelity, even while making appropriate adaptations. In addition, available cost-benefit data are certainly promising. The technology that could make a substantial positive contribution to the health of our nation is clearly available. What is needed most now is the political will for funding agencies to work together to help communities develop coalitions and implement scientifically sound resilience-building programs. The nation's mental health is not the sole responsibility of one or two federal, state, or local governmental departments or agencies. It is everybody's business.

REFERENCES

American Psychiatric Association. (1994). *Diagnostic and statistical manual of mental disorders-Fourth Edition (DSM-IV)*. Washington, DC: Author.

Aos, S., Phipps, P., Barnoski, R., Lieb, R. (2001, May). *The comparative costs and benefits of programs to reduce crime*. Olympia, WA: Washington State Institute for Public Policy.

Backer, T.E. (2001a). *Finding the balance: Executive summary of a state-of-the-art review*. Rockville, MD: Center for Substance Abuse Prevention, SAMHSA Model Programs. [On-line]. Available: www.samhsa.gov

Backer, T.E. (2001b). *Finding the balance: Program fidelity and adaptation in substance abuse prevention*. Rockville, MD: Center for Substance Abuse Prevention, SAMHSA Model Programs. [On-line]. Available: www.samhsa.gov

Botvin, G.J., Baker, E., Dusenbury, L., Botvin, E.M. & Diaz, T. (1995a). Long-term follow-up results of a randomized drug abuse prevention trial in a White middle-class population. *Journal of the American Medical Association, 273(14),* 1106–1112.

Costello, J.E., Erkanli, A., Federman, E., & Angold, A. (1999). Development of psychiatric comorbidity with substance abuse in adolescents: Effects of timing and sex. *Journal of Clinical Child Psychology, 28,* 298–311.

Curie, C. (2003). *Finding the common denominators: SAMHSA's strategic framework for prevention.* Paper presented at the Risk Avoidance Meeting, U.S. Department of Health and Human Services. Washington, DC: February 5, 2003.

Dryfoos, J.G. (1990). *Adolescents at risk: Prevalence and prevention.* New York: Oxford University Press.

Elias, M.J. (1997). Reinterpreting dissemination of prevention programs as widespread implementation with effectiveness and fidelity. In R.P. Weissberg, R.L. Hampton, & C.R. Adams & T.P. Gullotta, (Eds.), *Healthy children 2010: Establishing preventive services. Issues in children's and families' lives* (Vol. 9, pp. 253–289). Thousand Oaks, CA: Sage Publications.

Emshoff, J., Blakely, C., Gray, D., Jakes, S., Brounstein, P., & Coulter, J. (in press). An ESID case study at the Federal level. *American Journal of Community Psychology.*

Greene, R.W., Biederman, J., Faraone, S.V., Wilens, T.E., Mick, E., & Blier, H.K. (1999). Further validation of social impairment as a predictor of substance use disorders: Findings from a sample of siblings of boys with and without ADHD. *Journal of Clinical Child Psychology, 28,* 349–354.

Greenberg, M.T., Domitrovich, C., Graczyk, P.A., and Zins, J.E. (in press). *The study of implementation in school-based prevention research: Implications for theory, research, and practice.* Rockville, MD: Center for Mental Health Services, Substance Abuse, and Mental Health Services Administration.

Greenberg, M.T., Domitrovich, C., & Bumbarger, B. (1999). *Preventing mental disorders in school-age children: A review of the effectiveness of prevention programs.* Report submitted to The Center for Mental Health Services (CSMHA). University Park, PA: Pennsylvania State University, Prevention Research Center.

Hosman, C.M.H. (2002). Progress in evidence-based prevention and promotion in mental health. In P.J. Mrazek, & C.M.H. Hosman (Eds.), *Toward a strategy for worldwide action to promote mental health and prevent mental and behavioral disorders.* Alexandria, VA: World Federation for Mental Health.

Hussong, A.M., Curran, P.J. & Chassin, L. (1998). Pathways of risk for children of alcoholics' accelerated heavy alcohol use. *Journal of Abnormal Child Psychology, 26,* 453–466.

Kaplow, J.B., Curran, P.J., & Dodge, K. (2002). The Conduct Problems Prevention Research Group. Child, parent, and peer predictors of early-onset substance use: A multi-site longitudinal study. *Journal of Abnormal Child Psychology, 30,* 199–216.

Keenan, K., Loeber, R., Zhang, Q., Stouthamer-Loeber, M., & Van Kammen, W.B. (1995). The influence of deviant peers on the development of boys' disruptive and delinquent behavior: A temporal analysis. *Development and Psychopathology, 7,* 715–726.

Kumpfer, K.L. (1999). Factors and processes contributing to resilience: The resilience framework. In M.D. Glantz & J. Johnson (Eds.), *Resilience and development: Positive life adaptations.* New York: Kluwer Academic/Plenum Publishers.

Kumpfer, K.L., Alvarado, R., Smith, P., & Bellamy, N. (2002). Cultural sensitivity in universal family-based prevention interventions. In K. Kavanaugh, R. Spoth, & T. Dishion (Special Edition Eds.), *Prevention Science, 3* (3), 241–244.

McMahon, R.J., Collins, L.M., Doyle, S.R., & The Conduct Problems Prevention Research Group. (2002). *Relationship of kindergarten and first grade psychopathology to tobacco use in late childhood and early adolescence.* Manuscript submitted for publication.

Mrazek, P.J., & Haggerty, R.J., Eds. (1994). *Reducing risks for mental disorders: Frontiers for preventive intervention research.* Washington, D.C.: National Academy Press.

Murray, C.J.L., & Lopez, A.D. (1996). *The global burden of disease: Summary.* Geneva, Switzerland: World Health Organization.

National Institute of Mental Health. (1998). *Priorities for prevention research at NIMH: A report by the National Advisory Mental Health Council Workgroup on Mental Disorders Prevention Research* (NIH Publication No. 98-4321). Washington, DC: U.S. Government Printing Office.

New Freedom Commission on Mental Health. (2003). *Achieving the promise: Transforming mental health care in America: Final report* (DHHS Pub. No. SMA 03-3832). Rockville, MD: Author.

Olds, D., Robinson, J., Song, N., Little, C., & Hill, P. (1999). *Reducing risks for mental health disorders during the first five years of life: A review of preventive interventions.* Department of Health and Human Services, SAMHSA/CMHS. [On-line]. Available: www.sshsac.org/PDFfiles/ReducingRisks.pdf

Olds, D., Henderson, C.R., Cole, R., Eckenrode, J., Kitzman, H., Luckey, D., Pettitt, L., Sidora, K., Morris, P., & Powers, J. (1998). Long-term effects of nurse home visitation on children's criminal and antisocial behavior: Fifteen-year follow-up of a randomized controlled trial. *Journal of the American Medical Association 280*:1238–1244.

Scanlon, K., Williams, M., & Raphael, B. (1997). *Mental health promotion in NSW: Conceptual framework for developing initiatives.* Sydney, Australia: NSW Health Department

Sambrano, S., Springer, J.F., Sale, E., Kasim, R., & Hermann, J. (2002). The National Cross-Site Evaluation of High-Risk Youth Programs: Points of prevention overview, Monographs 1-4. United States Department of Health and Human Services & SAMHSA's National Clearinghouse for Alcohol & Drug Information. [On-line], Available: http://ncadi.samhsa.gov/govpubs/FO36/

Substance Abuse and Mental Health Services Administration. (2002a). *Results from the 2001 National Household Survey on Drug Abuse: Volume I. Summary of National Findings.* DHHS Publications No. (SMA) 02-3758. Rockville, MD: SAMHSA, Office of Applied Studies.

Substance Abuse and Mental Health Services Administration. (2002b). *Report to congress on the prevention and treatment of co-occurring substance abuse disorders and mental disorders.* Rockville, MD: Author. [On-line]. Available: www.samhsa.gov

Substance Abuse and Mental Health Services Administration. (2002c). *The National Cross-Site Evaluation of High-Risk Youth Programs* (DHHS Publication No. SMA 25-01). Rockville, MD: Center for Substance Abuse Prevention.

Taylor, T.K., Metzler, C., & Eddy, M. (2002, May). *Finding common ground in best practice lists: Top 21 evidence-based family-focused programs.* Paper presented at the meeting of the Society for Prevention Research, Seattle, Washington.

United States Statutes at Large, 102nd Congress, 2nd Session. ADAMHA Reorganization Act, July 10, 1992, 102 P.L. 321; 106 Stat.323. Potomac, MD: Potomac Publishing Company, Inc.

Webster-Stratton, C., & Taylor, T.K. (2001). Nipping early risk factors in the bud: Preventing substance abuse, delinquency, and violence in adolescence: Interventions targeted at young children (0–8) years. *Prevention Science, 2*(3), 165–192.

Werner, E. (1996b). How children become resilient: Observations and cautions. *Resilience in Action, Winter,* 18–28.

Index